MENTAL HEALTH CARE IN MODERN ENGLAND

MENTAL HEALTH CARE IN MODERN ENGLAND

THE NORFOLK LUNATIC ASYLUM/
ST ANDREW'S HOSPITAL c. 1810–1998

Steven Cherry

THE BOYDELL PRESS

First published 2003

Published by The Boydell Press
An imprint of Boydell & Brewer Ltd
PO Box 9, Woodbridge, Suffolk IP12 3DF, UK
and of Boydell & Brewer Inc.
PO Box 41026, Rochester, NY 14604–4126, USA
website: www.boydell.co.uk

ISBN 0 85115 920 6

A catalogue record for this book is available from the British Library

Library of Congress Cataloging-in-Publication Data
Cherry, Steven.
Mental health care in modern England : the Norfolk Lunatic Asylum/
St. Andrew's Hospital c. 1810–1998 / Steven Cherry.
p. cm.
Includes bibliographical references and index.
1. Norfolk Lunatic Asylum (Norfolk, England)–History.
2. St. Andrew's Hospital (Norfolk, England)–History. 3. Psychiatric
hospitals–Great Britain–Norfolk–History–19th century.
4. Psychiatric hospitals–Great Britain–Norfolk–History–20th century.
I. Title.
RC450.G72 N673 2003
362.2'1'094261–dc21
2002012482

Typeset by Keystroke, Jacaranda Lodge, Wolverhampton
Printed in Great Britain by St Edmundsbury Press Ltd,
Bury St Edmunds, Suffolk

Contents

Figures

Acknowledgements

I am not the first and will not be the last to refer to the help of many people in writing a book, but my acknowledgements and thanks are nonetheless heart-felt in regard to this one. I rapidly became absorbed in the history of 'madness', in its broadest and non-derogatory sense, and the changing concepts and boundaries of insanity and mental health care. For almost two centuries the Norfolk Lunatic Asylum/St Andrew's Hospital was a site for these. It opened as one of the very first county asylums and its closure featured among the last of the older psychiatric hospitals. From its establishment in 1814 it provided forms of care, some harsh and custodial, some compassionate and therapeutic, offering what was then considered to be 'fit provision' for its 'unfortunate patients'. The asylum/hospital was simultaneously a place for solace and relationships; a highly organised and controlled environment but also a living, working and therapeutic community. It embodied contrasting experiences, sometimes brutal but often kindly; it provides a case-example but also a place of many histories. This account cannot do justice to them all, particularly the hidden lives of literally thousands of patients, but this rationale informs what has been compiled here.

First and foremost, I thank the Norfolk Mental Health Care NHS Trust for its appreciation of the need for a researched history of St Andrew's Hospital and its willingness and generosity in making the necessary financial commitments. The Trust's staff at Drayton Old Lodge and Hellesdon Hospital have always been helpful and both Graham Shelton and Mark Taylor, respectively former and current chief executives, encouraged and allowed me considerable scope in accessing records, including confidential material falling within the '100-year rule'. Freda Wilkins-Jones, Jonathan Draper and other staff at the Norfolk County Record Office, where most of the extensive documentation relating to St Andrew's is now held, greatly facilitated this research. I also wish to thank staff at the Norfolk Local Studies Library and Norwich Health Authority for their assistance.

The University of East Anglia allowed and supported my period of research leave and colleagues in the School of History and the Wellcome Unit for the History of Medicine have willingly shouldered any burdens resulting from my absence. In particular, Roy Church, Edward Acton and Roger Cooter ensured a positive response to the Norfolk Mental Health Care NHS Trust's initiative. Carole Rawcliffe, Rhodri Hayward, Roger Munting and Richard Wilson offered constructive and enlightening comments on various draft chapters. I thank them for valuable advice whilst apologising for the few instances where I have remained obdurate. I also wish to thank current and former UEA students whose research on aspects of St Andrew's I have drawn upon, especially Helen Bettinson, Cathy Bowler, Margaret Hewitt and Wendy Plackett.

Impressions in the book concerning aspects of hospital life and experiences in the more recent past are based mainly upon interviews with former and current staff and patients, as indicated below. All those concerned willingly offered their time and hospitality and I regret that it has been possible to use only a fraction of the material that they provided. It is abundantly clear that many former staff had an emotional attachment to the hospital and its patients, far deeper than can be described in terms of employment. If this is not adequately conveyed, the fault is entirely mine. In addition to their own recollections Eric and Rita Browne, Edward and Mollie Middleton and Trevor Pull, just to name some, provided photographs and other materials. Vivienne Roberts, Clifford Graveling and Louise Fitt directly enabled me to form an impression of hospital life stretching back to the inter-war years.

In so many ways I have depended upon the work of Mary Fisher. She arranged and undertook exclusively several of the interviews, did a great deal of the research and compiled a data-base of patients over two centuries, only samples of which are offered here. I have a deep and especial debt to Mary as a research assistant and I will be the first publicly to acknowledge that this official description understates Mary's role as a fellow scholar and overstates mine as her supervisor. Using the records of St Andrew's and St Audry's Hospital, Suffolk, she is producing her own work and I look forward to the completed version, which will soon appear as a doctoral thesis on '"Getting out of the asylum": discharge and decarceration issues in asylum history c. 1890–1959'.

For the physical production of this volume and their enthusiasm for a new venture, I am grateful to Peter Sowden the commissioning editor, to the publishers Boydell and Brewer and to an anonymous but most encouraging and instructive external referee. To everyone mentioned here, I hope that my efforts will be considered a suitable reward. There is a private side to the book, which I must also acknowledge. It is impossible not to be touched by some of the experiences I have come across in the research, not least the consequences of that historically blurred and often socially constructed, changeable boundary between 'normality' and 'insanity'. Perhaps as a result, on the home front, Frances, Helen and Georgia have persevered for three years whilst the Cherrys' grumpiest family member struggled to link an inspirational project and the often grim mechanics of writing. Each has displayed a much better sense of when to stand back, humour, divert or cajole than their father and obviously they have acquired this from their mother, Joan.

Interviews

I wish to thank the following people, interviewed by Mary Fisher and/or myself. Each has been given a brief description showing their connection with St Andrew's Hospital and its duration.

Alan Adcock*	Garden manager 1950–90	20 April 1988
Wally Bond	Orderly/nurse 1956–85	23 March 2001
Molly Bond (Sexbery)	Student/nurse 1951–91	23 March 2001
Eric Browne	Hospital electrician 1941–88	19 February 2001
Rita Browne (Thomson)	Laboratory assistant 1960–7	9 March 2001
Jimmy Browne	Orderly/nurse 1957–89	21 March 2001
Olive Clarke*	Student/nurse/sister 1958–	3 May 1988
Professor Frank Curtis	Chairman NMHCNHS Trust 1994–9	14 September 2001
Mrs D—	Patient intermittently 1974–	29 August 2001
Michael Glasheen*	Estate management 1960–	20 April 1988
Clifford Graveling	Childhood, work at farm 1955–7	30 March 2001
Donald Hill	Student/nurse 1958–61	5 October 2001
Kevin Long	Student/nurse 1962–8, Director of Nursing Practice 1986–	4 April 2001
Mrs M—	Patient intermittently 1959–	29 August 2001
Cicely McCall	Psychiatric social worker 1953–7	19 March 1999
Edward Middleton	Junior clerk/senior administrative assistant 1941–81	2, 13 March 2001
Mollie Middleton (Blanchflower)	Student/nurse/nurse tutor 1940–64	2, 13 March 2001
Dr Ted Olive	Consultant 1979–	27 February 2001
Trevor Pull	Nurse/recreation officer 1953–83	4 May 2001
Dr Chris Reynolds	Consultant 1977– now Medical Director NMHCNHS Trust	30 April 2001
Vivienne Roberts	Daughter of, wife of, attendants	20 May 1999
Doris Rose	Student/nurse 1931–6	written testimony
Graham Shelton	Chief executive NMHCNHS Trust 1994–9	1 June 2001
Dr Elizabeth Taws	Consultant 1983–98	30 October 2001
Paul Thain	Director of strategic development	27 November 2001
Brian Watling	Facilities manager 1973–	27 November 2001

* interviewed by Wendy Plackett

1

Contexts: asylums, insanity and locality

James Thomas Secker, a pauper aged 36 from Aylsham, was among the first eight people, 'all of a very bad description of lunatic', admitted into the new Norfolk Lunatic Asylum in May 1814.[1] He suffered from fits but his noisy and violent behaviour appears to have led to his admission. Had he lived a century earlier, he might have been regarded as wild, 'furiously and dangerously mad' or worse: a century later, his epilepsy would have featured primarily in medical treatment. Thomas Caryl, the barely literate asylum master, reported early in June that Secker had been 'ordered to bed by Dr Wright for misconduct after which he knocked down a part of is sleeping cell'.[2] Helped by patient Richard Gent, Secker 'attempted to git away' on 17 June, after which Caryl 'put the chanes onto both of them'. Secker tried to hang himself on 8 July and was subsequently involved in a grim series of confrontations, restraints, and escape and suicide attempts before his death on 24 October 1821.[3]

Other early patients had different experiences. Sarah Newell attracted little comment or attention and within weeks was 'delivered . . . upto hir husbon', one of six people 'restored to their reason and discharged' by December 1814. The nature of her illness, treatment and recovery remained unclear. Hannah Harvey's release may have been temporary, as her admission was 'occasioned by excessive use of spirituous liquors . . . she would remain free from insanity if this habit could be conquered or prevented'. Amy Delf, aged 21, received greater attention as Dr Edward Rigby considered that her excitement stemmed from 'religious impression'.[4] In August Caryl reported that she had 'broken [a] window in the incurable yard upon which I locked hir up' and early in September she was one of three women patients who destroyed their stockings, shoes and gowns. Subsequently she was less disturbed and Dr Rigby persuaded the Committee of Visiting Justices which

---

[1] Under the 1714 Vagrancy Act the 'furiously and dangerously mad' could be confined by county magistrates. Norwich Quarter Sessions (NQS), c/s/4/2; 1812–19, 14 July 1814.
[2] Master's Journal, May 1814–Nov. 1815, SAH 123, 29 May and 17 June 1814.
[3] ibid., 14 Sept. 1814. Secker then had 'the straight wastecoat on which . . . he bit and pulled all to pieces and also broke 2 locks'. The day before his death he 'complained of a violent pain of the bowels' for which he had 'some drops . . . a small dose of salts every four hours and a powder at bed time'. Master's Journal, Dec. 1820–July 1832, SAH 126, 22 and 23 Oct. 1821.
[4] ibid., 3 Dec. 1814 (Newell); Physicians' Report Book 1814–17, SAH 147, 26 Sept. 1814 (Harvey); 7 Sept. 1814 (Delf).

ran the asylum that she was 'sufficiently recovered to be discharged'. Samuel Pestle, aged 70 and 'very melancholy; always alone' had meanwhile died from his 'diseased bladder' and John Payne's condition was causing concern: he had been 'in strong fits and is now in a very languid and torpid state'.[5]

These few examples suggest the complex role of the asylum from the outset. Secker had committed no crime but was seen as a danger to others and, after his suicide attempt, to himself. He experienced the asylum as a custodial environment, in which the unqualified Caryl was little different from a gaoler or workhouse master. Any treatment for Secker was indeterminate and secondary to the purpose of protecting society from his outbursts. Hannah Harvey's 'derangements' also led to her physical confinement and incurred moral approbation but, when they ceased, she was allowed to leave. Dr Rigby figured in her release, as in Amy Delf's case, but he did not determine it. At a time when the claims of medicine vastly exceeded its achievements he might influence the justices of the peace, but they constituted the local authority inside and outside Norfolk's lunatic asylum. Subject to statutory obligations, they made arrangements as they felt fit or proper. Thus control, help and treatment all featured within a common rhetoric of care. Secker's behaviour drew the first response but medical attention was procured for John Payne, who also had fits but was visibly exhausted, and for Samuel Pestle, whose melancholy was probably linked with infirmity and illness. If such caring was limited, conditional and paternalistic, so was that provided in contemporary voluntary hospitals and workhouse sick wards.

Examples of private asylums and early philanthropic provision for the insane could already be seen in and around Norwich before construction of the Norfolk Lunatic Asylum commenced in 1811 at the village of Thorpe St Andrew, three miles to the east of the city.[6] However, the county asylum was intended specifically for pauper lunatics and was only the second institution of its kind when completed early in 1814. Unlike its precursor, the Bedford Asylum which opened in 1812 but closed in 1860, the Norfolk Asylum utilised the same site and retained the original buildings virtually to the end of the millennium.[7] Bricks and mortar suggest continuity, although the use of

[5] Master's Journal, 12 Aug. 1814 (Delf); Physicians' Report, 20 March 1815 (Delf) 8 Sept. 1814 (Payne); 26 Jan. 1815 (Pestle).

[6] Norwich examples included the Bethel Hospital, a public charity from 1724, and the private Lakenham asylum, opened in 1807. There were roughly 50 private asylums and a handful of public subscription asylums, discussed below, in addition to metropolitan provision which included Bethlem (1247) and St Luke's (1751) hospitals.

[7] B. Cashman, A Proper House, Bedford Lunatic Asylum 1812–1860, North Bedfordshire Health Authority, 1992. Nottingham Asylum opened in 1811 but accommodated private and pauper patients and the original buildings had been demolished by 1899. H. Richardson (ed.), English Hospitals 1660–1948, Royal Commission on the Historical Monuments of England, Swindon, 1998, p. 160.

asylum buildings like any others may change markedly over time. Together with the asylum grounds and estate, they served to delineate a place for madness but this was not the only place available locally, nor was it entirely a closed space or a simple matter of geography.

As will become clear from subsequent chapters, the asylum and later hospital essentially comprised its staff and patients, their behaviour and relationships; all vital in any consideration of its history. Nor can this be separated from its wider contexts. The peopling of the institution arose largely from extraneous decisions; to commit patients to care, to appoint staff or to extend facilities and amenities. They and the institution were the subjects of external inspection and regulation by Norfolk and central government agencies and were visited by the relatives and friends of patients. As a living entity, the asylum provided multi-faceted forms of care with varying degrees of success. It served as a habitat and operated as a therapeutic and an economic community, controlled and tightly knit but never completely closed off. Internal boundaries changed as doors were unlocked, walls dismantled and ditches filled in but also in response to changing regulations, customs and practices. This was more obvious over time but, even in the short term, was never a wholly physical matter, precluding the discharge or temporary release of at least some patients. As a place for madness the nineteenth-century asylum did not obviate other forms of care for those deemed to be mad or categorised among the insane. Its functions might be radically revised in the light of twentieth-century national emergencies; for example, its transformation into a military hospital during the First World War, or use as a multi-purpose hospital in the Second World War. More consistently, twentieth-century mental health care arrangements increasingly operated across and then beyond hospital boundaries as the focus of care switched to the provision of services for patients rather than their accommodation.

The briefest of surveys will suggest the changing identities over two centuries of what began as the Norfolk Lunatic Asylum and the scope for an institutional study which recognises the changing contexts of care provision. With buildings initially readied for the reception of 40 male patients in April 1814 and females admitted from June, roughly 70 patients were present on average in the early years.[8] Modest extensions in 1831 and 1840 allowed this number to double but the asylum remained small by national standards. With more substantial additions in the late 1850s and the construction of an auxiliary asylum completed in 1881 some 700 inpatients could be accommodated. After 1845 the asylum was subject to the inspections and advice of national Commissioners in Lunacy, replaced from 1913 by the Board of Control, but the influence of professional medical knowledge

---

[8] Minutes of the Committee of Visiting Justices (CVIS) Oct. 1813–June 1816, SAH 2, 16 April and 25 July 1814.

increased after the rather belated appointment of a medical superintendent in 1861. However, formal control of the institution passed from a committee of visiting magistrates to one consisting of elected county councillors under the 1888 Local Government Act and in April 1889 it was re-titled the Norfolk County Asylum. There followed a process of modernisation into 'a hospital for mental disorders', with reorganisation into distinct male and female asylums offering combined accommodation for over 1,000 patients, shaped largely by medical superintendent Dr David Thomson.[9]

Although these developments were nationally recognised by the psychiatric profession their consequences in terms of patient care were disrupted by the outbreak of the First World War. Virtually all the asylum's usual patients were evacuated to other institutions across eastern England in 1915 as the Norfolk County Asylum was transformed into the Norfolk War Hospital for military casualties. On the asylum's peacetime re-conversion in 1920 the title 'Norfolk Mental Hospital' was adopted, although local use of the alternative 'St Andrew's Hospital' was officially recognised from January 1924. Whether this nomenclature indicates a genuine transformation in approaches to mental health care remains debatable. The inter-war period saw a resumed accumulation of more than 1,100 resident patients, seemingly restricted only by the overcrowding of existing facilities. Nevertheless, the use of parole and transfers to regulate patient numbers was also accompanied by voluntary admissions and outpatient treatments, offering services to patients beyond an institutional life and a glimpse of what 'community care' might represent.

There was no steady progress towards a defined goal, however. In the Second World War the hospital was greatly stretched in providing the additional functions of an Emergency Section hospital, receiving refugees, evacuees and civilian casualties in cleared wards whilst maintaining its complement of mental patients, cascaded into reduced accommodation. Its absorption within the National Health Service initially produced little relief from overcrowding or staff shortages and a demoralising loss of local control over the limited resources available. Although there were still more patients, there was no guarantee of better services. From the 1950s improved therapies and new medications, changing perceptions of patients' rights and increasingly critical assessments of the psychiatric hospital as an appropriate setting informed the delivery of patient care. Consequently, St Andrew's spent most of its years as an NHS hospital under threat of closure, first raised publicly in 1963. Alternative forms of mental health care in the community were always going to be easier to prescribe than to deliver, even had clear blueprints and sufficient resources been provided. Their establishment took

---

[9] D.G. Thomson, 'Presidential address on the progress of psychiatry during the past hundred years, together with the history of Norfolk County Asylum during the same period', *Journal of Mental Science*, LX, 1914, pp. 541–72.

longer than originally envisaged and, meanwhile, the hospital itself became a site for new services even as what were regarded as outmoded facilities were run down. A drawn-out closure process was ultimately resolved with the securing in 1994 of a separate NHS Trust for mental health care services in Norfolk. Although this could not guarantee the necessary resources, it arguably resulted in a coherent range of services and amenities, in the light of which the eventual closure of St Andrew's in April 1998 served a positive purpose.

Major objectives for this study are to provide a sense of what the Norfolk Lunatic Asylum/St Andrew's Hospital was like at particular times, to interpret changing emphases in its role over time and, wherever possible, to uncover the experiences of its patients and staff. These will underpin the value of an institutional study and embellish wider understanding of the rise and fall of the asylum/psychiatric hospital over two centuries. They also engage an important research question: 'how far do particular asylums correspond to or diverge from the picture drawn in an earlier generation of global histories.'[10] Yet all this in itself requires an appreciation of broader contexts, briefly surveyed in the remainder of this chapter.

'Madness' is used here as the broad lay term applicable at the establishment of the Norfolk Lunatic Asylum. It has also been claimed to cover 'certain kinds of unsocial behaviour which *everyone* recognises as unacceptable'.[11] In practice there was no such consistency and, though attitudes to madness changed sufficiently to generate reforming national legislation by the early nineteenth century, this in itself did not represent a universal indicator of perceptions of those considered mad, still less of approaches to their treatment. In the period reviewed madness was redefined and categorised into forms of insanity, primarily a legal concept, and then mental illness, primarily a medical one. Although the focus of this study is not insanity or its treatments as such, a broad framework for features examined in later chapters is offered.

Asylums and their role are considered as part of wider institutional reforms during a period of significant economic and social change and recent research covering their subsequent development can also be noted. There are also influences, some specific to Norfolk, which may have affected the development of its own asylum or the social composition of its patients. Standards of care or confinement locally and nationally were largely determined by socially dominant minorities and genuinely popular agitation on wider questions of health or welfare did not exist before the twentieth

---

[10] See A. Scull, 'Psychiatry and its historians', *History of Psychiatry*, 2, 1991, pp. 239–50, 245.

[11] J.L. Crammer, 'English asylums and English doctors', *History of Psychiatry*, 5, 1994, pp. 103–15, 104. Crammer's emphasis reflects a psychiatrist's frustration with critical commentators who have 'no first-hand experience of people regarded as mad or insane . . . realities about which something practical has to be done'.

century.[12] To variable degrees, social elites sought such improvements as they felt fit and proper, but they also attempted to maintain their influence and control. These were not considered to be contradictory motives, as was demonstrated in their application to the insane, but this also requires some further consideration.

Different perceptions of madness and of appropriate responses to it exist within any era and have altered radically over time. In later medieval societies, for example, madness was sometimes taken to indicate a sign of grace in sufferers enduring purgatory on earth but, more often, it was believed to reflect the dire consequences of sinfulness and the loss of divine protection. In these latter cases 'the madman seemed wilfully to have alienated himself from God by destroying his own reason: the one characteristic which distinguished him from brute animals and brought him closer to his Maker'.[13] Sin and exposure to malign cosmic influences, particularly that of the moon, were among the 'natural' causes of humoral imbalance which could produce insanity. Forms of madness were distinguished but none was likely to involve any separation of the mind from the body. Mania, for example, was for centuries attributed to excess heat or choler, while cold or black bile was associated with melancholia or, in excess, with stupor.

By the seventeenth century humoral approaches to madness coexisted with pioneering searches for its physical origins within the body, brain or nerves and distinct from any perceptions involving the mind. Yet views that the mad, having lost their humanity, required breaking, taming or chaining also persisted. Such brutal treatment was seen as a practical response to those 'as mad as wild beasts, nor do they differ much from them . . . (they) endure also the greatest hunger, cold and stripes without any sensible harm'.[14] Roughly a century later the loss of reason seemed all the more alarming in an age of enlightenment, as madness and disordering of the senses began to be disassociated from supernatural possession and from bestial or sub-human characteristics. Madness had various forms but was essentially a human condition and, whether resting upon bodily origins or a false association of ideas, it might therefore be manageable. With a rational view of 'unreason', further investigation suggested promising rewards, not least for an emergent medical profession and its clientele in the developing eighteenth-century medical market.[15]

---

[12] To oversimplify, aside from moral economy concepts involving rights and liberties, or their assertion in the face of specifics such as mechanised production or poor law reform, there was no *mass* agitation for public hygiene or systems of health care.

[13] C. Rawcliffe, *Medicine and Society in Later Medieval England*, Sutton, London, 1995, p. 10.

[14] William Salmon (1644–1713) and author of *System Medicinale* (1686), cited in A. Scull, *The Most Solitary of Afflictions*, Yale, New Haven, 1993, p. 57.

[15] K. Jones, *Asylums and After*, Athlone, London, 1993, p.13, considers ideas associated with the Enlightenment a better alternative than 'the splendid lucky dip' of selecting a specific date marking the establishment of the psychiatric profession (1535) or a European

This provided one reform impetus. Medical practitioners might claim superior knowledge in dealing with the humoral imbalances which produced insanity or they might justify attempted treatments as an extension of their attendance upon bodily ailments. Professional reputations were increasingly based upon specialised knowledge and territories marked out by specialisms. It was particularly important for doctors to establish physical causes of insanity in order to differentiate themselves from the clergy, or other healers of the mind, as impairments of the ability to reason were also being addressed by non-medical means, notably forms of 'moral' treatment.[16] Building upon anatomical traditions, some doctors simply equated the mind with the brain and focused upon organic disease. Others located the origin of nervous disorders and the symptoms of delusion within the brain, seeking to identify the different parts responsible for various aspects of behaviour.[17] In the early nineteenth century phrenologists believed that the organs within the brain which shaped personality were manifested as contours of the skull and could be read. These essentially somatic approaches, the suggestion of diagnostic aids and the prospect of treatment or cure increased the influence of other mad doctors and alienists as they occupied broader reform territory, notably moral treatment and later 'non-restraint', by claiming to synthesise moral–medical management or to be its most suitable practitioners.[18]

According to these views asylums offered appropriate and specific places for the insane where insanity itself could be better understood and treated, preferably under medical supervision. Responses to insanity and the reform of an established trade in lunacy also featured in broader humanitarian concern with prison conditions, hospital provision and arrangements for the poor by the late eighteenth century. However, any assertions of rights or liberties in these areas tended to be restricted or qualified. Thus the 1774 Madhouses Act, which produced the licensing of metropolitan institutions by the Royal College of Physicians and of provincial equivalents by local justices of the

'Great Confinement' (1656). M. Foucault, *Madness and Civilisation*, Routledge, London, 1967, ed., p. 39, saw the latter as an imposed order based on work or incarceration: 'what made it necessary was an imperative of labour. Our philanthropy prefers to recognise the signs of a benevolence towards sickness when there is only a condemnation of idleness' (p. 46).

[16] Moral treatment, associated with Samuel Tuke and the York Retreat (1792), built on the principle that madness in some respect did not completely destroy the patient's ability to reason. It focused upon the patient's 'desire for esteem' to promote self-restraint within a family-like model which involved submission to authority and work but not physical coercion. A. Digby, *Madness, Morality and Medicine: A Study of the York Retreat*, Cambridge University Press 1985.

[17] M. Neve, 'Medicine and the mind' in I. Loudon (ed.), *Western Medicine*, Oxford University Press, 1997, pp. 232–48, cites William Cullen 1710–90 and Franz Gall 1758–1828 as the respective instigators.

[18] Non-restraint (associated with Drs Charlesworth and Gardiner Hill at Lincoln and John Conolly at Hanwell asylums 1835–9) avoided the physical immobilisation and coercion of patients.

peace, did not anticipate the release of the insane or address the wider associations of poverty and lunacy. Excepting its focus upon those wrongfully incarcerated, reform was seen in terms of better care and treatment within improved asylums.[19] More ambitious reformers argued for the remodelling of people using a range of specific institutions to maintain social control.[20] Yet this is not to see social control as an all-pervasive feature, nor merely 'to impute completely cynical and hypocritical motives to individuals whom an earlier tradition counted as humanitarian reformers'.[21]

Why were reformers so committed to institutional models? The rapidity of population growth and economic change associated with the growth of market production had unsettling social consequences. Unrest and protest featured as more public manifestations of displacement or the breakdown of families or individuals unable to cope. Wealth creation was accompanied by heightened concern for property and public order generally, but social tensions were further aggravated by the French Revolution, by fears of an English radicalism or of threat sharpened by the additional economic dislocations consequent upon wars with France.[22] In such contexts, questions of order might arise within various reform causes as well as in repressive measures. Thus variants of the Speenhamland system of poor relief, which offered bread allowances as income supplements in times of inflation, also served to restrain wages and to offset social disturbances. A reform agenda for private asylums already existed but, apart from the earliest voluntary 'public subscription' examples, they had yet to feature as a specific alternative to workhouses, family or domestic environments for greater numbers of the poor.

Problems posed by the 'furiously and dangerously mad' were recognised within the Vagrancy Acts of 1714 and 1744, which allowed justices of the peace to order their detention. Eighteenth-century law held such persons responsible for any criminal acts and prisons or bridewells (houses of correction) were the main form of secure accommodation. Poorhouses or workhouses offered no special provision for lunatics. From the 1790s Evangelical concern with abuses of the insane and Utilitarian urges to

---

[19] A. Scull, 'Rethinking the history of asylumdom' in J. Melling and B. Forsythe (eds), *Insanity, Institutions and Society 1800–1914*, Routledge, London, 1999, pp. 295–315, 300.
[20] Thus Dr James Currie felt that the labouring poor 'demand our constant attention. To inform their minds, to repress their vices, to assist their labours, to invigorate their activity, and to improve their comforts: these are the noblest offices of enlightened minds in superior stations.' Cited in R. Porter, 'Was there a medical Enlightenment in England?', *British Journal of Eighteenth Century Studies*, 5, 1, 1982, pp. 49–63, 57.
[21] W.F. Bynum, R. Porter and M. Shepherd (eds), *The Anatomy of Madness*, Tavistock, London, 1985, Vol. 2. Institutions and Society, pp. 1–16, 6. The Bethel Hospital, Norwich is a case in point.
[22] Viz. the French Revolutionary Wars, 1792–1802, and the Napoleonic Wars, 1803–15. See the 'Norfolk Notes' section below.

systematise arrangements produced greater emphasis upon asylum as the specific procedure and place for insanity, where recoveries might be effected and proper supervision guaranteed.[23] In addition, the 1800 Criminal Lunatics Act allowed the longer-term detention of the criminally insane and also those regarded as potential criminals because of their 'derangement of mind'.[24] This was the immediate background to inquiries by the Commons Select Committee of 1807 which revealed great discrepancies in the perception, classification and treatment of criminal and pauper lunatics. The resulting legislation of 1808, *An Act for the better Care and Maintenance of Lunatics, being Paupers or Criminals in England*, empowered justices of the peace to establish and maintain county asylums from local rates, with those in Norfolk among the very first to respond positively.[25]

Asylum implied space for madness, in which the process of 'retreat' might itself be healing or could be combined with therapy. However, no particular model was prescribed and local authorities were under no compulsion to provide such accommodation prior to the 1845 Lunatic Asylums Act. Eighteenth-century philanthropic effort had already produced some asylums, including the Bethel, Norwich (1724) and in Newcastle (1765); others originated in conjunction with voluntary general hospitals (Manchester 1765) or were founded via public subscription (St Luke's, London 1751, York County 1777). County asylums for Nottingham (1810), Bedford (1812), and Norfolk (1814) were the first to be provided under the 1808 Act. That at Nottingham headed a new wave of public subscription asylums, five of the nine actually constructed by 1828, involving voluntary donations and a social mix of patients.[26] The remainder, at Bedford, Norfolk, Lancaster (1816) and Wakefield (1818), were funded by ratepayers and intended only for county paupers. Many other areas continued to rely heavily upon poor law accommodation or payments meant to cover the care and supervision of lunatics in private lodgings.[27] A relatively small number of asylums and variable forms of provision, sometimes involving places secured within private asylums, reflected the permissive legislation and the particular

---

[23] English emulation of Philippe Pinel's 'breaking of the chains' at the Bicetre 1793 or Salpetriere 1795 in Paris did not lead to general release but to greater confinement. Pinel himself was an advocate of asylum. E. Shorter, *A History of Psychiatry*, Wiley, New York, 1997, pp. 10–13.

[24] K. Jones, *Lunacy, Law and Conscience 1744–1845*, Routledge, London, 1956, pp. 68–9.

[25] 48 George III, *An Act for the Better Care and Maintenance of Lunatics, being Paupers or Criminals in England*. Also known as Wynn's Act after Charles Williams-Wynn, chairman of the 1807 Select Committee. See Chapter 2.

[26] Viz. Nottingham, Stafford (1818), Lincoln (1820), Cornwall (1820) and Gloucestershire (1823) asylums.

[27] P. Bartlett, 'The asylum and the poor law' in Melling and Forsythe, *Insanity, Institutions . . .*, pp. 48–67.

influence of local elites in decision-making.[28] This suggests that asylum care, whether custodial or therapeutic, was not yet clearly differentiated from other institutional provision.

Interpreting the asylum

Yet virtually throughout the period considered, increasing numbers and proportions of the whole population were regarded as insane and placed in asylums, notwithstanding changes in attitudes, the terminology of care or any different emphases within these institutions. This process began relatively slowly – less than 5,000 people were in county asylums when the 1845 Act was passed – but the number and size of asylums soon increased. By 1880 some 40,000 people, perhaps two-thirds of those 'of unsound mind', were accommodated. During the next fifty years asylum or mental hospital patients tripled in numbers while the institutions themselves and the proportion of the whole population in them each increased by 50 per cent (see Table 1.1).[29] Excepting wartime emergencies, this institutional emphasis was sustained until the 1950s. Then a simultaneous rise in treatments and fewer long-term committals, associated with the costs and closure of former asylum accommodation, improvements in rehabilitation therapy and new drug treatments, heralded major changes. Attempts to provide care in the community began with de-institutionalisation rather than with the provision of alternative services but, by the 1980s, the ratio of people in psychiatric hospital accommodation again approximated to that for asylums in the 1850s.[30]

A patient's admission to an asylum was usually triggered by some event or deterioration sufficiently at variance with conventions of normality, in terms of public order, and the ability to cope in work situations, domestic or family life. Alternatively, it might involve transfer from another institution, such as a general hospital or the workhouse. There were no absolute or unchanging criteria and any digressions were considered subjectively by other individuals, even those who claimed objectivity in accordance with the state of recognised medical knowledge or in their official capacity. Under the legislative and regulatory framework then operating, admission usually followed some form of reporting by family, neighbours or public official, variously a poor law

[28] Some have suggested that this anticipated purchaser/provider arrangements. L. Smith, 'The county asylum in the mixed economy of care' in Melling and Forsythe, *Insanity, Institutions . . .* , pp. 33–47.

[29] The workhouse remained a place for madness, as did the antecedents of community care. See P. Bartlett and D. Wright (eds), *Outside the Walls of the Asylum: the History of Care in the Community 1750–2000*, Athlone, London, 1999.

[30] J. Raftery, 'The decline of asylum or the poverty of a concept' in D. Tomlinson and J. Carrier, *Asylum in the Community*, Routledge, London, 1996, pp. 18–30.

Table 1.1 Insanity, mental illness and the rise of the county/borough asylum (CBA)

	Persons of unsound mind (000)	% rise over 10 years	Per 1,000 population	Numbers of CBAs	Patients in CBAs	% of patients in CBAs	of whom %M	%F
1807	2.2		0.2					
1827								
1837				9	1,046	21 (of paupers only)		
1842	20.0 +		1.3		2,850			
					5,098 (1847)	29 (of paupers only)	51	49
1850				24	7,140			
1860	31.4		1.6	41	15,845	42	46	54
1870	46.7	48	2.2	50	27,109	50	46	54
1880	61.6	32	2.4	61	40,088	58	45	55
1890	75.6	23	2.7	66	52,937	66	45	55
1900	95.6	26	3.0	77	74,004	73	45	55
1910	128.2	34	3.7	91	97,580	79	46	54
	inpatients*							
1920	116.7		3.1	94	93,648	80		
1930	141.1	21	3.6	98	119,659	85		
1938	157.4	12		100	131,952	84	44	56
1949	144.7	1	3.3					
1959	133.2	−8	2.9					

Sources: 1837, 1842 derived from R. Hodgkinson, 'Provision for pauper lunatics 1834–71', *Medical History*, 10, 1966, pp. 138–54, p 141–2. 1850–1910 from 67th *Report of the Commissioners in Lunacy*, HMSO, 1913, Appendix A, Table 1. 1920–59 from BoC Reports cited in Jones, *Asylums*, pp. 116. 1939 n/a and 1938 is from 1 January 1938, BoC Report 1937, p. 12.

* Inpatients includes relatively small proportions in general hospitals and mental nursing homes.

officer, clergyman, doctor or justice of the peace.[31] Practicalities such as the availability of care or accommodation, its cost relative to alternatives and estimate of risks involved, including violence, infection and death, were considered by asylum authorities, usually the medical superintendent. Thus, economic and social influences defining and bearing upon responses to insanity were strong. What applied to asylum admission might similarly feature in perceptions of recovery and discharge procedures, particularly when the patient was allowed only a passive role and his or her account was likely to be discounted, if not excluded.

Although diagnosis, treatment and prognosis increasingly involved medical expertise, decisions were made within wider contexts and it remains debatable whether, historically, 'psychiatrists may on the whole be better equipped to interpret these events than the majority of historians and sociologists'.[32] It is also recognised that 'the definition and conceptualisation of "asylum", "community", "care" and, for that matter, "'insanity", varied both over time and between regions'.[33] Asylum was only one remedial measure and its differing role and guises over two centuries have already been suggested by the changing institutional titles employed in Norfolk. Similarly with other terminology: in addition to the particular associations already introduced, different connotations were likely to be attached to the broad use of 'madness' in the eighteenth century, compared with nineteenth-century 'insanity' or with those surrounding twentieth-century 'mental illness'.[34] This may also apply to the transformation of 'inmates' into patients and clients; or of keepers and attendants to nurses and carers.[35]

'Insanity', a term covering a wide range of conditions, can be seen, to take polarised views, entirely as a social construction or merely a matter of epidemiology.[36] In the latter approach particularly, there is a danger that present-day knowledge or values affect interpretations of outlooks, terms and

---

[31] From 1890 this normally involved a justice's order and two medical certificates (one for existing poor law cases after notification from the PL relieving officer).

[32] G.E. Berrios and H. Freeman (eds), *150 Years of British Psychiatry 1841–1991*, Gaskell, London, Vol. 1 1991, intro., p. x.

[33] Bartlett and Wright, *Outside the Walls*, p. 5.

[34] From a professional vantage point Crammer argues; 'Not all those people with a mental illness are insane (lunatics); not all the insane are mad. Though the placing of a given individual in one of these categories or in "normal" may be difficult or impossible, in very many cases there is no doubt at all.' Crammer, 'English asylums', p. 104.

[35] Here I do not attach specific meanings, or assume steady progression and improvement, or corresponding alterations in public perceptions of asylum or mental illness. For example, 'patient' was used at the Norfolk Lunatic Asylum from 1814 and late nineteenth-century 'attendants' were male and 'nurses' female.

[36] Thus Shorter, *Psychiatry*, pp. 48–9 castigates historians and others for failing to disaggregate 'madness' and distinguish between different forms of 'real' psychiatric illnesses, which were on the increase. His own early examples are 'neurosyphilis, alcoholic

practices which contemporaries at different times assumed to be facts of life or self-evident. Was eighteenth-century melancholy really the equivalent of late twentieth-century depression, for example? Similarly, rudimentary classifications and provision for the 'mad' or 'idiots' may appear less harsh when considered in the context of standards then available.[37] Conversely, well-meaning intent and progressive improvement cannot simply be assumed. Moreover, from the 1808 Act to 'care in the community', policy declarations could be delayed, subverted or simply fail to materialise at grass roots levels.

Yet the transformation of asylum conditions through humane social reform, state regulation and the influence of medical practitioners, remains a powerful theme.[38] Inevitably, much research has been shaped by the succession of landmark legislative changes cumulatively suggesting progress. Asylum regulation generally involved inspections and requirements that institutions compile appropriate information in a reporting process which held them accountable to informed public representatives. The results provide copious source material – most certainly for this study – almost all of which presented official supervisory or institutional viewpoints. Any contrasting, grass roots or unofficial information was much less frequently compiled or preserved. Patients in particular do not feature as central figures: their ability to contribute or report was discounted more or less by definition, even on the rare occasions when they had an official opportunity to request discharge or to complain.[39] Further complications involve the undoubted need to protect patients and their relatives and the practice of censorship, either of which can still the patient's narrative.[40] Medical case notes invariably view individual

psychosis, and apparently, though this is less certain, schizophrenia'. There is a wider debate on the viral origins of schizophrenia and whether this existed in ancient or different forms. If such illnesses existed before they were first diagnosed they evidently involved only small minorities at the NLA, which had few 'paralysis' or alcohol-related cases of any description.

[37] Thus arrangements for hot baths at the NLA matched those at the Norfolk and Norwich hospital in the 1830s and the diet probably compared favourably with that of the Norwich poor.

[38] D.G. Thomson, 'Presidential Address ... History of Norfolk County Asylum', pp. 541–72. See also A. Walk, 'Mental hospitals' in F.N.L. Poynter (ed.), *The Evolution of Hospitals in Britain*, Pitman Medical, London, 1964, pp. 123–46. R. Porter, 'History of psychiatry in Britain', *History of Psychiatry, 2*, 1991, pp. 271–9 surveys the erosion of this position.

[39] Scull, 'Psychiatry and its historians', p. 245, cites David Ingleby's comment that, until recently, the historiography of psychiatry, 'like the histories of colonial wars, [tells] us more about the relations between the imperial powers than about the "third world" or the mental patients themselves'.

[40] Norfolk Mental Health Care NHS Trust very kindly allowed access to two current patients and, with the Norfolk Record Office, the examination of asylum/hospital case notes, including those falling within the '100-year rule', details from which are anonymised in the text.

patients through the eyes of their doctors. They constitute a valuable source, subject to inference by doctors and researchers alike, which can all too rarely be compared with patients' own powers of recall.[41]

Other recent research has examined issues of rights and interests within asylums, and the role of the asylum/hospital in the context of shifting boundaries of care. Nineteenth-century institutional studies have suggested that the asylum was not a monolithic institution but a site for conflicts. Disputes between lay and medical authorities over the management and treatment of patients seem to have been rare in Norfolk but the failure to appoint a medical superintendent at Norfolk Lunatic Asylum before 1861 became a national professional issue for the Medico-Psychological Association.[42] Tensions between local justices, responsible for running county asylums until the Local Government Act of 1888, and the central lunacy commissioners who inspected and regulated them before 1914 were more obvious. Early instances in Norfolk included levels of medical provision and dietary standards in the early 1840s. Almost a century later, the committee of county councillors which had managed the mental hospital since 1889 faced sustained criticism from the inspectors of the post-1914 Board of Control over inadequate facilities for new admissions.

Asylum and poor law authorities often disputed the appropriate site and expense of treatments and the need to assuage Norfolk ratepayers may well have undermined the quality of asylum care locally.[43] For much of the nineteenth century the workhouse remained part of the greater system of care of the insane.[44] Paupers comprised the great majority of county asylum patients and the process of committal largely operated through the poor law and its officials, suggesting the considerable influence of that system's mentality and medical standards. With the relative costs of care a pressing concern, potential asylum patients may have been in the workhouse or on outdoor relief for some time and only the most unmanageable, violent, helpless or suicidal were likely to by pass this stage before their transfer. There was the further possibility that paupers regarded as uncooperative, idle or intemperate might be disciplined by a transfer to the asylum, justified by the 'structuring' of their insanity. However, the persistence of workhouse or out-relief for the insane can be inferred from Table 1.1. As late as 1890 less than two-thirds of the insane poor had been relocated to asylums in England, although the proportion then increased, and one in ten was still being cared

---

[41] See D. Gittins, *Madness in its Place, Narratives of Severalls Hospital 1913–97*, Routledge, London, 1998.

[42] See *The Asylum Journal*, London, 15 Aug. 1854, p. 104. The issue is explored in Chapter 3 below.

[43] L.D. Smith, *Cure, Comfort and Safe Custody*, Leicester University Press, 1999, p. 77.

[44] P. Bartlett, 'The asylum and the poor law: the productive alliance' in Melling and Forsythe, *Insanity Institutions . . .*, pp. 48–67.

for under outdoor relief arrangements.[45] The practice of boarding out patients 'with friends' also continued, notably in Scotland, while some in north Wales were literally 'farmed out', working on the land.[46] Norfolk had 1,005 people classed as pauper lunatics in 1900 yet, despite the growth of asylums for the county and city of Norwich, nearly 15 per cent of these remained with relatives and friends and over 7 per cent were retained within workhouses.[47]

Whether or not household and family care directly corresponded to 'informal' care in the community, it preceded, persisted throughout and post-dated the asylum era. The role of patients' families and friends in their admission and release has also attracted considerable research interest. Suggestions that family breakdown triggered usage of the asylum have been modified to encompass proactive resort by families with unmanageable relatives, which implies either that asylums were no longer seen as wholly repressive institutions or that they represented a last line of care.[48] In some instances asylum care may even have been used by non-paupers 'who could utilise its provision without acquiring the stigma of illness and improvidence associated with workhouse residence'.[49] Some of this research may be unduly influenced by present-day concepts of medical markets and the language of consumerism. County asylums were stigmatised institutions. Although separately funded, administered and regulated, they were often identified with the poor law system and, certainly in Norfolk, most of their patients were paupers. The early asylums imposed top-downwards reform and, well-intentioned or otherwise, they were not initially demanded by the poor, even if they were later utilised by them. Relatives of the pauper insane were rarely in a position to negotiate with poor law or asylum authorities or, initially at least, to exert leverage from their own sense of entitlement or rights.

However, there is evidence of relatives or friends seeking the release of asylum patients in Norfolk throughout the period reviewed. It appears that,

[45] P. Bartlett, *The Poor Law of Lunacy*, Leicester University Press, 1999, Figure 4, p. 263.

[46] H. Sturdy and W. Parry-Jones, 'Boarding out insane patients: the significance of the Scottish system 1857–1913' in Bartlett and Wright, *Outside the Walls*, pp. 86–114; D. Hirst and P. Michael, 'Family, community and the lunatic in mid-nineteenth century North Wales', ibid., pp. 66–85.

[47] A major feature was the cost of such help: even with a subsidy on asylum patients at least 4/- each per week, asylum charge of 8s 9d exceeded cf. 3s 6d workhouse. Ninety-five per cent of those with relatives cost under 4/- and 80 per cent cost 3/- or less. Norfolk Quarter Sessions, C/Saa/6/1/1–24, Guardians' Returns of Pauper Lunatics, 1 Jan. 1900.

[48] J. Walton, 'Casting out and bringing back in Victorian England: pauper lunatics 1840–70' in W.F. Bynum, R. Porter and M. Shepherd (eds), *The Anatomy of Madness* Vol. 2, Tavistock, London, 1985, pp. 132–46; R. Adair, B. Forsythe and J. Melling, 'A danger to the public? Disposing of pauper lunatics in late Victorian and Edwardian England', *Medical History*, 42, 1998, pp. 1–25.

[49] J. Melling, 'Accommodating madness; new research into the social history of insanity and institutions' in Melling and Forsythe, *Insanity, Institutions . . .*, p. 7. The Devon County Asylum (1845) was not restricted to pauper patients.

from the justices onwards, asylum authorities sometimes approved of such demonstrations of family support and saw economic advantages in the discharge of suitable patients. They were also quick to develop and support financially systems of leave, parole or probation. Although this terminology suggests a custodial outlook, its practice often led to release and was associated with institutional benefits involving lower costs of maintenance or the relief of overcrowding. Alongside the limited numbers of patients cured or relieved and subject to considerable rates of readmission, these developments indicate that the nineteenth-century asylum was not merely a place of incarceration.[50] However, demonstrations of flexibility in the asylum system over time do not mean that short-term rigidities were unimportant, or that the long-term restraint of threatening individuals and forms of behaviour was diminished. Processes of change should not be telescoped and most asylum patients found their own confinement marked by physical and procedural boundaries that were all too apparent. Moreover the circumstances in which asylums were initially constructed still require explanation by those who focus upon their operation and utilisation. The economic and social context offered earlier may be too general but to suggest that changes in family feelings or behaviour and responses by asylum authorities were decisive, but somehow independent of this background, seems even more problematic.

Economic considerations have been relatively neglected in asylum history and hospital history in general. They feature strongly here because they largely determined the working of the institution as a community and were a critical factor in its eventual closure. The early justices were fully aware of the need for tight household management and soon adopted perspectives which involved income generation and the pursuit of institutional self-sufficiency. Long before the development of rehabilitation therapy, 'work therapy' at the asylum/hospital was enthusiastically supported by lay and medical authorities and there was much overlap in their respective rationales. Experiences in the Great War confirm the importance attached to economic matters, even when an asylum's own patients had been dispersed, and the pursuit of 'economy' became a still more daunting task amidst the financial uncertainties of the inter-war years. A new National Health Service brought no release from these particular labours. Changes associated with the growth of voluntary patients, particularly their legally granted 'informal' status after 1959, and the reorganisation of the St Andrew's patient clientele under the NHS, did end the long association of asylum accommodation with work. But at the macro-economic level, demoralising shortages of resources within the NHS affected the hospital as a therapeutic community well before the sale of the hospital estate and buildings to secure wider service improvements graphically confirmed the shifting boundaries of mental health care.

[50] D. Wright, 'The discharge of lunatics from county asylums in mid-Victorian England' in Melling and Forsythe, *Insanity, Institutions . . .*, pp. 93–112.

Therapeutic regimes?

Norfolk Lunatic Asylum initially admitted a handful of lunatics from prisons or bridewells and some of the most difficult or dangerous poor law patients, the others remaining where they were. Hopes for the asylum combination of custodial framework, medical skills and moral treatment probably explain why this facility developed: otherwise, prison reform might have sufficed for some, cases of brain diseases could be addressed in general hospitals and examples of moral shortfall corrected through workhouses. The asylum's successive master and superintendent were long-serving officials, as were each of the medical superintendents who wielded considerable power even into the NHS era.[51] Similarly, the longevity of the Norfolk Lunatic Asylum/ St Andrew's provides opportunities to consider whether their respective 'regimes' reflected contemporary national standards of practice and new thinking. The ensuing chapters are largely delineated by these regimes, except for those dealing with wartime experiences and the greater external influences associated with the hospital's reorganisation and closure. Each chapter offers a commentary on treatment records but also attempts an interpretation of asylum conditions or hospital life, looking at nursing staff and using available information on the social composition of patients, their own case experiences and the fragmentary evidence concerning pastimes, exercise and leisure.

National models of asylum development suggest that medical officers and reformers were optimistic but vague about moral treatment and its benefits, hoping that asylum would provide a space for recovery aided by exercise, recreation, hygiene, diet and medical attention to bodily ailments. Their individual attention to relatively small numbers of patients was soon undermined by more admissions, overcrowding and the increased scale of the asylum undertaking, which necessitated more rigid systems of organisation and supervision.[52] Restrictive conditions initially predominated at Norfolk Lunatic Asylum (NLA) but may have eased by the 1830s, not least because the asylum remained relatively small. As Chapter 2 also indicates, doctors focused upon the physical body and, although patients were discharged, readmission rates were considerable. However, an air of optimism accompanied the introduction of work therapy and the belated appointment of resident medical officers, although the lack of a medical superintendent

---

[51] Medical superintendents had a direct relationship with 'their' Committee of Justices (later councillors) until the NHS, when Regional Hospital Boards became the authority on most financial matters. The office of medical superintendent was abolished in 1971 (see Chapter 10).

[52] J. Walton, 'The treatment of pauper lunatics in Victorian England: the case of Lancaster Asylum 1816–70' in A. Scull (ed.), *Madhouses, Mad-doctors and Madmen*, University of Pennsylvania, Philadelphia, 1981, pp. 166–97.

before 1861 earned the NLA a notorious and rather undeserved reputation, explored further in Chapter 3.

Although asylum doctors nationally had little to show from their investigations and classification of inmates, they succeeded professionally by offering explanations of insanity which focused upon its complexity and the need for inmates' management. Thus 'the optimistic aspects of moral management had to be exchanged for a bleaker prospect for psychiatric therapies which none the less demanded the presence and the skill of the trained medical psychiatrist'.[53] As Chapter 4 reveals, one of the earliest actions of the NLA's first medical superintendent, William Hills, was to combine practical improvements with a more pessimistic assessment of the possibilities of asylum treatments. Yet he also claimed that the chronic insane, the handicapped and even the elderly and infirm could be most effectively managed and cared for within an auxiliary institution. This approach reflected national developments and was soon reinforced by reference to theories of evolution and natural selection. Increasingly, the various deficiencies detected in patients were cited as proof of regression from higher functions and linked with heredity and environmental influences, notably poor diet and a range of 'toxins' varying from alcohol to sexually transmitted diseases.

The accelerating growth of late nineteenth-century asylums was fuelled by an apparent surge in those of 'unsound mind', numerically and as a proportion of the national population (see Table 1.1). Further differentiation of forms of mental defect, from idiocy to the 'weak-minded', was beginning to be reflected in separate institutional provision from the 1860s, though not in Norfolk.[54] Increasing numbers of people were found to be living on 'the borderland of insanity' and consigned to asylums by general practitioners and poor law relieving officers.[55] Although new mental illnesses were detected and explanations advanced for these, the Medico-Psychological Association and its members could claim few therapeutic achievements. A not unsympathetic summary acknowledges: 'There was no organising principle, no doctrine comparable in power to the germ theory of disease, no consistent approach to treatment.'[56] However, in the search for underlying causes of insanity, degeneration and idiocy, 'heredity was increasingly seen lurking behind an assortment of merely superficial moral and environmental

[53] Neve, 'Medicine and the mind', p. 243.
[54] J. Saunders, 'Quarantining the weak-minded: psychiatric definitions of degeneracy and the late-Victorian asylum' in W.F. Bynum and R. Porter (eds), *The Anatomy of Madness*, Routledge, London, 1985, Vol. 3, pp. 273–95.
[55] See M. Jackson, *The Borderland of Imbecility*, Manchester University Press, 2000, pp. 1–20.
[56] R.E. McGrew, 'Psychiatry', *Encyclopedia of Medical History*, Macmillan, London, 1985, pp. 279–84, 280.

causes'.[57] Signs of 'hereditary predisposition' featured increasingly in patient admissions and in diagnostics, the latter having its own uncertain parentage involving scientific, social and cultural values. Whilst claiming objective detachment, medical superintendents such as David Thomson were themselves heavily influenced, as will be seen in Chapter 5. Evolution, science and nature were also evoked in presentations of women mentally unbalanced by their bodily functions, sexuality or vulnerability.[58] However, if local experience in Norfolk or the evidence of Table 1.1 is any guide, these developments had little effect on the gender balance among the mainly working-class patients in county asylums.[59]

Early twentieth-century asylum responses to manic depressive psychosis or schizophrenia, illnesses with no obvious physical cause, were limited. Developments involving individualised therapy for patients diagnosed with these illnesses or hysteria were seen as impractical in asylums with a thousand or more patients and small medical staffs.[60] Even when such conditions were diagnosed, they were often initially incorporated within existing classifications or explained in terms of hereditary features.[61] Similarly the modernisation of the Norfolk County Asylum (NCA), now described as 'a hospital for mental diseases', involved essentially infrastructure improvements and the reorganisation of services around work and sexual divisions. Amenities for patients were enhanced and laboratory testing provided safeguards against infectious diseases but innovations such as malarial treatment for syphilis, the use of Phenobarbital to limit epileptic seizures, and of barbiturates in continuous narcosis were not applied until the 1920s. By then the experience of war neuroses had contradicted earlier 'scientific' generalisations concerning hereditary predisposition, or the physical or feminine origins of mental illnesses. War also proved a stimulus to therapeutic regimes and in changing public attitudes to mental illness, though these developments can be exaggerated.[62] NCA patients had a hidden and

[57] J. Andrews, 'Notes on mental health care and prophylaxis in late 19th century Britain', *Health Care Discussion Papers*, 1, Oxford Brookes University, 1998, pp, p. 20

[58] e.g. L. Hall, *Sex, Gender and Social Change in Britain since 1880*, Macmillan, Basingstoke, 2000, pp. 26–8.

[59] See also J. Busfield, 'The female malady? Men, women and madness in nineteenth-century Britain', *Sociology*, 28, 1994, pp. 259–77.

[60] e.g. psychoanalysis, hypnosis or free association to resolve subconscious conflicts and 'release' patients.

[61] Official classifications in 1912 included primary dementia (dementia praecox), but mania, confusional and delusional insanity were wide labels. Physical or degenerative approaches were also retained: thus schizophrenia was 'the quiet collapse of jerry-built brains under the strain of their own weight or on the first contact with the social responsibilities of adult life'. Dr Hayes Newington at the 1909 RMPA Conference, cited in P. Barham, *Closing the Asylum*, Penguin, Harmondsworth, 1992, p. 76.

[62] R. Cooter, 'War and modern medicine' in W. Bynum and R. Porter (eds), *Companion*

altogether different war experience; they were removed from the asylum prior to its conversion as the Norfolk War Hospital and dispersed around regional asylums with considerable loss of life, a neglected issue investigated in Chapter 6.

In the reopened, renamed St Andrew's Hospital systems of parole were promoted in the 1920s, voluntary patients were admitted under the 1930 Mental Treatment Act and outpatient clinics were established in conjunction with local general hospitals. Nationally these developments have been interpreted as the relaxation of former asylum regimes and a new emphasis upon treatment, although they may also have extended systems of surveillance beyond hospital walls.[63] Yet, as Chapter 7 shows, the majority of patients remained unaffected. Economic uncertainty and strict financial controls, coupled with a traditionalist emphasis upon the physical fabric of the hospital, restricted innovations in treatments locally. For all the emphasis upon voluntary patients and outpatients, more suitable admission, observation and clinical facilities were not provided.[64] Most patients still led limited lives based upon echoes of moral management: work therapy, a bare diet, outdoor walks and modest entertainments. More invasive measures began in the late 1930s with insulin coma treatment, followed by ECT and neurosurgery. These were delayed by the Second World War which, as Chapter 8 shows, placed great stresses upon hospital resources and patients. Yet they were operative and indeed were cited as proof of the hospital's modernity and capabilities even in rather outmoded settings at the inception of the National Health Service.

From then on two broad therapeutic features at St Andrew's became more pronounced. More outpatient attendances and short-term admissions, with steady improvements in assessments and psychotherapy, suggested changes even before the onset of new drug treatments led to unlocked wards, greater freedom for patients and more rehabilitation. Chapter 9 also shows that, at the same time, ageing and ultimately dwindling groups of chronic patients were provided essentially with continuing care. Undergoing one local NHS reorganisation in 1965, St Andrew's was already scheduled for a reduction in the range of services it provided when the hospital was caught up in national closure campaigns and the development of community care provision, the theme of Chapter 10. Even then the process of closure lasted over thirty years and was not without twists, but ultimately the hospital's longevity proved a

---

Encyclopaedia of the History of Medicine, Vol. 2, Routledge, London, 1993, pp. 1536–73, 1550–1.

[63] Compare Jones, *Asylums*, pp. 35–6 with Bartlett and Wright, *Outside the Walls*, pp. 13–14.

[64] The need to provide separate facilities for the mentally handicapped, particularly children, was a complicating feature as it inevitably meant competition for limited resources (see Chapter 7).

disadvantage. Its physical associations with the asylum era and, less fairly, with older practices and an inflexible 'hospital culture' rather masked the long-term relative neglect still affecting psychiatric hospitals and their patients under the NHS. New and more appropriate services were developed elsewhere, though their sufficiency remains an issue, particularly with respect to those 'who need something rather more than short-term therapy for an acute phase of their illness'.[65] These are questions for clinicians and politicians, but interviews with former St Andrew's staff reveal very differing perceptions and experiences of change in the hospital's final years.

Norfolk notes: the local context

Most of the county asylums constructed by 1828 served rural areas, suggesting that there were local dimensions to affirmative decisions by county justices. Stresses arising from the generalisation of market production and industrial-isation, compounded by the additional dislocations of the French and Napoleonic wars, certainly caused them concern.[66] However, the immediate response to perceived threats to property, if not the social fabric, in Norfolk was to establish forces of loyal volunteers rather than prisons, workhouses or asylums. Volunteer units were proposed from 1794 and a number of pro-government Tory families later associated with the governance of the NLA were actively involved. Concern over radicalism in Norwich was also expressed in public subscriptions to relieve the industrious poor but determined efforts were made to build volunteer forces loyal to the local establishment rather than for the purpose of resisting any French invasion.[67] Social distress led to increased spending, particularly on public works and foodstuffs to relieve the poor, but 'reform' was more typically posed in terms of restriction and economy, in which timing rather than desirability was the critical question.[68]

Did the NLA and workhouses provide 'a convenient way of getting rid of inconvenient people . . . the difficult and troublesome sorts'?[69] An emphasis on workhouse provision in the reformed post-1834 poor laws enhanced such

---

[65] P. Sedgewick, *Psychopolitics*, Pluto, London, 1982, p. 213.

[66] Scull, *Afflictions*, p. 28.

[67] C.B. Jewson, *Jacobin City*, Blackie, Glasgow, 1975, pp. 30–2. Prominent county families whose members commanded volunteer forces and who were also involved in the asylum included the Harveys, Beevors and Wodehouses (see Chapters 2 and 3).

[68] Robert Harvey, Mayor of Norwich in 1792, was prominent in organising poor relief and volunteer forces in 1797. A contemporary investigation into the cost of poor law feeding arrangements featured one prominent critic, Dr Edward Rigby, who became mayor in 1805 and was appointed to the NLA. F.M. Eden, *The State of the Poor*, Warrington, 1797, pp. 477–522. Poor law spending in the city peaked at almost £18,000 in the early 1800s, perhaps three times the normal level. F. Blomefield, *History of Norfolk*, 1806, Vol. III, p. 432.

[69] Scull, *Madhouses, Mad-doctors and Madmen*, p. 17.

possibilities but this occurred fully two decades after the asylum was established. Meanwhile, the slow growth of asylum admissions was not suggestive of systematic and general incarceration, even though potentially dangerous insane or sick prisoners were transferred there, as were some unmanageable workhouse inmates. Yet nineteenth-century indications in Norfolk seem to confirm the related point that asylum expansion was not a proportionate response to population growth but to economic dislocation and other stresses upon the rural poor. Roughly two-thirds of the Norfolk population lived outside Norwich, Great Yarmouth and King's Lynn and the NLA focused upon pauper lunatics beyond the city and borough towns. Population growth in rural Norfolk was only half the national average and rather uneven, slower in western districts, rising from 294,000 in 1831 to 327,000 in 1851. A prolonged decline then occurred, to 276,000 in 1901, followed only by limited recovery to 301,000 in 1931.[70]

Why was this? Nineteenth-century Norfolk labourers were not favoured with jobs or pay. Military or civilian employment opportunities in the French wars were partly offset by the rising cost of living and reversed by post-war arable recession in the county. This aggravated economic stagnation in Norwich where, by 1851, one-third of adult males were migrants from elsewhere in the county. Agriculture still provided the bulk of employment and in 1861 roughly four-fifths of working adult males in Norfolk were farm labourers. Arable farming was labour intensive but involved seasonal underemployment and was undermined by repeal of the Corn Laws in 1846. Diversification in the era of high farming was associated with greater labour productivity, reduced arable acreages and fewer jobs: there was a 30 per cent reduction in male farm labourers from 1861 to 1891 and women had still fewer opportunities.[71] Norfolk's limited and patchy industrial development failed to offset the decline of rural crafts and occupations such as worsted weaving, papermaking and woodworking. The fortunes of others, such as brickmaking, often remained tied to agriculture and local markets. Railway development meant enhanced markets for agricultural goods but was also associated with more competitive industrial products and the undermining of local employment. As the continuing emigration of younger, economically active people exceeded rates of natural increase, the population declined.

Landowners and farmers could pay very low wages to those who did not emigrate or who were unskilled. As ratepayers or poor law guardians, they sought to balance the convenience of temporary labourers at harvest time with the overall costs of poor relief. Particularly in the early nineteenth century these were comparatively high, as Table 1.2 suggests, and any additional charges arising from poor law services, including those provided at

[70] A. Armstrong, *The Population of Victorian and Edwardian Norfolk*, Centre of East Anglia Studies, Norwich, 2000, p. 11.
[71] ibid., p. 15.

Table 1.2 Poor Law spending per head per annum, 1803–43

	Norfolk	% Norfolk 'excess'	Average for England and Wales
1803	12s 5d	42	8s 11d
1813	20/–	58	12s 8d
1824	14s 5d	57	9s 2d
1833	16s 3d	72	9s 9d
1843	9s 2d	43	6s 5d

Sources: Based on R. Taylor, 'The development of the old Poor Law in Norfolk 1795–1834', UEA MA dissertation 1970, and Digby, *Pauper Palaces*, p. 84. The Norfolk figure for 1813 would be partly inflated by the levy for the asylum (see ch. 2).

the county asylum, would be unwelcome. Supplements to wages, the tied cottage, small allotments and scraps of work for women and children all featured in Norfolk rural life but, characteristically, 'wages were determined by social assumptions about what was needed to provide a subsistence income, and this led to a deterioration in real wages after 1814'.[72] One response by the labouring poor was social disturbance, including riots and incendiarism from 1815 to the early 1830s, followed by protest against the new poor laws. Such threats exercised local magistrates but, to judge from its admissions, the asylum was not used as an instrument of containment. Instead, distress committees and poor law sponsored emigration schemes acted as a social safety valve, with over 8,000 people emigrating in 1835–6 alone.[73] Some of the fervour of primitive Methodism in Norfolk arose from perceived injustices and economic hardship, as with early forms of agricultural trades unionism and political Liberalism, although the latter tended to be more restrained.[74] Sufferers from 'religious mania' were among the increased admissions to the NLA in the 1840s but otherwise were not systematically confined.

It was the grinding effects of poverty that took a more general toll. Official statistics of pauperism, a dismal understatement of poverty, indicated Norfolk levels well above national averages.[75] Although the growth in asylum

[72] A. Digby, *Pauper Palaces*, Routledge, London, 1978, p. 22.

[73] Armstrong, *Population*, p. 23. Net overseas emigration from Norfolk exceeded 30,000 in 1861–1901 and heavy migration into Norwich, London and north-east England continued.

[74] See N. Virgoe and T. Williamson (eds), *Religious Dissent in East Anglia*, Centre of East Anglia Studies, Norwich, 1993. George Edwards, methodist lay preacher and leader of the farmworkers' union was inclined to be 'Lib-Lab' in his political outlook and became a Labour councillor and MP and a member of the NCA/St Andrew's hospital committee (see Chapter 7).

[75] e.g. Norfolk average of 6.7 per cent 1851–80, c.f. national 4.8 per cent. Late nineteenth-century Norfolk averages always exceeded 4 per cent, with national averages below 3 per cent. Digby, *Pauper Palaces*, p. 84.

admissions was nowhere unusual, its Norfolk context was within a declining rural population. This may indicate the inability of stressed rural families and individuals to cope, either with prolonged economic hardship or with relatives regarded as unmanageable. It also hints at the 'medicalisation' of individuals and their problems and of extended usage of the asylum by poor law authorities.[76] Returns in 1847, for example, indicate slightly higher percentages of people in Norfolk classed as 'pauper lunatic/idiot' than nationally, with a greater proportion placed in the county asylum.[77] Less controversially, close affinities between the asylum as a working community and Norfolk lifestyles persisted well into the twentieth century and contributed heavily to hospital culture and staff–patient relationships, the 'kindly' atmosphere frequently remarked on even by critics who saw both as outmoded.

None of this explains why Norfolk justices decided to proceed with asylum building at the comparatively early date of 1814. It would be surprising if the need for suitable custodial provision did not enter their deliberations – they were magistrates – but there were immediate and more positive features. One was the upward trend in agricultural prices and demand, which made an asylum a more affordable proposition for the county's landowner and farmer ratepayers. Public provision for the insane in eighteenth-century Norfolk was limited to houses of correction (bridewells), workhouses and outdoor relief. County justices could detain the 'furiously and dangerously mad' and those 'disordered in their senses' under the Vagrancy Acts of 1714 and 1744. In the mid-1770s the prison reformer John Howard had noted one lunatic among the five inmates at the Swaffham bridewell but did not specifically identify others among 53 'felons, debtors etc.' in his tour of Norfolk.[78] Persons acquitted at trial on the grounds of insanity could also be detained under the 1800 Criminal Lunatics Act. However, the 1744 Act allowed for treatment as well as incarceration, raising the possibility of separate facilities for such cases and for those who were particularly difficult to manage under poor law arrangements. In Norwich the Corporation workhouse, established in 1711, had a separate infirmary although no distinct provision was made for lunatic inmates until 1828.[79] County provision was inadequate: even in 1863, only

---

[76] Scull, *Afflictions*, p. 375, argues that doctors 'medicalised' behaviour previously seen as socially 'problematic' thereby extending their professional influence. Thus asylums first dealt with 'some of the frenzied' but later with 'the routine consignment of the deranged, the depressed and the distracted'.

[77] Lunatic Paupers chargeable to Parishes in Norfolk, Suffolk and England and Wales on 1st Jan. 1847. Poor Law Commission, *Official Circulars of Public Documents and Information*, London, 1851, No. 10, 1 Oct. 1847. Thirty-six per cent of these were in the NLA, compared with the national equivalent of 28.6 per cent.

[78] J. Howard, *The State of the Prisons*, 1777, p. 260, 257–62.

[79] These were adjacent to the infirmary in St Augustine's. Provision remained appallingly bad in Norwich until the City asylum opened at Hellesdon in 1880. S. Cherry, 'Responses to Illness: health and health care in modern Norwich' in C. Rawcliffe and R.G. Wilson (eds.), *The History of Norwich* (forthcoming).

four Norfolk workhouses had separate lunatic wards and, although some individuals were boarded out, 13 of the 22 poor law unions mixed sane, insane and 'weak-minded' patients.[80]

If the asylum was judged affordable and necessary, there was also some confidence about its prospects. Locally, the Bethel and Norfolk and Norwich hospitals, opened in 1724 and 1772 respectively, embodied the expression of civic pride and institutional therapeutic achievement. The Bethel was a pioneering provincial institution for the treatment of mental disorders, stemming from the personal experience and concern of its founder, Mary Chapman, in 1713. From 1724 it was administered as a public charity, expressly for those 'afflicted with lunacy or madness, not such as are fools or idiots from their birth'.[81] Its forty beds were mainly for private patients, although charitable cases and paupers charged to the Norwich Corporation comprised roughly one-quarter of the 500 admissions before 1800.[82] As England's third largest city Norwich also represented a developing medical market, in which professional reputations were made on the basis of claims to special knowledge. Mad doctoring, which synthesised moral and medical management, was already established. In addition to the Bethel, the private asylums founded at Loddon in 1782, Framlingham in 1807, Heigham Hall in 1836 and Heigham Retreat before 1840 suggested medical entrepreneurship and an identifiable need. The physicians or surgeons involved retained their broader work but those such as Edward Rigby, founder of another private asylum at Lakenham in 1807, or William Dalrymple, surgeon to the Bethel, were closely associated with asylums.

Arguably Britain's first cottage or village hospital opened in Shotesham, Norfolk in the early 1730s and attempts beginning in 1744 to provide a larger and more durable institution succeeded when the Norfolk and Norwich Hospital admitted its first patients in 1772. Like most eighteenth-century voluntary hospitals, it focused upon the treatable and non-pauperised sick poor and it specifically excluded 'persons disordered in their senses'.[83] If this admissions policy acknowledged the Bethel hospital, it also recognised the local medical market and reflected contemporary lay and medical opinion on the difficulties surrounding the treatment of mental disorders. Eighteenth-century examples of public subscription asylums or voluntary hospitals with wards for mental disorders were not pursued in Norwich. Yet the success of the Norfolk and Norwich and the Bethel hospitals as civic projects probably strengthened and shaped efforts to establish a county asylum.

---

[80] Digby, *Pauper Palaces*, p. 172.

[81] F. Bateman and W. Rye, *The History of the Bethel Hospital*, Norwich, 1906, p. 5.

[82] M. Winston, 'The Bethel at Norwich: an eighteenth-century hospital for lunatics', *Medical History*, 38, 1994, pp. 27–51.

[83] S. Cherry, 'The role of a provincial hospital; the Norfolk and Norwich Hospital 1772–1880', *Population Studies*, XXVI, 2, 1972, pp. 291–306, 295.

A more direct impetus was provided by the 1807 Select Committee on the state of criminal and pauper lunatics, chaired by Charles Williams-Wynn, which raised the cause of lunacy reform and envisaged the provision of successful, cost-effective treatments offered within regulated asylums. Andrew Halliday, compiling evidence for the committee, visited Norfolk that year. He concluded that there were 112 lunatics and idiots, 27 of whom were detained in poor law or penal institutions, in comparison with the county's own estimate of 22 pauper and criminal lunatics in 1806.[84] The ensuing Act made outline proposals but was permissive in tone: local justices were empowered to raise a rate to establish and maintain a county asylum, but much depended upon their own inclinations. Those in Norfolk were not unanimous and probably had a variety of motives but they were likely to be influenced by their observations of already existing provision and a sanguine assessment of the asylum's utility as a custodial and therapeutic institution.

[84] K. Jones, *Lunacy, Law and Conscience 1744–1845*, Routledge, London, 1955, pp. 73, 131.

2

Norfolk Lunatic Asylum: plans, problems and patients, 1814–43

Although the 1808 Act encouraged county justices to establish lunatic asylums, it provided few specific instructions and there was no compulsion to build until additional legislation was passed in 1845.[1] A complex of national and local influences, outlined in the previous chapter, may have featured when the Norfolk Quarter Sessions first discussed this possibility in October 1808 but the dominant contributions were not recorded.[2] This chapter examines the establishment of the Norfolk Lunatic Asylum and its physical features, its medical and lay personnel, the patients and treatments, focusing upon local records but drawing upon contemporary surveys and accounts. It suggests that considerable efforts were made to ensure that the relatively novel institution incorporated good practices as they were then understood. The grim beginnings of the NLA, particularly as experienced by its patients, were not wholly intentional and there were signs of improvement over time, although there was much to be desired when reform standards of the early 1840s were applied by the inspecting Commissioners in Lunacy.

With an eye to wider contexts, two issues emerge. The Norfolk justices, in building at an early date and to plans which involved considerable cost – more than they intended – responded to the reforming intent of permissive legislation. Yet they were not wholly compliant, which may indicate local motives and a desire for autonomy. Research findings on other asylums suggest that, 'as states sought to exert greater control over the classification and treatment of lunatics by the elaboration of administrative regulations and statistical information, local agents and professional bodies asserted their own capacity to identify and manage the insane'.[3] In Norfolk, the committee of visiting justices was involved in close supervision of the asylum, rather than relying upon indirect control, and they evidently resisted its medical superintendence, although medical influences began to feature more prominently in the 1840s. Moreover, the asylum's management suggests awareness

---

[1] 8 and 9 Vict. *An Act to amend the Laws for the Provision and Regulation of Lunatic Asylums for Counties and Boroughs, and for the Maintenance and Care of Pauper Lunatics, in England.* (1845) c.126.
[2] Norfolk Quarter Sessions minutes (NQS) 1805–1811, c/s/1/17; 11 Oct. 1808.
[3] B. Forsythe, J. Melling and R. Adair, 'Politics of lunacy. Central state regulation and the Devon Pauper Lunatic Asylum 1845–1914', in J. Melling and B. Forsythe (eds), *Insanity, Institutions and Society 1800–1914*, Routledge, London, 1999, pp. 68–92.

of the need for economy and a sound reputation with ratepayers and poor law guardians.[4] This persisted over the nineteenth century whether the justices or the medical superintendent predominated, as seen in their later dealings with the lunacy commissioners as the representatives of central authority, examined in subsequent chapters. The second question involves the NLA's standing in contemporary and recent comparative studies, which appears to be better than as portrayed.[5]

Planning for the asylum

Having considered the propriety of establishing an asylum on 11 October 1808, the Norfolk justices ordered a further survey of 'idiot and lunatic paupers' in the county hundreds in January 1809.[6] A slow response was reported at the April and July quarter sessions but the numbers mentioned were regarded as exaggerated and relating to persons 'not within the intention of the legislature'. Some 153 'lunatics and dangerous idiots', 76 men and 77 women, featured on a revised list presented on 30 September.[7] As the justices were divided over their next step the decision to build an asylum was deferred. Costs were a major consideration for some and the permissive terms of the 1808 Act offered a prospective escape route. Others wished to reflect further on the 1807 Select Committee recommendations, particularly on the possibility of a combined asylum for Norfolk and Suffolk. The option of a county public subscription asylum, then being adopted in Nottinghamshire, may also have been considered as a year elapsed before the justices took a majority decision to provide a rate-funded lunatic asylum 'for the County sole'.[8]

The committee of nine which considered the best means of building and managing the asylum was a body of considerable social standing. Its members included two baronets, Sir Edmund Bacon and Sir Thomas Beevor. Edward Stracey of Rackheath, the chairman, had been the County Sheriff in 1785, a position held in 1796 by Thomas Browne Evans of Kirby Bedon. Sigismund Trafford Southwell of Wroxham later became the Sheriff in 1816, as did Edmund Bacon in 1826.[9] Although it was concerned with costs, the

---

[4] This was at times parsimonious, but the Suffolk justices excelled in such respects. M. Fisher, 'Getting out of the asylum: discharge and decarceration issues in asylum history', a Ph.D. thesis to be submitted to the University of East Anglia, Norwich in 2003 (chapter 3).

[5] e.g. John Conolly, *The Construction and Government of Lunatic Asylums*, Churchill, London, 1847; L.D. Smith, *Cure, Comfort and Safe Custody*, Leicester University Press, 1999.

[6] NQS, 11 Jan. 1809.

[7] NQS, 12 April, 12 July and 30 Sept. 1809, p. 208. The list bears the last date.

[8] NQS, 4 Oct. 1810.

[9] H. Le Strange, *Norfolk Officials Lists, from the earliest period to the present day*, Norwich, 1890, pp. 26–7, 38. Other members included Thomas Beevor (younger), Thomas Blake and Thomas Preston.

committee was sensitive to considerations of social order, medical opinion and standards of care. A certain amount of deference to its social standing and the association with public order enhanced the committee's ability to push through what was seen as a desirable reform measure.[10] Agriculture in Norfolk was still sufficiently prosperous to bear additional rates and the apparent success of philanthropic projects which had involved considerable financial outlay on buildings probably counted in the asylum's favour. A public subscription asylum established collaboratively with philanthropic effort was discounted, as were developments involving the Norwich Bethel hospital. The result was a non-compromised county-wide reform initiative, focused upon a pauper clientele and retaining a custodial element. Evidently, the association of reform with order, affordability and due acknowledgement of responsibilities to county ratepayers was sufficient to obtain general endorsement or, at least, to avoid open opposition.

Select Committee recommendations incorporated in the 1808 Act included the need to 'fix upon an airy and healthy situation with a good supply of water, and which may afford a probability of the vicinity of constant medical assistance'.[11] In November 1810 a sub-committee of five justices duly sought a healthy rural location, where a site might be obtainable at lower cost, though it considered that communications and medical facilities required close proximity to Norwich. An advertisement resulted in the purchase of five acres of suitable land from John Harvey at Thorpe St Andrew.[12] This site contained a good springwater source; it was south facing and slightly elevated, offering views over the River Yare and marsh-meadows. A chalky sub-soil favoured drainage and provided good brick earth, features which seemingly outweighed concerns over potential flooding or difficulties with sewerage.[13] Immediate access to the Norwich–Yarmouth turnpike road was a further advantage and the surrounding area was considered favourable, indeed fashionable. Thorpe Hamlet contained 'many delightful residences and some very elegant and convenient villas' and Thorpe village, a mile to the north-west, was described as 'a beautiful and picturesque place containing numerous neat cottages and mansions for the gentry'.[14] If prospective asylum patients were to be marginalised, they were not deliberately hidden or placed into a threatening environment.

As yet there was no distinctive asylum architecture, though the experience of larger private institutions, provincial public subscription

---

[10] J. Walton, 'Casting out and bringing back in Victorian England: pauper lunatics 1840–70', in W.F. Bynum, R. Porter and M. Shepherd (eds), *The Anatomy of Madness*, Tavistock, London, 1985, Vol. 2, pp. 132–46, 133–4.

[11] 48 George III, *An Act for the Better Care and Maintenance of Lunatics, being Paupers or Criminals in England* (1808), Section XVI, c. 96.

[12] NQS, 10 Nov. 1810, and 25 April 1811.

[13] See Chapter 5 below.

[14] G.K. Blyth, *Norwich Directory*, 1842 edn, p. 211.

asylums and Bethlem and St Luke's in London could be drawn upon.[15] Variations on linear, 'E', 'H', 'L' and 'U' shaped designs mirrored hospitals for the physically sick, workhouses and prisons. However, particular features which began to be associated with asylums included a central administrative block with wings, seen at St Luke's, which incorporated a long corridor accessing the cells and day rooms, as in the examples of Bethlem and Nottingham. These allowed for supervision, the sexual segregation of patients and a rudimentary classification of illness, often based upon little more than tendencies towards violent behaviour.[16] A combination of security and substance, confining inmates and protecting society, using buildings which were imposing and even forbidding, was to be expected when at least some patients were seen as dangerous or criminal.

Yet asylum buildings had another public face: the expression of reform effort, specialist provision, and civic achievement. Initially the Committee of Justices considered schemes providing accommodation for 180 patients but capable of enlargement for 300, the respective costs envisaged as £16,500 and £29,000. Money was to be raised by an additional quarterly rate of £1,200 which, it was hoped, 'would inconvenience the inhabitants of the County as little as possible'.[17] Designs were submitted in competition but the Committee did not select a clear winner and instead asked the county surveyor, Francis Stone, whose own plans had not been approved, to incorporate the best features from two successful entries.[18] This procedure reflected a desire for economy and utility and the convenience of Stone's presence and supervision during building operations. No time was lost taking possession of the site and in purchasing bricks, but building work was affected by the inflation associated with the Napoleonic war. In October 1811 the justices were informed that the projected costs were 'no less than £23,138 exclusive of furniture'.[19] Possibly reflecting also upon Halliday's own findings on lunacy in Norfolk, they concluded that accommodation 'for 104 patients is now deemed sufficient', although provision for an additional 50 patients had been costed at £5,000.[20] The quarterly levy was increased to £3,900 from

---

[15] e.g. respectively Brislington House, Bristol (1804) and York Lunatic Asylum (1776). St Luke's was rebuilt in 1787.

[16] H. Richardson (ed.), *English Hospitals 1660–1948*, Swindon, 1998, pp. 154–82.

[17] NQS, 25 April 1811 (p. 279).

[18] ibid., 10 Nov. 1810 (p. 260) and 25 April 1811 (p. 279). William Browne (Ipswich) received 70 guineas and Good and Lockaby (Hatton Gardens) 30 guineas for their designs. As county surveyor Stone (1770–1835) had supervised repairs to Norwich cathedral and castle.

[19] NQS, 10 Oct. 1811.

[20] ibid., 10 Oct. 1811. Halliday's investigation for the 1807 Select Committee had indicated 112 lunatics and idiots in Norfolk, 27 of whom were already detained in poor law or penal institutions. The additional provision was made by extensions undertaken in 1831.

Men's side   Women's side

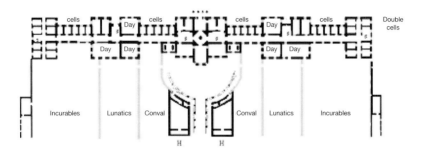

Figure 2.1 1814 plan of Norfolk Lunatic Asylum. Walls and ha-ha arrangement extend on south side. (H) marks additional small 'hospitals'. See text for detailed description of central administrative area.

November 1812 in the hope that the construction and financing of the buildings could be completed by Christmas 1814.

Having consulted the authorities at York asylum and Bethlem, the final NLA plan reflected considerable attention to current knowledge and matters of detail. The asylum buildings were finished in white gault brick with stone quoins, which must have appeared quite striking when new, and were topped with a hipped roof of grey Welsh slate. Their design combined the 'asylum features' mentioned in an early form and the external appearance may be regarded as restrained and functional, neither ornate nor austere, and imposing rather than intimidating. They were described in contemporary guides as 'a noble and extensive structure' and as 'spacious and handsome'.[21] A determination to avoid a block plan or the rather cramped 'E' shape seen at Bedford resulted in a linear and symmetrical building, some 430 feet long, with a raised central portion but for the most part of two storeys. It had an east–west orientation, offering a southern aspect and views to most of the day rooms. As the turnpike road ran immediately to the north of the building, this was the 'public' side, incorporating the main entrance, with the 'private' south-facing rear overlooking a succession of terraces down to meadows, marshland and the river Yare.

The complex was initially dominated by a central, domed three-storey administrative block, with a double roof and pediment. Visitors and admissions were received under a portico with columns through the entrance into an octagon-shaped hall, flanked by the main corridor to the wings and

[21] Blyth, *Directory*, 1842, p. 146. For detailed discussion, see Cathy Bowler, 'The importance of architectural and medical theories in the planning and construction of Norfolk County Lunatic Asylum, 1808–14', unpublished M.A. dissertation, UEA, Norwich, 1997.

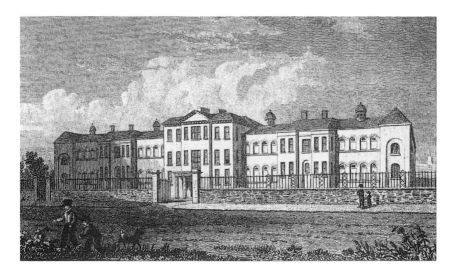

Figure 2.2 Norfolk Lunatic Asylum in its original state: an engraving by T. Barber in 1825. Note the compressed length of the building, its proximity to the turnpike road and the unglazed lower cell windows

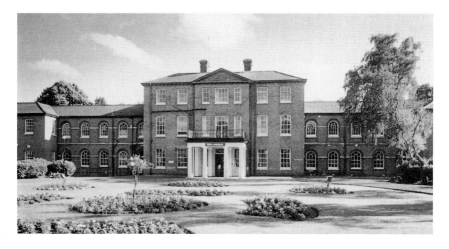

Figure 2.3 The same buildings in 1998 (Norfolk Mental Health Care NHS Trust)

staircases. At the front were rooms for a porter and visitors, with kitchen, scullery and an eating room across the corridor to the rear.[22] On the first floor the principal feature was the committee room and balcony, with the master's

---

[22] Description based on the adopted plan of 1814, held at Drayton Old Lodge (hence DL), headquarters of the Norfolk Mental Health Services NHS Trust. The positioning of baths suggests that new admissions were bathed on arrival.

room flanked by visiting doctors' and matron's offices at the rear. Five of the six rooms on the second floor were marked as staff bedrooms, with no indication for the sixth. Supervisory concerns were reflected in the stairways, which gave access to open galleries, and views obtained along the corridors. Similarly, a bay window provided the master with a view over the airing courts, with the matron able to see eastwards along the women's wing and the physician looking along the men's wing to the west. A brick vaulted basement with stone flags contained a well and cellars for beer, meat, bread and coals. A steam boiler for baths above was included at the outset and pumps for the cold water supply were soon added. Iron grille work let into at least one cellar roof may suggest the supervision of confined patients, but was probably an aid to ventilation as there were already cells, including dark cells, at ground-floor level.[23] To the south of the administrative block a semi-circular courtyard with arcades led to buildings which included isolation rooms, a nurse's room, wash house and drying room.[24]

Recommendations under the 1808 Act concerning the sexual segregation of patients, the provision of 'dry and airy cells', separate day rooms and airing courts were closely followed in the layout of the wing buildings.[25] Similarly patients were divided into the convalescent, incurable and a third category, soon referred to as 'approbation'. Each wing had two floors, with rows of five single cells lining the north side of the corridor and arranged either side of a projecting block, which contained three day rooms, a staircase, and two keeper's rooms on each floor. This also incorporated a central arched doorway with rectangular windows each side, so echoing features of the administration block (see Figures 2.1–2.3).[26] Initially rooms with two baths stood at the administrative end of each wing corridor and eight larger double cells, one without a window, a stairway and a furnace were located at the wing extremes, which projected slightly to align with the administration block frontage and the south-facing day rooms. Thus 104 patient inmates could be accommodated if all cells were fully used.

Cell windows were recessed within round arched brickwork, with the arch glazed but the lower part shuttered and barred on the inside. Although patients might be confined, the cells were intended primarily as sleeping quarters, the day rooms giving controlled access to exercise yards and airing courts. Wing corridors allowed movement and supervision from the extreme

[23] As discovered during re-flooring work, which also revealed iron rings set in the walls of ward 3 at floor level, the likely anchor points for chains.
[24] Marked as male and female 'hospitals' on the 1814 plan. Both buildings were replaced by the octagon church, built between them in the late 1850s, which incorporated a basement mortuary.
[25] 48 George III, 1808, Section XVI.
[26] NB: the 1825 engraving distorts the building's proportions, compressing its length, cf. 1990s photograph.

staircase to the octagon hall, where locked doors prevented access to more public space. Convalescent patients were grouped nearest to these exits, with 'lunatics' beyond the day rooms and staff rooms and incurables at the extremities. If this arrangement aimed to confine levels of disturbance away from visitors, it also signalled to patients their physical route to recovery and release, for which orderly conduct was a precondition. Significantly, the only day rooms which faced north and looked to the public road were for convalescent patients. External yards and airing courts were similarly divided, controlling those interactions between patients which were seen as harmful and facilitating closer contact with asylum staff.

Whether or not the asylum buildings can be considered a fully-fledged example of 'moral architecture', their layout was conducive to the movement of segregated groups of patients through environments suggesting improvement, convalescence and eventual discharge and not mere incarceration.[27] They stood comparison with Samuel Tuke's influential *Practical Hints*, published as the asylum was completed. Tuke identified as good design features the separation of male and female patients, with further segregation according to their state of mind, the easy supervision of patients and attendants, and provision of cheerful accommodation 'as is compatible with security'.[28] The extended frontage, linear corridors with cells at one side and a maximum of two storeys were still identified as essentials in good construction by reformers thirty years later.[29] Other features at Norfolk Lunatic Asylum included full-length sash windows in the day rooms and a ditch and 'ha-ha' arrangement at the rear of the building, which maintained the view across the river from each day room whilst meeting security concerns. Similarly a low front wall with iron railings and gates was adopted for the more public north side of the buildings. As with other choices of building materials and design, these indicated considerations beyond the cheapest forms of mass confinement. With completion costs eventually exceeding £35,000, the NLA was no monument to cost-effective provision: its capital costs of £343 per inmate considerably exceeded the £262 incurred at Nottingham or £192 at Bedford.[30]

Expressions of reforming intent and civic pride may have been purely 'external', the solidity of the buildings signifying security to county ratepayers in a period when Norfolk agriculture was enjoying great prosperity. However, some expense was incurred on features which softened an otherwise

[27] The patient's awareness of the importance of his or her own conduct was critical to moral management and there are some parallels with the regime of Samuel Tuke at the York Retreat.

[28] S. Tuke, *Practical Hints*, 1815, pp. 10–11, 51–4.

[29] Conolly, *Lunatic Asylums*, pp. 14–15.

[30] Jones, *Asylums*, p. 60. Lower comparative costs at post-1815 asylums reflected general economic recession and price deflation. Bowler, 'NCLA', pp. 40–1, notes that the use of white rather than red bricks added almost £700 to building costs.

intimidatory environment for asylum patients or at least suggested some duality of function. Small paned cell windows reduced the escape risk and were relatively cheap to replace. They were primarily intended to admit light rather than to afford a view, although this was a feature of the day rooms, but the barring of windows, like the later raising of walls, was a reaction to patient behaviour rather than part of an initial containment strategy. A network of under-floor steam-heated pipes proved ineffective, but its provision suggests rejection of older ideas that the insane were insensitive to cold and recognition that warm air and hot water were part of expected standards and had therapeutic value. The principle of cross ventilation of corridors and the additional use of perforated plates in the ceilings of patients' cells served to lower temperatures further, though both measures were intended to reduce the risk of infection and to promote health and hygiene.

The early regime: arrangements and patients

As work on the asylum buildings progressed those magistrates charged with its establishment increasingly turned their attention to matters of administration and regulation. An initial announcement that the first 40 male patients could be received was accompanied by acknowledgements that the county lunatic population 'considerably exceeded that number'.[31] This suggested a priority system: patients in the asylum would certainly be mad, but this was not the only place for madness. There were few sources of specialist knowledge or national guidelines and additional Select Committee reports on madhouses and their better regulation did not appear until 1815 and 1816.[32] A committee of visiting justices was appointed under the chairmanship of Jerimiah Ives and the authorities at Bethlem and York asylums were again contacted. By October 1814 it had produced Rules and Regulations which officially determined the asylum regime and reconciled the twin objectives of economy and reforming intent. Reflecting the spirit of the new legislation, the asylum was described as a hospital 'where every means may be employed to restore the patients to their reason and to sanity'. 'Gentlemen of the medical department' had assured the committee of their 'every endeavour' and other staff had been given 'the most positive directions' to achieve this objective.[33]

The initial medical staff of four was soon reduced to two physicians, Doctors Edward Rigby and Warner Wright, and a surgeon, William

---

[31] Minutes of the Committee of Visiting Magistrates (CVIS) SAH 2, Oct. 1813–June 1816, 16 April 1814. The first three women patients were admitted by 25 June 1814.

[32] These appeared following scandals and excesses at asylums, including York County and Bethlem.

[33] NQS, 1812–14, c/s/1/18, 20 Oct. 1814.

Dalrymple.[34] All held prestigious honorary posts at the Norfolk and Norwich hospital and each had a local reputation as a mad-doctor. Rigby was co-proprietor of the private asylum at Lakenham and Wright was physician to the Bethel hospital, where Dalrymple was the surgeon-apothecary. The two physicians each received 50 guineas annually and the surgeon 80 guineas; payments rather in advance of contemporary poor law doctoring and indicative of more than the simple 'sensible precaution' of a medical officer.[35] Plans for joint physicians' visits were quickly superseded by their demarcation of patients, based upon weekly visits and agreed arrangements for emergency attendance. Early physicians' journals refer occasionally to individual treatments but indicate their attention to general features in the asylum, notably its cleanliness, order, security, temperature, ventilation and dietary.[36] This approach reflected contemporary theories of contagion, as seen in prisons, workhouses, ships and barracks as well as hospitals and asylums. It assumed that, in offering security and a degree of comfort and rest supported by adequate diet and medicaments, asylum care was itself a form of treatment.

Potential conflicts between medical and lay authorities lay ahead but it is questionable whether the doctors' general approach in their evaluation of a well-regulated institution differed markedly at first from that of visiting magistrates or other public figures. A specific medical contribution represented only part of the wider reform agenda, which recognised the essential humanity of the asylum patient and held that 'madness' in some respect did not necessarily imply complete destruction of the patient's ability to reason. Terms and their meanings were open to differing interpretations but this approach excluded notions of madness as bestial or evidence of some possessive force and it discounted responses based upon excessive physical coercion. Yet 'moral' approaches, based upon acceptable behaviour and appeals to the patient's self-esteem, clearly imposed upon the patient, requiring conformity and self-control as evidence of the improvement necessary in order to return to society. Further, the approving authority consisted of the same justices who were a major force in local government, responsible for prisons and an integral part of the political and social establishment.

Responsible to the Quarterly Sessions Court, the Committee of Visiting Justices had its own treasurer and clerk, William Simpson, and could call upon the services of the county surveyor. It met monthly, requiring a quorum of five, and somewhat unusually did not delegate powers to a house committee or equivalent body. Instead, it retained active control of the

---

[34] The first physician, Henry Reeve (1780–1814), died prematurely and was succeeded by Edward Rigby (1747–1821) who had a specialist interest in obstetrics.

[35] cf. Jones, *Asylums*, p. 39.

[36] Rigby, Visiting Doctor's Journal, Nov. 1814–Jan. 1817, SAH 151, pp. 1–7. Wright, Physician's Report Book, June 1814–Oct. 1817, SAH 147, 4 Aug. 1814.

asylum's finances and general conduct, including the admission and discharge of patients. Chairman Edward Stracey personally and formally advised patients considered for release to 'guard against a return of their disorder'.[37] However, the admissions process depended heavily upon the initiatives of poor law guardians, overseers and doctors and the treatment of patients, though not the power to discharge them, was directed by the asylum medical officers. These officials had other interests to consider, as will be seen, in decisions which were often to the detriment of the asylum and its patients. Weekly inspections were made by deputed Committee members, with the master accountable for day-to-day matters and supervision of non-medical staff. Thomas Caryl, appointed master on an annual salary of £125, had already taken up residence in April 1813. He and Mrs Caryl formed a master and matron combination often seen in workhouses and she received £25 annually. They were assisted by a staff comprising two porters, paid 16 guineas, two housemaids each earning 10 guineas, and a cook, who received 12 guineas.[38] The Reverend J. Maxwell was 'officiating minister' in 1814 but his was likely to have been a part-time appointment initially.

Considering its planning and expense, the working of the asylum building was beset by early problems and its rather bare interior contrasted with its external appearance. Flagstones were used throughout in floors and staircases and an austere atmosphere was hardly dispelled by the limited illumination afforded by oil lamps, which initially lacked reflectors and used fish or whale oil. Because the under-floor heating system was ineffective 'german' stove fires, each surrounded by a heavy metal guard or cage, were installed in day rooms and corridors. However, the typical single or double cell was unheated and, with the emphasis upon fresh air and cross-ventilation to combat smells and the miasmas thought to be the cause of disease, there could be marked variations in temperature within the building. On a cold November morning in 1814, for example, Dr Wright recorded temperatures of 58 and 59 degrees Fahrenheit respectively in the men's and women's day rooms, but 'in rooms without fires 45 degrees . . . the external air 39 degrees'.[39]

The carrying or hand-pumping of water from the central basement well to the upper floors and roof tank was quickly seen to be impractical and piped water to the dark cells in the wings was belatedly installed, the rooftop supply being fed by improved and later hydraulic pumps.[40] Hot water for the large copper baths was still carried from the central steam boiler. Patients were bathed on admission, but it is not clear whether early reporting that 'all the

---

[37] CVIS, SAH 2, 4 Aug. 1815.
[38] CVIS, 1816–22, SAH 3, 30 Sept. 1816. A gardener was also employed shortly afterwards.
[39] ibid., 25 Nov. 1814. From Dec. 1816 additional stoves were fitted in wards and corridors but heating arrangements were not satisfactory until the 1840s.
[40] Respectively in Sept. 1814, 1819 and 1825.

female patients were yesterday washed in the warm bath' referred to a routine observation or a noteworthy event.[41] Additional baths were provided in 1818, but two or three patients were still expected to use the same bath-water. An underground rainwater reservoir supplied the separate wash house, which initially relied upon copper boilers to heat water then poured manually into wooden troughs. Early sanitary arrangements consisted of a gulley set in the floor of each cell, which also had a chamber pot, with large earthenware pots in the main buildings and external privies at some distance off the airing courts. The first water closet for patients was installed in the women's wing in 1815, but no others appear to have been added for thirty years. Dirty water was often thrown on to the grass outside and left to run, via ditches and settling tanks, to the river before a full drainage system was installed in 1833. Incontinent patients were provided with straw and their cells regularly sluiced to avoid miasmas, accentuating the problems of damp and cold.

Each cell had plastered walls, a fixed wooden seat and bedstead, to which locks or chains could be fitted, with a straw mattress, sheeting, pillow and blankets. Day room furniture was also heavy and cumbersome, suggesting that rough usage was envisaged. Heavy locks, bolts and guard doors between sections on the wings remained in use until 1830 and more windows were fitted with wire guards on the outside, in response to breakages by patients in the airing courts. The latter combined grassy areas and gravel paths and were the scene of several escape attempts. Consequently chairs and handrails were repositioned and the walls raised by two feet 'in such parts as may be deemed necessary' in 1817.[42] Such measures contributed to a custodial environment, though the asylum remained less prison-like than some and, after a troublesome start, it avoided the chaotic conditions and abuses associated with open galleries.[43]

All patients were provided with shoes and clothes on admission. Women had an undercoat and uppercoat, neckerchief, cap and apron, while the men wore breeches, a rough shirt, waistcoat and overcoat. Nightwear consisted of a shift and cap for women and shirts for men. Although the physicians regularly commented upon 'sweet and clean' cells, 'airy' house and 'comfortable warmth', they frequently requested that stoves in the passages be kept alight to combat dampness.[44] Staff were further instructed to ensure that patients' feet were dry before they were put to bed; the incontinent patients

---

[41] Physician's Book, 26 May 1816. The rivet heads in these baths caused problems and were all knocked down in 1821.

[42] CVIS, SAH 3, 5 July 1817. Most were raised to a height of 13 feet.

[43] e.g. Cornwall Asylum, Bodmin had cast iron windows and doors throughout and was located next to the prison. Smith, *Cure, Comfort*, p. 34.

[44] D.G. Thomson, 'Presidential address on the progress of psychiatry during the past hundred years, together with the history of Norfolk County Asylum during the same period', *Journal of Mental Science*, 60, 1914, pp. 541–72, 568. But see Physician's Book, 19 Feb. 1817, for example.

'on straw' were to be wrapped up in flannel in cold weather. In addition, the master and matron had produced a form of sleeping bag or 'large warm sock' for most of the infirm and disordered patients by December 1814.[45]

An adequate, well-regulated diet was seen as essential to physical health and the treatment of insanity by the medical staff, who monitored the food served and their patients' appetites closely.[46] The Committee not only accepted this advice but overruled suggestions from the Bethel hospital in favour of the master's own proposals for a dietary which included beef, mutton, cheese, table beer, potatoes and bread, all of which were to be 'good'.[47] Breakfast normally consisted of milk broth, with bread and cheese or butter on two days. Beef and potatoes were served as dinner three times per week, with suet pudding or rice pudding on other occasions. Supper consisted of bread and butter or cheese with beer, although meat broth was available on two days when dinner had not included meat.[48]

This early dietary did not specify the portions of food to be served or the measures to ensure that all patients received proper quantities, but it compared favourably with that available in workhouses or to most Norfolk labourers and their families. An apparent lack of fruit and vegetables other than potatoes possibly stemmed from the initial absence of asylum farmland and gardens, but also reflected contemporary practice. Special diets prescribed by medical officers, for example, were usually of 'good broth with rice', supplemented by wine or spirits. Adverse comments centred not upon the dietary but concerned eating utensils – bone knives and forks and metal platters – and the shortage of dining space as patient numbers increased.[49] Suspicions that physically fit patients obtained food from the less able-bodied suggested either that the asylum was understaffed or that attendants were neglectful. Time was found to feed 'by forse' those patients like James C—, who refused to eat, but others whose behaviour was unacceptable were sometimes punished by the order 'to go without'.[50]

Sixty-two patients aged between 18 and 75 years were admitted in the first year. Detailed case notes were not kept but references to 57 of the patients in the master's journal and physicians' report books suggest that nearly 60 per cent were male and a similar proportion were between 30 and 49 years old.[51]

---

[45] Physician's Book, 30 Nov. and 9 Dec. 1814.

[46] ibid., 21 Aug. 1814; 'meat and dumplings remarkably good': the physicians' frequent investigations included sampling.

[47] ibid., 12 Sept. 1814. 'Seconds flour' was allowed, providing this was also 'good'.

[48] Admissions Register, SAH 171, May 1814–Sept. 1836.

[49] The diet had possibly deteriorated when it was criticised by the Lunacy Commissioners in 1842–3.

[50] Master's Journal, Dec. 1820–July 1832, SAH 126, 10 Oct. 1821 (C—); 10 July 1815 (S— punished for destroying clothing).

[51] Twenty were discharged within two years of admission; the rest remained and at least 33 eventually died in the NLA.

From the outset the optimism of the reform strategy was severely tested. Apart from the 'very bad' cases, such as James S—, the pauper patients were often already institutionalised or had presented such difficulties in their management or care that parish overseers were prepared to sanction the additional cost of asylum charges. At the Bethel hospital, which accommodated some charitable and pauper cases, the governors had also taken 'an opportunity to discharge a number of their patients; notice was given to the parishes concerned, who promptly arranged their admission to the county asylum'.[52] Sarah F—, sent directly from the Norfolk and Norwich hospital, was 'afflicted with diabetes and . . . in a dying state'.[53] She died at Thorpe within three days, though others took a little longer. Mary A— was 'extremely emaciated and is obliged to be fed' on admission and, in successive weeks, she was 'very weak', 'low' and 'sinking' before her death.[54]

In instances where patients were elderly or 'feeble' in body and mind, or where cases of breakdown or neglect were belatedly discovered, the asylum was a place of last resort, offering little scope for therapy and few hopes of improvement or cure. Aware that such distressing admissions also harmed the image of the asylum, the justices requested in August 1815 that other magistrates and poor law overseers should ensure 'a sufficient state of bodily health' in any patient being transferred.[55] On his admission four months later Isaac S—, aged 56, was 'scarcely able to stand and is altogether in a deplorable state . . . this poor man ought not to have been sent here as he was not in a fit state to be removed'.[56] He also died within three days. The severity and, at the time, criminality of suicide often ensured that such cases were also promptly transferred to the asylum, where they posed particular problems. Elizabeth W— was 'religiously insane and she has more than once made attempt on her life', while 'Phoebe L— made three different attempts to destroy herself yesterday . . . ordered that somebody sleep in the same room with her and that extraordinary precautions be observed regarding her'.[57]

Broader interpretations of insanity by poor law officers, doctors or justices had dramatic consequences, particularly for women, who sometimes attracted a degree of sympathy within the NLA when their misfortune was obvious. Thus, 'her insanity came upon her . . . through disappointment of marriage with the man who she had a child by'; or 'her husbon did keep another woman and take her home to his house'; or 'her insanity came from her lying-in. She has been insane once before from a similar cause'.[58] These

---

[52] Winston, 'Bethel at Norwich', pp. 27–51, 49.

[53] Physician's Book, 10 and 13 April 1815.

[54] ibid., 12, 15 and 23 May; 4 and 11 June 1815.

[55] CVIS, 4 Aug. 1815.

[56] Master's Journal, 16 Dec. 1814, Physician's Book, 30 Nov. and 3 Dec. 1815.

[57] Physician's Book, 7 July 1815. Similar measures failed to prevent Samuel Vincent from hanging himself on 20 Sept. that year.

[58] Master's Journal, 1815–16, SAH 124, 15 Dec. 1815; Physician's Book, 26 June 1815.

cases suggest more to the asylum than purposes of control, though whether it offered an appropriate setting and forms of care remained questionable. Other patients were given less consideration, though their cases again illustrate variable definitions of insanity and recovery. Like Hannah H—, referred to in the previous chapter, Thomas D— was 'perfectly sane since . . . his complaint was occasioned by habitual drunkenness'.[59] William Waters' recovery was less obvious, since he had been 'low and unsettled and had wandered away from his work'.[60] The problem of recurring illness quickly became apparent when the medical staff recognised Mary A— and Mary H— as former patients at Norwich Bethel hospital and Phoebe S—, discharged 'recovered' from the NLA in July 1815, was readmitted 'low and desponding' that November.[61]

According to one critic, 'the Norfolk justices, having constructed an expensive building, went to the other extreme with minimal staffing, low wages and salaries, and a poor standard and quality of diet for the patients . . . a harsh regime based on financial stringency was perpetuated'.[62] Over a period when pressure from ratepayers and others to curb expenditure on the dependent population culminated in reform of the poor laws, the justices were required to manage the asylum efficiently. They initially charged appropriate poor law authorities 14 shillings per patient per week but the reduction in patient admissions which then followed in 1816 dictated a rate more aligned with workhouse costs. Charges had been reduced by 25 per cent, to 9s 6d, by 1818 and they were pared down to a low point of just 4s 9d in March 1835.[63]

Full value was also expected in contracts for asylum provisions. In an era when the average asylum patient consumed two-thirds of a large loaf per day the quality of bread was carefully monitored. One supplier was soon reprimanded and then faced with 'a proper deduction . . . from his bill', 'in consequence of the hardness of the bread'.[64] Quantity and wastage caused greater concern. Anonymous accusations concerning the master and matron had been investigated and dismissed in 1816, but both were reprimanded for 'great neglect' two years later. Although the medical officers testified on the Caryls' behalf, arguing that waste and destruction were only to be expected in an asylum, the Committee felt that the Caryls had been 'frequently and unnecessarily absent' and their lack of supervision had led to thefts. One porter was convicted for stealing bread but the failure to mark hospital clothing and sheets had undermined further prosecutions.[65] Subsequently, the master's conduct, his availability, inventories and purchases came under

---

[59] Physician's Book, 26 Sept. 1814, 23 May 1815.

[60] ibid., 23 May and 10 July 1815.

[61] ibid., 12 and 23 May 1815 (A— and H—); 30 July and 12 Nov. 1815 (S—).

[62] Smith, *Cure, Comfort*, p. 77.

[63] Reductions exceeded the fall in the cost of living. Cheshire charged just 4 shillings in 1836, Smith, *Cure, Comfort*, p. 74.

[64] CVIS, 29 July, 29 Sept. and 20 Oct. 1816.

[65] CVIS, 20 Sept. and 24 Oct. 1818. The Caryls, 'frequently and unnecessarily absent'

greater scrutiny, which may have contributed to an emphasis upon economy but also to changes in Caryl's regime.[66]

Both features were achieved by keeping additional staff to a minimum. Apart from the appointment of a gardener and the occasional assistance of the Caryls' housemaid, neither the asylum staff nor their wages were increased during the 1820s. By 1834 another maid and a porter had been appointed but patient numbers had doubled (see Table 2.1). The NLA had probably the highest ratio of patients to attendants seen in late 1830s asylums and twice that of the best-practice examples.[67] More patients justified the asylum's role and costs, assisting economies of scale, but the justices recognised that positive endorsements rested upon treatments and recoveries, rather than mass confinements or parsimonious displays on their part. A therapeutic regime was suggested by early announcements that 'the better sort of patients both male and female have now been separated from the others and now occupy different day rooms and wards'.[68] References to patients in the 'approbation ward' suggest periods of transition and possibly of assessment prior to discharge. Nor was confinement to the incurable rooms seen as indefinite: Daniel H—, sent there following 'disappointment in marriage' in 1815, was discharged after eight months.[69]

It was not long before efforts were made to attract patients who were not paupers or Norfolk residents. An 1815 amendment to the 1808 Act specified that private patients could be admitted to county pauper asylums if there was sufficient room and the committee offered to accommodate these as 'boarders' at 13s 6d per week, soon raised to 15s 6d. Suffolk had no public asylum as yet so its county magistrates were informed that their pauper patients could be sent to Thorpe 'upon the terms prescribed by the last Act of Parliament'.[70] In both instances the higher charges obtained were earmarked as subsidies for Norfolk pauper patients and ratepayers; thus, standard Norfolk charges might be less than the true cost of maintenance. In this early demonstration of the political economy of care, patients without the prospect of matching funds were not welcome. After Caryl sought advice concerning a patient 'brought from London', a magistrate visited with instructions to 'have nothing to do with the man . . . he might take the patient back to London as [inquire] what parish or what place he belongs to'.[71]

---

from the asylum, were saved by medical staff testimonies. Caryl's allowance for a horse and gig was cancelled: he was 'desired to discontinue with them'.

[66] CVIS, 22 Feb. 1819.

[67] The NLA ratio increased from roughly 1:14 1815–20, to 1:18 1820–9 and 1:27 1830–9. 'Best practice' examples were 1:15 at asylums in Maidstone, Stafford and Gloucester, where work therapy was already established. (See Smith, *Cure, Comfort*, pp. 234–6 and Chapter 2, below).

[68] Physician's Book, 25 Aug. 1814.

[69] Master's Journal, 29 May 1815.

[70] CVIS, 29 July and 20 Oct. 1816.

[71] Master's Journal, 19 Dec. 1814.

Treatments, care and restraint

It is rarely possible to differentiate treatment from care and restraint in early nineteenth-century asylums. Patients presented a variety of conditions, including physical ailments, and their experiences of what has been called 'the rhetoric of care' diverged considerably. NLA inmates were always referred to as 'patients', but those who threatened fellow patients or staff were subjected to custodial control. In offering refuge, care, treatment and the prospect of recovery to the patient, the asylum also represented a safeguard to society, where the uncontrollable or strange might be contained. It was never assumed that all patients would recover or that all were socially disruptive, though early experiences soon suggested that potential difficulties had been underestimated.

The asylum was established before a distinct 'moral management' approach began to inform the practice of medical staff and was under the daily direction of Caryl, who had no medical qualifications.[72] He believed that patients were responsible for their actions and that misconduct without apology or contrition deserved reprimand, which might include restraint and physical coercion. With a family of his own, he may have adopted a parental attitude to some patients; for example, sending a young woman with his children to be 'churched'.[73] Over time Caryl's approach focused increasingly upon care and non-violent restraint, but his was not a total conversion and there are few signs of a progressive medical staff determining it.[74] Its consequences, as reflected in mortality and recovery rates, suggested the need of further improvement but that the selection of the NLA specifically for criticism is not wholly justifiable.

When patients arrived the master was instructed to inquire into their family histories and circumstances and to record information for the medical staff prior to a preliminary assessment of the prospects of cure.[75] Thus R.W. was high and violent but 'his sister died about five weeks back in the Bethel . . . and his brother think that was what hurt his mind'.[76] A.C. had been 'in a dispondent way for about 6 months from the account of her husborn – but she say it come from the change of life'.[77] Judgements, rather than the semblance of prognosis, were generally based upon social criteria, the patient's ability to conform with accepted rules and standards of human

---

[72] This was unexceptional; the West Riding asylum at Wakefield was the first to be run by a medical superintendent, William Ellis, in 1818.

[73] Master's Journal, 23 July 1815. This is not to confuse early nineteenth-century perceptions of 'the child' with those of the early twenty-first century.

[74] cf. interpretations of improvement under a developing medical profession or the depiction of the NLA as a particularly bad asylum.

[75] CVIS, 13 Oct. 1814.

[76] Master's Journal, 26 Nov. 1816.

[77] ibid., 6 Dec. 1816.

behaviour. Although the term 'moral insanity' was not used initially, the notion was applied in a number of cases including alcohol abuse, 'religious insanity', vagrancy and stress. Evidently, William R—'s insanity had 'come on by studying and learning & musick'.[78] Often the evidence of physical neglect or severe 'disorders of the senses' was all too apparent and the experience of a head injury was readily accepted as an indication of insanity. 'Idiots' whose condition stemmed from 'hereditary disposition' or a 'family complaint' were included with 'dangerous lunatics' among the 'incurables'.

Treatments were based only partly upon a limited medical knowledge and available medication. Medical officers employed variations of traditional humoural theory and physical therapies predominated, their attention directed towards 'exercise, health, security and even . . . comfort'.[79] Purgatives and emetics were used to remove bodily impurities associated with mania or hysteria, with 'opening' mixtures, 'steel pills', rhubarb medicine, peppermint drops, or Epsom salts generally given as laxatives. Patients with failing heart conditions or the 'dropsical' symptoms of oedema were also purged, though phlebotomy was less regularly employed. Opium was occasionally administered as an analgesic to dying patients rather than as a sedative or cure for insanity. Treatment for 'noisy' or 'high' patients centred upon confinement to bed until their conduct was considered to be acceptable, though warm baths were given to soothe and relax patients following fits or outbursts of mania. Thus Mary P—, admitted with 'religious insanity', was prescribed 'brest bath with some lotion' and discharged after only six weeks at the asylum.[80] Bathing was also an act of simple humanity; on his arrival the tragic Isaac S— was placed 'in the hot barth . . . being so dirty from his riding to long in the cart'.[81]

Less than £30 was initially allocated for the cost of drugs, which included malt beer, wines and spirits given as tonics. Ammonia was also used as a stimulant for patients exhausted by epileptic fits or those who were 'sinking'.[82] A set of surgical instruments 'for use of the asylum' was soon purchased and the particular needs of individual patients were attended to, with the relevant poor law guardians billed for additional expenses, for example, 'a truss for John M—'.[83] The most interventionist measures were usually carried out for traumatic or pathological rather than psychological reasons. When John L— pulled out his own eye Dalrymple ordered one dozen

---

[78] ibid., 29 March 1815.
[79] ibid., 17 Oct. 1816.
[80] ibid., 5 Jan. 1816.
[81] ibid., 24 Nov. 1815. After Secker, the master and Mrs Caryl bathed Elizabeth L— and Mary G—. Same sex bathing was soon enforced, e.g. 20 July 1816.
[82] Early physicians' journals referring mainly to lotions, pills or mixtures rather than specifics.
[83] CVIS, 29 July 1816 (instruments); 30 Sept. 1816 (bill to the Attleborough guardians).

leeches to be applied to the eye socket.[84] L— survived this double trauma, but others were still less fortunate. The suffering of a patient with 'violent paine of the bowels' was probably aggravated by Dalrymple's triple combination of bleeding, purging and blistering, used to draw impurities and as a 'counter-irritant', before he died the next day.[85] Grim though such interventions were, they reflected standard procedures, as George III found to his own cost.[86]

Roughly one quarter of the patients admitted in 1814–15 were 'feeble' or epileptic and at least a similar proportion were regarded as incurable. Under pressure to produce positive results, the justices referred regularly to the asylum's 'beneficial effects . . . NINE of these unfortunate persons have been restored to their reason and discharged . . . others we expect are approaching to convalescence'.[87] Twenty of the first patients had recovered by 1816, leading to hopes that one-third of new admissions could regularly be cured. In common with asylum doctors everywhere the NLA medical officers recommended the prompt admission of patients showing signs of mental disorders to enhance their prospects of recovery. Yet they were continually presented with patients suffering from long-term neglect, chronic or advanced illnesses. On attending the elderly Mary G— in October 1816, Dr Rigby noted: 'It was surely very improper to bring such a patient to the asylum and this is not the first instance in which patients have been brought in a dying state.'[88] By then the doctors were already commenting on the increasing proportion of 'incurable' cases which, they anticipated, would become a long-term feature.[89]

Table 2.1 shows that the average number of patients more than doubled by the 1830s, although annual admissions had not increased until then. Roughly one half of those admitted each year were discharged, recovered or otherwise but, with the increase in residents, the percentage of all patients discharged rapidly declined. Interpreting their 'recovery' was hazardous; there were no subsequent monitoring procedures although the proportion of those discharged patients who were later readmitted tended to rise, from one-fifth towards two-fifths.[90] If the suggestion is of very limited success as a therapeutic regime, there was greater movement out through the asylum gates than might have been expected, even as the proportion of cases

[84] Master's Journal, Dec. 1820–July 1832, SAH 126, 21 July 1821.
[85] ibid., 22 and 24 Oct. 1821. Note that this patient was treated by a surgeon not a physician.
[86] I. MacAlpine and R. Hunter, 'The "insanity" of King George III: a classic case of porphyria', British Medical Journal, 8 January 1966.
[87] NQS, c/s 4/2, 1812–19, 6 April 1815
[88] Doctor's Journal, 11 Nov. 1816.
[89] ibid., 17 Oct. 1816; 16 Jan. 1817.
[90] CVIS, SAH 5, 1830–9, March 1836.

Table 2.1 Patients at Norfolk County Asylum, 1814–39

	Average no. resident			Admissions			Discharged as % adms			Mortality %		
	Total	M	F	Total	M	F	Total	M	F	Total	M	F
1814–19	71	37	34	44	21	23	49 (34)	40 (22)	56 (38)	11.2	12.1	9.7
1820–29	110	55	55	42	18	24	54 (21)	53 (17)	56 (24)	13.4	13.6	13.1
1830–39	159	72	87	52	26	26	45 (15)	40 (15)	50 (15)	17.0	20.7	13.8

Notes: The hospital year ran from 18 May until 1833, with May–Dec. 1833 presented as a whole year. From 1834 the full calendar year was used.

Figures in parenthesis refer to the percentage of all patients who were discharged.

regarded as chronic or incurable increased. Death rates appeared to be rising, possibly reflecting the accumulation of patients over time but suggesting shortfalls in their diet or medical care.

Whether the asylum's poor comparative standing was justified is more questionable. According to national information for the period 1835–45, the NLA had the highest mortality (19.1 per cent), and a rate of 'cures' (13.1 per cent) which placed it in the lowest third of county asylums.[91] Such figures do not appear to tally with information compiled in Table 2.1 (nor with that in Table 3.1 in the following chapter), and cannot be considered a sound indicator of standards at the asylum. Whatever its faults, the NLA data was regularly presented and may be more reliable than that offered by other asylums. As the lunacy commissioners acknowledged, their comparative statistics 'have unfortunately not been compiled upon any fixed plan' and contained some extraordinary variations.

Eventually, the need to expand accommodation at the NLA was added to other objectives; sound economic management, the prospect of cure for a minority, care for the majority and custody for a few. These were associated with increased awareness of the need for more sympathetic environments. Cells began to be converted into small wards, for example for eight of the 'quietest male patients' in 1821, and a waiting room and a physician's room were adapted for similar purposes.[92] In 1831 extensions to the wing ends, each incorporating cells and a day room, increased the number of available beds to 150. More sinks were installed and a full drainage system completed

[91] Conolly, *Lunatic Asylums*, Table III, p. 151 and notes, p. 150. These were based on returns to the Commissioners in Lunacy. Some 'cure rates' were clearly spurious: Liverpool Asylum claimed 63.4 per cent, compared with Chatham's 3.4 per cent. The NLA mortality figure cited may have been distorted by an 1843 peak of 26 per cent.
[92] CVIS, 20 April and 25 July 1821.

in 1834. Replacement cell windows, capable of opening, also began to replace the fixed glass and wooden shutter arrangement once they had been successfully demonstrated in day rooms.[93] In October 1840 plans were announced for north/south projections, providing 32 additional beds at the wing ends and producing a cruciform shape which required the repositioning of staircases.[94]

Although they relied upon assessments by the medical staff, the visiting justices held formal responsibility for the discharge of patients. Family applications for the release of an inpatient relative were normally refused unless they were endorsed by medical staff: only one of the four family appeals in 1815 was approved.[95] The likely effectiveness of a cure was difficult to establish so the justices focused upon the conditions for a patient's discharge. These included medical evaluation of improvement or the availability of alternative care, but patients thought liable to harm themselves or others were not recommended, regardless of cost considerations or the appeals of their relatives. Thus John L—'s requests for the release of his wife Frances were refused 'as she was continuing in a dangerous state'.[96] Yet the justices recognised that patient release signified some success for the asylum and, increasingly, they were aware of periodic overcrowding within it. Early recoveries included Sarah N— and Mary H—, released to their husbands in December 1814, and one patient was granted 'trial out of the house' or probation in July 1815.[97] By 1818 the justices were discharging 'perfectly harmless' patients such as John H—, 'a dumb lunatic', along with 'three recovered patients'.[98] They also requested greater notice from the physicians of likely recoveries so that poor law overseers could be summoned to the committee meetings to collect discharged patients.[99] With an eye to overcrowding Dr Wright went 'carefully' through the house in August 1829 but found no one whom he could 'safely recommend to be sent away'.[100]

In public statements the visiting justices played down the use of mechanical restraint within the asylum and expressed their intentions

---

[93] This prolonged process began after Dalrymple reported that the combination of closed windows, window boards and hot weather 'had occasioned patients to be restless' in south-facing day rooms. CVIS, 31 Aug. 1818.

[94] CVIS, SAH 6, 1840–8, 26 Oct. 1840. These unsigned plans at Drayton Old Lodge are in the style of Francis Stone's design and pre-date John Brown's office as county surveyor. The northern walls of the extensions were now very close to the turnpike road and plans were made for its diversion in 1850.

[95] CVIS, 25 March 1816. A critical factor was a local landowner's offer to keep the patient in 'a state of security'.

[96] ibid., 29 July 1816.

[97] ibid., 3 and 27 Dec. 1814; 30 July 1815.

[98] ibid., SAH 3, 6 Jan. 1818.

[99] ibid., 27 April 1818.

[100] Physician's Book, SAH 149, May 1829–Feb. 1835, 28 Aug. 1829.

'of keeping the unhappy patients free from manacles or other fetters except in the violent paroxysms of their disorder'.[101] Officially, the medical officers limited its application to violent or suicidal patients and an unspecified category exhibiting 'outrageous' habits but frequently gave instructions to secure, lock or chain patients. Thus 'Mr Dalrymple . . . ordered P.G. to bed and M.R. for emproper behaviour and dirtying the day room also M.J. to be cross locked as a punishment for distroying so manney clothing'.[102] Caryl added his 'punishments' for those failing to control themselves or behave as he thought fit but the sick and infirm were treated more compassionately and suicidal patients received round-the-clock attention, albeit accompanied by restraint to avoid self-harm.

Attacks upon staff, window breaking, damage to furnishings, clothing and bedding, and fighting in airing courts and day rooms were extensive in the first years. These were usually punished and asylum porters and maids went beyond restraint on several occasions, even though physical abuse was officially frowned upon and the staff were periodically reminded that 'they are answerable for their conduct to the medical men'.[103] One maid was reprimanded by Dalrymple and Caryl for striking a female patient but a porter was fortunate to escape with a similar rebuke after an incident in which a patient lost sight in one eye, following which the visiting justices issued a general reminder that 'all violence should be avoided'.[104] The committee was more sensitive to escapes and suicides, which compromised the status of the asylum as a secure institution, and in 1815 a maid who left a key unattended was dismissed as an example to other staff. Culpable staff were usually fined one month's wages when a patient escaped, although they were liable under the 1808 Act for the full cost of any retrieval.[105]

In 1815 fully two-thirds of male and one half of female patients were subjected to instances of mechanical restraint, either as a direct control or to serve as a 'check to other patients', as indicated in Table 2.2. Abraham L—, for example, was punished 'for making a noise' during Dr Wright's visit.[106] That year 123 instances occurred in which patients were locked to chairs in the day rooms or outside in the airing courts, 'chained down cross' to their beds, put into 'the dark cell', confined to bed, ordered 'to go without', or put in straitjackets or handmuffs. Each was meticulously recorded by Caryl, who invariably added 'till [she or he] behave better', and was generally endorsed by

---

[101] CVIS,16 Jan. 1817.

[102] Master's Journal, 23 Nov. 1816.

[103] ibid., 14 Oct. 1818.

[104] ibid., 30 Sept. 1816, 27 Nov. 1827.

[105] CVIS, 20 Dec. 1815. Suicides, viz. the patient who hanged himself in a privy on 22 Sept. 1815, involved public investigations and suggested shortcomings in asylum management.

[106] Master's Journal, 28 Dec. 1815. Semi-starvation, periods of 'going without' also featured.

Table 2.2 The Caryl regime: punishment in 1815 and 1834

	1815 Male	Female	1834 Male	Female
Punishments given	73	50	2	15
Patients involved	20	16	2	8
Patients at NLA	30	30	95	105
% of patients punished	66.7	53.3	2.1	7.6

Source: Master's Journals, May 1814–Nov. 1815, Nov. 1815–Dec. 1816, July 1832–Mar 1843.

the visiting doctors.[107] Patients who were aggressive or violent, particularly towards fellow inmates, were locked to chairs or left to wander in 'day chaines', 'stright westcoats' or 'leather muffs' in communal areas of the asylum as a visible deterrent. Caryl's early zeal was possibly influenced by the murder of James Bullard, Master at the Norwich Bethel Asylum, by a patient in 1813.[108] Women patients were treated similarly; the unfortunate Jemima D— was locked down to her bed by both hands and one leg 'with a box of the face in the bargain' for abusing a housemaid.[109]

Yet Table 2.2 also shows that punishments were reduced by a factor of six, affecting less than 5 per cent of all patients, within twenty years. 'Restraint' increasingly meant confinement to rooms, with only one instance of chains being used. Well before Caryl's retirement, the management of patients had changed considerably, with a preliminary inspection by the Metropolitan Commissioners in Lunacy reporting that they 'are obviously kindly treated'.[110] In the early 1840s the asylum did not feature among eleven in England and Wales where coercion 'still appears to remain in force', nor among five others 'which profess the non-restraint system while they practise the reverse'.[111]

How did such changes come about? Although Caryl held patients responsible for their actions, he often withdrew punishments following an explanation or apology. When Amy H— 'completely destroyed her bed and blankets . . . I asked her in the morning why she did so and she said that she could not help it but would not do so any more. I therefore said no more to her'.[112] He also routinely allowed those under physical restraint 'time up' for exercise. However, his general conduct came under increased scrutiny following his reprimand in 1818. When Dr Rigby died in 1821 no

---

[107] Recorded in the Master's Journal for inspection by Committee. See also Doctor's Journal, 3 Nov. 1816.

[108] Bateman and Rye, *Bethel Hospital*, p. 77.

[109] Master's Journal, 6 Dec. 1815.

[110] Reports of the Commissioners in Lunacy, (CiL) Aug. 1844–Apr 1925, 22 Aug. 1844.

[111] Conolly, *Asylums*, pp. 175–6. The York Retreat was named among the latter.

[112] Master's Journal, 5 Dec. 1815.

replacement was appointed and Dr Wright's visits did not increase to compensate for the shortfall. As patient numbers increased and staff appointments lagged, greater responsibilities for patient care fell upon Caryl and his wife. Noticeably from the middle 1820s, following Mrs Caryl's death at an early age, Caryl seemingly dedicated himself to attending sick patients, particularly the elderly or feeble, using stock-in-trade medicines. He gave 'fever mixture' to those with high temperatures and offered hot spirit drinks, warm baths and blankets to those with 'shivering fits'. He dispensed 'Reads Calm Pills' to 'feeble subjects' and poulticed swollen limbs. From his enquiries into the circumstances of patient admissions he occasionally attempted to diagnose causes of insanity.[113] Dr Wright's own journal in the 1820s also contained more observations on individual patients but it indicated very few medical treatments and the routine remarks upon the 'sinking' or 'declining' condition of dying patients were testimony to Caryl's workload.

It is possible that Caryl made some response to the growing influence of 'moral management', which embodied the doctrine of non-restraint, as this system was employed in 1829 by John Kirkman, medical superintendent at the Suffolk County Asylum. It is unclear when Reverend Lubbock became NLA Chaplain but his £60 annual salary suggests a regular presence, if not full-time involvement with patients, and some association with Caryl.[114] The latter sought to extend his reformed views to asylum porters and maids, even refusing the visiting Reverend Day access to a woman patient because he had come 'by himself'.[115] Staff were more frequently warned about 'drinking and using foul language', rough handling of patients or 'making use of bad language to the patients', all of which became grounds for dismissal, not least because they might be emulated by patients. As more individual cells were opened into shared sleeping rooms and fewer patients were locked down for the night, a changed atmosphere within the asylum may have produced fewer occasions necessitating restraint. With greater responsibilities Caryl may simply have become less zealous over punishments, although bread and water 'low diet as punishment' persisted.[116]

On balance, significant change occurred at the NLA not because non-restraint was applied wholesale but because repressive methods were simply used less often. In this respect Caryl's 'regime' was not unlike that of many of his lay and medical contemporaries.[117] Almost everywhere, asylum

---

[113] cf. Smith's assertion that he had 'no role in the implementation of treatment', *Cure, Comfort*, p. 55. For a Caryl diagnosis, see Master's Journal, 12 Feb. 1829 (Martha T—).

[114] CVIS, SAH 5, 30 Dec. 1833.

[115] Master's Journal, 28 May 1827.

[116] Master's Journal, SAH 126, Aug. 3 1830. Punishment diet was still in use in 1884, see Case Books, Mar 1883–Sept. 1884, SAH 271 (Christmas S— and Arthur B—).

[117] R. Gardiner Hill developed the non-restraint system at Lincoln Asylum in 1835, closely followed by John Kirkman at the Suffolk Asylum, but only five county asylums employed this approach by 1844.

treatments were still criticised in the 1830s by advocates of 'moral management'.[118] It is also questionable whether the NLA 'had a particularly poor recovery rate'.[119] This had fallen by the 1830s but an average approximating to 45 per cent of new admissions were discharged, most apparently recovered, even though readmissions increased. However, an upward trend in patient mortality, which peaked at 26 per cent in 1843, was only partly explained by the presence of more elderly patients, some already inmates of twenty years' standing. Even if they were more 'kindly treated', earlier deficiencies in diet and sanitation may have left patients vulnerable to asylum diseases such as tuberculosis and dysentery, a severe test even if sufficient qualified medical attention had been available.

L.D. Smith's comparative study of early nineteenth-century asylums has little praise for the NLA. The therapeutic regime was allegedly poor, the justices were 'notoriously parsimonious' and the asylum was 'consistently the worst managed of all'.[120] While the relative merits of other asylums cannot be assessed here, there is little evidence that the early NLA regime was exceptionally bad or unusual, even if it was no exemplar for reforming agendas. It was only the third county asylum to be constructed and considerable effort and expense went into building plans, which may be seen as a proto-example of moral architecture. Defects, notably in heating and drainage arrangements, were exposed in use and remedial measures were taken, albeit belatedly. As a pauper asylum, the NLA offered a bare environment but this was arguably no worse than existed in many poverty-stricken households and poor law institutions in early nineteenth-century Norfolk or elsewhere.

All asylums had a custodial role, with its associated excesses, in which security accompanied the provision of care. However, coercion at the NLA initially reflected inexperience and responses to patient behaviour rather than pre-planned measures, and physical forms of restraint featured less over time. The comparatively small size of the asylum by the late 1830s suggests that local justices had not resorted to mass confinement or 'warehousing' the mad.[121] Undoubtedly driven by a keen sense of economy, they sought to justify the asylum during a period when agricultural depression and demands for restraint on all forms of poor law expenditure were predominant. Diet, levels of care and medication at the NLA may have suffered but were probably no worse than that available to other Norfolk paupers or the non-

---

[118] J. Conolly, *An Inquiry Concerning the Indications of Insanity, with Suggestions for the Better Protection and Care of the Insane*, Taylor, London, 1830, p. 29.
[119] Smith, *Cure, Comfort*, p. 173.
[120] ibid., pp. 133, 172.
[121] Only the Cornwall, Dorset and Bedfordshire asylums were smaller then. The expression is associated with Andrew Scull, *The Most Solitary of Afflictions*, Yale, New Haven, 1993, p. 303.

pauperised poor. Asylum care cannot be evaluated on the basis of current day standards, nor identified as the sole preserve of an emerging branch of the medical profession. Until the 1830s the NLA was unexceptional in lagging on the appointment of a medical superintendent, whose true expertise might be questionable. Moral management was not strictly medical. It may be considered progressive in asylum contexts but the same hardly applies to that range of therapeutic innovations which included the 'swing chair', the 'bath of surprise' and mechanical devices associated with force-feeding.[122]

Contemporary commentators on asylums often had their own agendas or confined themselves to routine blandishments and superficial observations. Local visitors to the NLA were frequent but few made thorough inspections and their comments rarely ranged beyond 'cleanliness, order and comparative comfort'.[123] Thomas and Mrs Caryl were described in complimentary terms in 1825, though their good reputations may have been spurred by earlier and more private criticism.[124] However, Andrew Halliday's comprehensive survey of asylums also found the NLA 'upon the whole . . . a well-arranged and ably-conducted establishment'.[125] In Caryl's last years visiting Metropolitan Commissioners in Lunacy also concluded that patients were 'obviously kindly treated'.[126] Yet both investigations raised reform issues, including staffing levels to cope with increasing patient numbers whilst improving standards of care and the need for a resident medical officer, if not a medical superintendent. Similarly, the NLA lacked sufficient space to meet rising expectations concerning exercise and leisure coupled with a new emphasis upon work therapy.[127] As such criteria became the benchmarks for state-endorsed inspection and regulation, the NLA committee, staff and patients in their various ways would all have work to do.

---

[122] The swing chair nauseated and disorientated unruly patients; the bath of surprise involved a cold plunge/douche to counter mania; oral locks used a key which forcibly opened the mouth.

[123] *History of Norfolk, Norwich, Yarmouth, etc. Or Supplement to Excursions in the County.* Norwich 1825, Vol. 2, 'The Norfolk Lunatic Asylum', pp. 46–50, 46.

[124] Mrs Caryl, described as 'intelligent, humane and active . . . was first and last on every occasion where duty and humanity needed her presence'. ibid., p. 50. (cf. the 1818 allegations).

[125] (Sir) Andrew Halliday, *A General View of the Present State of Lunatics and Lunatic Asylums, in Great Britain and Ireland, and in some other kingdoms*, London, 1828, pp. 19–23.

[126] CiL, 22 Aug. 1844. The Commissioners had also visited the NLA on 9 Sept. 1842 and 23 Aug. 1843.

[127] Halliday, *General View*, pp. 21–3. The NLA then had little horticulture and no agriculture.

3

A superintendent and 'work therapy', 1843–61

Thomas Caryl had begun his twenty-ninth year as master at Norfolk Lunatic Asylum when the justices advertised for a new appointment in February 1843. Their decision, prompted by Caryl's ill-health and advancing years, also reflected plans to extend the asylum and an inspection by the Metropolitan Commissioners in Lunacy. They sought an unmarried man, aged under 45 years, 'able to read and write and do accounts'.[1] Ebenezer Owen, former master of Malmsbury Union workhouse and one time attendant at the Hanwell Asylum, was selected from twelve applicants in rather unusual circumstances.[2] He was offered the post from 24 April 1843 at a provisional salary of £100 with board and lodging, raised to £150 in August 1844 when Caryl died and thereby ceased to draw his annuity. Owen and matron Houghton evidently made a practical couple; they married and were granted leave of absence at the end of August, while his brother Hugh temporarily became acting superintendent.[3]

Ebenezer Owen's tenure as master and then superintendent at the NLA coincided with greater national emphasis upon the asylum as the appropriate place for madness. By 1859 there were 17,608 patients in county asylums nationally, more than five times the 1843 figure and twice the number of lunatics then in workhouses.[4] His period of office began and ended with expansionary phases in NLA buildings and facilities and during it patient numbers more than doubled. Although Owen had no medical qualifications, these were also years of growing medical influence and external regulation. Each suggested minimum safeguards for asylum patients, although the impact of medicine can be overstated and legalistic concern often focused upon the rights of richer patients who might be confined in asylums.[5] 'In compliance with the statute 8 & 9 Vict. c.126', the 1845 Lunatics Act, the first resident

---

[1] Committee of Visiting Justices (CVIS) Minutes, SAH 6, Jan. 1840–Dec. 1848, 6 Feb. 1843.

[2] Owen was selected from twelve applicants. After his brother Hugh (later chief clerk of the Poor Law Commission 1853–72) arrived with a sickness certificate for Ebenezer, the Committee waited seven weeks to confirm the appointment.

[3] In July 1845 Mrs Owen's new baby was minded by her sister (possibly Louisa Houghton, head female attendant in 1854). During Ebenezer's illness in January and February 1847 Hugh returned to keep the books.

[4] Viz. county asylum patients 3,274 in 1843 and 17,608 in 1859 and, in workhouses, 3,829 to 7,963. Poor Law Commission, Official Circulars, 23, 13 Feb. 1843 and 68th *Report of the Commissioners in Lunacy*, 1914, Part Two, Appendix A, Table 1.

[5] K. Jones, *Asylums and After*, Athlone, London, 1993, pp. 75, 90. From 1842 Poor Law

medical officer, surgeon T. Morison was appointed at an annual salary of 80 guineas, the expense partly offset by the death of Dr Wright, the visiting physician, in February 1845. G.W. Firth remained as visiting surgeon and Morison, who resigned in August 1847, was replaced by another surgeon, Charles Broughton. As the last English asylum to appoint a medical super-intendent, the NLA nevertheless adopted an optimistic outlook by the early 1850s, with a medicalised approach added to earlier emphases upon work as therapy and an economically more self-reliant community.

The nine justices who appointed Owen consisted of three clergymen, four landowners, a colonel and a Member of Parliament. Of these, the Reverends Charles Wodehouse, Thomas Blofeld and Edward Postle were still on the committee when Owen resigned in 1861, Blofeld having replaced Wodehouse as chairman. Just two of the 1843 committee members had retired by 1850 but the remainder departed over the next decade and their successors came from all over Norfolk, rather than the environs of Norwich.[6] Their initial response to criticism from the new Commissioners in Lunacy was rather defensive, couched in the language of cleanliness and economy. It reflected their continuing attention to county ratepayers and their need to persuade poor law authorities to make extensive use the asylum's facilities. Of the 401 'idiots, lunatics and insane persons chargeable to parishes' in Norfolk in 1843, for example, only 164 were lodged in the NLA itself; 91 others were in work-houses, 140 'with friends' and 6 in private asylums.[7] Yet this situation was to alter considerably by 1861.

The national inspection of asylums and other accommodation for the insane was first undertaken by the Metropolitan Commissioners in Lunacy in 1842, preceding their report of 1844 and more systematic arrangements under the 1845 Lunatics Act. The latter implied some movement away from the narrowest of cost considerations in the care of the insane and their retention within the workhouse system. Three medical officers and three members of the legal profession became responsible for the annual inspection of each county asylum, workhouse, private licensed establishment and those hospitals or gaols that housed the insane. Normally a doctor and a barrister would visit provincial institutions but five additional lay officers helped within the metropolitan area. Under the chairmanship of Lord Shaftsbury, the lunacy commissioners operated in the spirit of the 1828 County Lunatic

Commissioners urged that lunatics should receive 'proper medical treatment . . . in a well-regulated asylum' and this featured in the 1845 Lunatics Act.

[6] The ten justices in 1860, including five clergymen, were from King's Lynn, Aylsham, Hoveton, Wroxham, Cantley, etc., cf. the localised Thorpe, Norwich, Catton membership of 1844.

[7] Poor Law Commission, *Official Circulars*, 23, 13 Feb. 1843. 133 persons were 'dangerous to themselves and others'.

Asylums Act and left routine asylum administration in local hands.[8] They had few compulsory powers but asylum authorities were legally required to compile detailed information for their examination. This related to the processes of certification, admission and discharge, to the use of restraint and seclusion, and to escapes, suicides and injuries. Inspection was seen as the key to good order and as a safeguard against abuses but the commissioners also served as an information bureau and generally encouraged the justices in greater accountability and reform initiatives.

Two commissioners had visited the NLA in the autumn of 1842. Their report criticised the amount of mechanical restraint used on patients, insufficient heating, the poor dietary, and the shortage of tables and utensils for meals. However, they felt that 'the most serious defect in this institution . . . is the want of a resident medical officer'.[9] This became a legal requirement under the 1845 Act, though only the Norfolk, Bedford and Pembroke asylums had yet to make such provision. The commissioners' remarks reflected the contemporary influence of the non-restraint movement but also the rising importance of asylum doctors. In 1841 the Association of Medical Officers of Asylums for the Insane, later the Medico-Psychological Association, was established and it published from 1853 *The Asylum Journal*, precursor to the *Journal of Mental Science*. This journal publicly criticised the NLA first, because the new resident medical officer remained under Owen's superintendence and second, because from 1854 it was the only county asylum without a medical superintendent.[10] Nevertheless, a process of 'medicalisation', initiated by surgeons and focused upon bodily ailments within a therapeutic regime of hygiene, work and exercise, was noticeable at the NLA. The potential of new therapies and a broad non-restraint policy was endorsed and arrangements involving probation and allowances for recovering patients out 'on trial' were rapidly adopted.[11]

Expressions of reforming intent cannot be isolated from their economic and social context, however. Agricultural depression and a toughened poor law had already been associated in Norfolk with social disturbances and considerable emigration in the 1830s. Norwich, traditionally a destination and a source of employment, suffered with the decline of the local textile industry until economic diversification, associated with railways and

---

[8] 9 Geo IV (1828) c. 40 and c. 41. This legislation established a framework inspection and regulation of metropolitan asylums, extended to the provinces in 1845.

[9] As later reported in *The Asylum Journal*, 7, 15 Aug. 1854, pp. 99–102.

[10] In 1843 Norfolk, Bedford and Pembroke were the only county asylums without a medical officer. This became a legal requirement in 1845. After Bedford appointed a medical superintendent in 1854, the NLA was the only English example without one.

[11] The NLA was an early claimant for non-restraint methods by the late 1840s: as in 'moral therapy', solitary confinements, 'deterrent' attendants and occasional restraint incidences occurred. Suffolk County Asylum (SCA) adopted non-restraint before 1840 but not probation before 1914.

engineering, occurred in the 1850s. Yet railways resulted in competition for many rural industries and trades, with the result that parts of Norfolk became still more reliant upon the land. Agricultural diversification increased after repeal of the Corn Laws in 1846 but the era of high farming was associated with greater labour productivity, reduced arable acreage and fewer jobs. According to the 1851 Census, 7 per cent of the Norfolk-born population already lived in London and 55,000 others left the county over the next two decades.

Economic hardship led to greater dependence upon the poor law. More than 10 per cent of the Norfolk population was classed as paupers in the 1840s, and still 7 per cent in 1861, with an increasing proportion subjected to workhouse relief.[12] These higher than national levels understate the real incidence of poverty and say nothing of the grinding hardship which drove some men and women, particularly those with children, to their wits' end. Popular responses in the county during the period ranged from quasi-revolutionary incendiarism to agricultural trade unionism, primitive methodism, interest in suffrage extension and political Liberalism. There was also a marked apparent increase in lunacy, particularly during the 'hungry forties'. Poor Law Commission returns suggest that the number of lunatic or idiot paupers in Norfolk rose by 150, or 37 per cent, in just four years, reaching 551 in January 1847. Norfolk then had above average proportions of people considered 'dangerous to themselves and others' and 63 per cent of the insane were in, arguably, the most active age groups between 20 and 50 years. Not all could promptly be placed in asylums but a higher proportion than the national average was accommodated in this way as NLA patient numbers almost doubled, from 167 to 304, in the decade after 1843.[13] No doubt more people experienced forms of breakdown in periods of economic stress and social disturbance, but it appears that their behaviour was more likely to be construed as insane by county poor law and asylum authorities at such times.

Developing the asylum

How did external and internal influences affect the asylum and its patients? Although the initial building costs were high these were covered by the county rate and levies, which meant that the justices were not burdened with

---

[12] Anne Digby, *Pauper Palaces*, Routledge, London, 1978, pp. 13, 84.
[13] Poor Law Commission, lunatic paupers chargeable to parishes on 13 Feb. 1843 and 1 Jan. 1847, *Official Circulars of Public Documents and Information*, No. 10, London, 1851, p. 23. In 1847 this represented 1.36 per 1,000 in Norfolk (cf. 1.15/000 for England and Wales), 29 per cent of whom were considered dangerous (cf. 26 per cent). Less than 11 per cent were aged under 20 years or over 70 years.

debt and could contemplate further expansion.[14] After extensions in 1831 the asylum could accommodate 150 patients, but this capacity was exceeded within the decade. Women's rooms were 'inconveniently crowded by a greater number of beds than they were originally designed to hold but the hospital also . . . is completely filled'.[15] In 1841 work began on 'airy, capacious and convenient' wing extensions to the main building, using iron girders and wooden floors, each providing 32 beds and additional bathrooms.[16] Construction was straightforward and the cost of £2,300 relatively modest but the justices pressed for rapid completion of the project as the patients had become 'more disturbed and uncomfortable'.[17] Additional room was considered necessary and was achieved 'at a very trifling expense by taking down partitions in sleeping rooms', with expansion also reflected in extensions to the cemetery and plans for a new octagon-style chapel in 1848.[18]

Although asylum weekly charges of 5s 9d per patient were declared 'the lowest in the Kingdom' in 1844, compared with the 1845 national asylum average of 7s 3d, this was more than double the national workhouse average of just 2s 7d.[19] The average number of patients, 174 in 1844–5, was close to the asylum's capacity of 180 but the justices sought to attract more and to expand its facilities. Having appointed a resident medical officer, they moved from cost comparisons to warn of increased staffing and other costs and to focus upon the asylum's therapeutic role. Thus:

> we have reason to believe that the cure of Lunatics is often prevented or retarded by delaying too long to send them to an Asylum . . . as cure is the first object . . . care of these unfortunate persons is entrusted to the Magistrate . . . we believe that a considerable increase of accommodation may be made at a small expense by some different arrangements in the House.[20]

The language of care and cure, the concept of asylum as an appropriate environment, and the possibilities of reorganisation in securing greater efficiencies were now emphasised.

Simultaneously, the justices responded directly to criticisms. They explained that:

---

[14] *Report of Commissioners in Lunacy* (CiL) 1844–1925 SAH 141, 1845–6, p. 29. It took 20 years to clear SCA establishment costs of £30,273. ibid., p. 33.

[15] CVIS, 1840–8, SAH 6, Jan. 1841.

[16] ibid., 26 April 1841, 30 May 1842. These were provided at a cost of £1,838.

[17] ibid., July 1841.

[18] CVIS, 5 Sept. 1846, 6 Jan. 1842 respectively; CiL, 24 Nov. 1847, 26 Oct. 1848. Chapels were required at all asylums under the 1845 Act.

[19] Annual Report NLA (AR), 1844–76, SAH 28, 1844–5, Cttee, p. 7; Jones, *Asylums*, p. 75.

[20] AR, 1844–5, Cttee. p. 7.

owing to the situation of the Asylum near the low meadows of the river, the House is sometimes filled with a damp foggy air, and some means . . . are desirable for occasionally drying and warming the whole building . . . the Medical officers . . . consider such a plan desirable for the health and comfort of the Patients.[21]

New stoves added in the galleries from 1843 were ineffective, so work installing new heating pipes commenced. This involved considerable upheaval and the opening of walls, making the asylum still colder: in January 1845 temperatures on the men's side of the asylum did not exceed 50 degrees Fahrenheit, according to visitors' report books.[22] A year later, with the work completed, temperature readings were rarely below this level, even with windows open for ventilation.

On their second inspection in August 1844 the lunacy commissioners were pleased that 'all the leg-locks and chains have been removed from the seats and benches in the dayrooms and airing courts', and only one male patient was under restraint. Although the dietary remained 'less liberal' than in some asylums, it had improved and better cutlery and tables were provided. However, 'the very inadequate extent of the land so essential to the due occupation of the patients' remained 'a great defect'.[23] The justices responded that one acre of land served as frontage between the road and the asylum and should be retained for this purpose but they recognised that the remaining land was now fully occupied by buildings, exercise yards, the kitchen garden and cemetery. Three acres of 'land for employment of patients' had been purchased in 1844 and 2.75 acres more were added in 1846, 'partly as pleasure ground in which the females may enjoy air and exercise'.[24]

By January 1846, the commissioners 'observed a very decided improvement . . . since the Asylum was first visited . . . the house remarkably clean and well warmed and ventilated throughout' and the food 'sufficient and of a fair quality'.[25] Another female attendant and a house servant had been appointed and surgeon Morison was in post. Major Richard Wood 'was much struck in the improved order . . . the cheerfulness of everything . . . the kindness shown towards the unfortunate patients' since his previous visit in 1840.[26] With additional bathrooms installed, patients were bathed individually from 1850 and daily rather than twice weekly laundry was now provided. A new day room and smaller female wards providing 24 beds, additional indoor recreation space and two male workshops were added

---

[21] ibid., pp. 6–7.

[22] Visiting Justices Report Books (Visitors), 1844–68, SAH 138, 8 Jan. 1845, 13 Dec. 1846. Flues, pipes and grates circulated hot air from basement furnaces.

[23] CiL, 2 Aug. 1844, p. 9.

[24] CiL, 1845–6, p. 29; 24 Feb. 1847. Three acres on the west side were purchased for £160 in 1844, land and property on the east side cost £31,200 in 1846. CVIS, 5 Sept. 1846.

[25] CiL, 27 Jan. 1846, p. 3.

[26] Visitors, 5 May 1847.

by 1852, with gas lighting installed in 1853.[27] More ambitious expansion was already contemplated, contingent upon a diversion of the turnpike road to allow more space, with 30 acres of farmland purchased in 1853 and six more as plans became clearer by 1855.[28]

According to the asylum's first published annual reports, income for 1844 and 1845 averaged £2,600, 93 per cent of which was provided by county poor law unions for their patients, accommodated at a weekly charge of 5s 9d. The rest came from additional 'boarders' and 'criminal and vagrant' patients, charged at ten shillings per week respectively to those boroughs not paying the county rate and to the Chancery. Food was the major item of expenditure, costing £1,068, followed by salaries of £611 and fuel £305. The £283 spent on beer, tobacco and snuff exceeded the £224 on bedding and clothing, suggesting a curiously uneven approach to the patients' comforts.[29] By 1850 standard weekly charges were further reduced to 5s 3d and those at higher rates for outcounty and criminal patients produced more significant income, £795 out of a total £4,508, than previously.[30] An increase in patient numbers was thus accompanied by a degree of cross-subsidisation. There was no evidence that 'outcounty' or criminal patients represented higher costs to the asylum, certainly not proportionate to the higher charges made, and income from these sources helped to restrain the standard county charge.[31] In turn, this enhanced the asylum's claims to be an economic institution and benefited Norfolk ratepayers.

With the establishment of gardens and a farm, food could be produced directly, using the patients' labour. From 1852 the asylum had its own slaughter house with live animals brought in as a safeguard against 'inferior' meat supplies. Farm accounts, beginning in 1854, show that an initial grant of £250 for livestock purchases was quickly repaid. In each of the next ten years livestock sales averaged approximately £150, with stock and vegetables produced for asylum use valued at over £210. This comfortably exceeded the expenditure on seeds, new livestock and the annual £48 land rent paid to the asylum. Surplus funds, transferred to the asylum for refurbishments, exceeded £150 per annum, with small amounts of cash in hand retained in the farm account. It appears that receipts averaging £45 for 'extra labour' referred to the external employment of asylum farm horses and a farmhand, but patients were clearly contributors to the asylum economy.[32]

---

[27] CVIS, 1849–56, SAH 7, July 1851, April 1852.

[28] A plan of the proposed diversion, dated 1850 (at Drayton Old Lodge), indicates a route south of the asylum, passing through Thorpe common. This also shows the original chapel, west of the octagon church.

[29] AR, 1844, Cttee, p. 6. The master received £150, the matron £50, medical officers £135, servants £153, clerk £63 and chaplain £60.

[30] AR, 1850, Cttee, p. 8.

[31] A modest number of private patients later had marginal privileges and more 'treats'.

[32] AR, Farm Accounts, 1854–64. The method of book keeping changed in 1863–4.

The justices also reassessed patient amenities and standards of care. From June 1853 Owen began to visit a number of asylums 'reputed for their appropriate construction and management'.[33] He reported that sanitary arrangements at the NLA lagged in respect of provision of water closets on the wards and that the proportion of single bedrooms, one quarter, was lower than the one-third average in the asylums he had visited. The combination of straw, hair and flock mattresses used in the asylum was not unusual, nor were the arrangements using strong dress and padded rooms for refractory patients. Clothing issued to patients was also typical, though the NCA had recently introduced a softer grey cloth for women, in addition to flannel undergarments and cotton dresses. In terms of recreational land and farmland the asylum fared comparatively well for its size, although it noticeably lacked home brewing and baking facilities. As these issues were addressed the weekly charges for patients increased markedly and the 8s 8d figure for 1860 was almost identical to the national asylum average of 8s 9d.[34]

With inputs from the farm and cross-subsidies from the outcounty patient charge of 14 shillings continuing at the NLA, these increased weekly charges suggest considerable upgrading of patient facilities in the 1850s. More ambitious modernisation plans commenced in 1854 with the construction of the dining hall, immediately to the south of the central administration block and leading to the proposed new church. Three acres of land, purchased from the Earl of Rosebery for £439, accommodated a northern diversion of the turnpike road, providing additional frontage space and room for new buildings. Considerable earthworks were involved for the new road was to be level: it ran through a cutting 16 feet deep, spanned by a new bridge giving safe access to farmland on the north side. By making extensive use of patients' labour to remove excavated earth, these roadworks appear to have been completed at small cost to the asylum and the county.[35]

Revised proposals for additional extensions to the main asylum buildings were announced in 1857. These were built in matching style on an east–west orientation, turning outwards again from the northern spurs to the existing wings, and were to accommodate 60 male and 60 female patients (see plan on page 118). Steam pumps and the construction of two water towers would facilitate more general use of springwater and reduce dependence upon filtered river water for cooking purposes. The labelling of water taps was an

[33] Master's Journal, 1849–60, SAH 129, 4 June 1853. Owen visited county asylums at Stafford, Wakefield, York, Lancaster, Rainhill and Denbigh, and Birmingham borough asylum.

[34] AR, 1860, Superintendent, p. 2.

[35] An 1854 plan showing the bridge directly to the front of the asylum was revised in 1856, moving the bridge eastwards for maximum clearance (at Drayton Old Lodge). AR, 1857, Superintendent, p. 2 mentions costs of £400. The cutting also helped to screen part of the asylum.

insufficient precaution in an asylum environment and only a marginal improvement on previous designations of 'h', 'c' or 'r'. One tower was the central feature in a new laundry, located between the women's wing and the new road. Conversion of the former laundry rooms provided an additional twenty-bed ward, raising the overall capacity to 440 beds.[36] A second water tower stood in a complex of buildings which included the boilerhouse, converted workshops and improved stores, north of the men's wing and east of the stables and road bridge. Finally an octagon church, incorporating a basement mortuary, was constructed on the site of a former washroom and dead house south of the dining hall. This allowed most patients to attend religious services whilst maintaining their sexual segregation.

The physical expansion of the asylum suggested not only a hospital but a distinct community, in which male and female patients lived separated lives and performed gendered work-roles geared to the objectives of efficiency and greater self-sufficiency. Yet the building costs seemed to contradict such goals and incurred the wrath of the county Quarter Sessions. The committee requested the county surveyor, John Brown, to explain why original estimates of £19,926 had grown to £23,140 before fittings were added.[37] Brown, an architect of some repute, had faithfully maintained the original design features in the new wards. He responded that modifications over a six-year construction period, including the provision of additional offices, alterations to existing buildings and engineers' work, had all added to the expense. Less than satisfied, the justices decided to borrow £26,000 to cover all costs in June 1859 and their subsequent correspondence with Brown was acrimonious. His threat of litigation to safeguard plans which he regarded as his own intellectual property, rather than belonging to the county, may have speeded his retirement, as he was described as 'the former county surveyor' in 1861.[38]

In the new and renovated buildings each ward was equipped with bath and water closets, remedying one deficiency noted by Owen and the justices' previous views that, 'not being found suitable to the patients . . . no increase of them found requisite'.[39] Despite the extra capacity, the medical officers drew attention to a shortage of infirmary provision, particularly for the

---

[36] An excess of female accommodation developed from this point. Women were now on the west side, with the new laundry: earlier plans suggest they were originally accommodated in the east wing.

[37] CVIS, 30 Nov. 1858. Brown designed several churches in Norfolk and Suffolk 1832–51 and workhouses at Colchester, Sudbury and Docking 1836–8. He also supervised the restoration of Norwich Cathedral's central tower. H.M. Colvin, *Bibliographical Directory of English Architects 1660–1840*, John Murray, London, 1954, p. 100.

[38] CVIS, 30 Nov. 1858 and 29 June 1859. Brown had refused to hand over working plans and was threatening legal proceedings (20 May 1859) but settled out of court (28 Jan. 1861).

[39] CVIS, 26 April 1847.

many elderly and 'feeble' women patients.[40] However, annual admissions immediately increased by forty on the average for the middle 1850s and the boroughs of Great Yarmouth, Thetford, King's Lynn were advised that the asylum was ready to receive their patients.[41] Clearly the justices wished to develop the cross-subsidy of county patients, but other authorities also sought to bargain. For example, the Yarmouth guardians requested the NLA 'to determine the lowest sum per head for 22 patients – 11 male, 11 female, the numbers to be increased until determined by notice, payment to be made quarterly'.[42] Those in Norwich, constantly urged by the lunacy commissioners to improve their own accommodation, tried to minimise their expense by delaying the temporary transfer of patients to the NLA.[43]

By 1860 the asylum had an average of 340 patients and was able to accommodate 100 more. As was to be expected, this expansion had implications for maintenance accounts, summarised in Table 3.1. Income doubled over the 1850s and though earnings from 'outcounty' patients increased by 1860, the potential of this source was not yet realised. A greater than proportionate increase in spending on food, allowing also for the contribution of the asylum farm, suggests improvements in the patients' diet. Salaries amounted to a reduced portion of expenditure and the combined wages of an enlarged staff (£552) still lagged behind those of the superintendent, matron, medical officers, treasurer and chaplain (£710). Fuel costs were almost £750 and spending on clothing and bedding, which had been very low in 1850, just exceeded that on beer and spirits by 1860. Beer featured prominently in provisions and as a bonus for working patients and spirits were the principal medication, if the £37 spent on other drugs and medicines is any guide.

In many asylums staff shortages have been linked with the overuse of physical restraint and patients' seclusion or with overt forms of abuse. The NLA was understaffed with just four male and five female attendants plus three women house servants for upwards of 160 patients in 1844. As there was little outdoor work beyond gardening, it is likely that patients undertook cleaning and ward work, possibly including nursing, which was standard poor law practice. Although the lunacy commissioners made no criticism of NLA staff in 1844, patient Sarah B— complained of ill treatment in September and another patient died of violent cause the following month. In both cases the justices decided that the evidence was 'inconclusive'.[44] The same year a visitor, noting that 45 patients were out of doors exercising with their

---

[40] AR, 1858, Medical Officer (MO), p. 6.

[41] CVIS, 25 Oct. 1859.

[42] ibid., 31 Dec. 1859.

[43] ibid., 25 June 1860. The committee replied that standard outcounty charge was 14 shillings. Fifty Norwich patients were involved. 27 Nov. 1860, 30 April 1861.

[44] CiL, 22 Aug. 1844; Visitors, 30 Sept. and 26 Oct. 1844; 11 Sept. 1845.

Table 3.1 Income and major items of expenditure at the Norfolk Lunatic Asylum, 1844–60

	1845	1850	1860
Net annual income	£2,687	£3,632	£7,723
'Norfolk' %	89.4	85.1	93.7
'Outcounty. etc.' %	10.6	14.9	6.3
% Expenditure on:	£2,768	£3,012	£8,117
officers' salaries	16.8	14.1	9.2
attendants/wages	5.6	7.7	7.1
food	39.1	42.0	50.3
beer, spirits	10.4	13.5	9.1
fuel	12.3	9.4	8.0
clothing, bedding	8.2	6.6	9.7
drugs, surgery	0.7	0.5	0.5
sundries	3.1	3.4	3.6
Brought forward from previous year	£813	£108	–£1,582
Carried forward	£734	£738	–£1,976

respective keepers, reported that this left 'only one porter in charge of the whole interior of the building'.[45] After a woman patient drowned in September 1845 the matron complained of inadequate staff supervision, but the appointment of a single male gardener/keeper in 1846 did not satisfy the lunacy commissioners, who requested more staff in 1847.[46] However, a staff complement of six male and six female attendants, plus six others and the occasional hire of additional nurses in 1850, suggested an incremental response by the asylum committee.

'The entire absence . . . of all kinds' of mechanical restraint in the asylum was proclaimed by the medical officer in 1853 but a year later he made allegations, not unconnected with his own removal, that 'blows, bruises and injuries to patients were not reported to him and that . . . the attendants treated the patients with harshness and severity'.[47] Meanwhile the commissioners also expressed concern that five patients had died overnight in their beds, with no attendant reporting this until the following morning, and that six further deaths had occurred from pneumonia.[48] They recommended the appointment of night attendants and improved sleeping rooms and bedding. Now the justices responded more positively and medical officers planned for

[45] Visitors, 19 Aug. 1844.
[46] CiL, 24 Nov. 1847.
[47] AR, 1853, MO, p. 26; *Asylum Journal*, 15 Aug. 1854, p. 101.
[48] CiL, 10 May 1853.

staff ratios of one to ten for noisy or dirty patients and one to twenty or twenty-five for convalescent or quiet patients. By the mid-1850s, when the average number of patients was almost 300, there were eleven male and eleven female attendants, plus laundresses, a cook and three other servants.[49]

It is generally accepted that 'asylum work was of low status and not popular, and the stigma of the insane rubbed off on those who worked with them'.[50] Such work was also poorly paid but this was perhaps less obvious in the Norfolk labour market. Male attendants' weekly wages ranged between 7s 8d and 10 shillings with board and lodging in the 1850s, according to seniority, the amount of night-watching and the shaving of patients undertaken. This compared with a Norfolk farm labourer's wages of roughly 8 shillings in the 1840s, and 9–11 shillings a decade later. Day labourers earned more at harvest time but could not be sure of regular work throughout the year.[51] Asylum work guaranteed this in abundance, with a 6.00 a.m. start, no time or opportunities for leisure at night and very few days off. Female attendants were paid between 4s 6d and 5 shillings, again with supplements for night nursing. Although staff turnover was a problem, some attendants had apparently settled to their work: of the 21 who had completed their probationary period by 1856, one-third had worked at the asylum for over four years, one-third for between two and four years and one-third from six months to two years.[52]

However, the behaviour of attendants remained a cause for concern. One woman was dismissed for ill-treating a patient in 1853, but this produced little exemplary effect.[53] A major incident occurred in 1854 when William S—, a patient aged 36 who slept in a single room, suffered a broken sternum and eight fractured ribs and died. Investigations by the commissioners and the local coroner concluded that S—'s injuries had been inflicted, though the medical officers suggested that he had previously injured himself throwing his bed about and the six male attendants called gave contradictory evidence. A jury concluded there was 'some mystery in this case' but, after a further commissioners' meeting, three attendants were dismissed 'for prevarication in several material points of statement'.[54] There were no similar scandals for

---

[49] Ten male attendants received 20 guineas annually and the head attendant 22 guineas. An assistant matron received £18 annually and ten female attendants between £12 and £13, according to seniority, with extras for night work. There were two laundresses, a cook, a gatekeeper, a house lad and an office boy. NLA Wages Book, 1854–90, SAH 75, 1854–6.

[50] P. Nolan, A History of Mental Health Nursing, Chapman & Hall, London, 1993, p. 48; M. Carpenter, 'Asylum nursing before 1914' in C. Davies (ed.), Rewriting Nursing History, Croom Helm, London, 1980, pp. 123–46.

[51] ibid., 1854. Wages were unchanged by 1860. Farm wages from Digby, p. 23.

[52] Based on wages data, 1856.

[53] AR, 1853, MO, pp. 11, 20.

[54] AR, 1854, Cttee, pp. 6–7; Asylum Journal, 15 Oct. 1854, pp. 143–4.

four years but close supervision was necessary. While Owen was away from the asylum in March 1859, Hannah B— was dismissed for being intoxicated on duty, Maria F— was fined 10 shillings for abuse and bad language and Samuel T— escaped with a caution after kicking a patient only because his victim would not identify him.[55] Another attendant, John E—, was dismissed for violence towards patient William S— a few months later.

Work therapy and recreation

Until the early 1840s the employment of patients was restricted by the absence of suitable occupations and an officialdom which looked no further than limited forms of domestic service. As in workhouses, suitable women were expected to do washing and cleaning and a few did needlework, which was partly offered as an amusement, along with drawing boards and wooden bricks. Little outdoor work could be provided without farmland and, though the importance of physical exercise was understood, the lack of space and supervisory staff limited this to dull rounds in the airing courts. Andrew Halliday's 1828 asylum survey, looking for evidence of genuine outdoor work and physical exercise, had found 'almost none at Norfolk'.[56]

Although medical and other reformers began to promote the concept of work as therapeutic or rehabilitative, local justices initially felt that its provision at the NLA was beyond their remit.[57] Later, they claimed:

> the necessity of more land not only as an airing ground but also to provide employment as the likely cure, has long occurred to us, and has been recommended by our medical officers, though at the same time there were in some quarters doubts and objections.[58]

However, the post-1834 poor law involved the expectation of work and the asylum was a pauper institution. When urged by the commissioners to buy land in 1844 the justices complied but whether therapeutic or political economy considerations determined their response is unclear. Owen's past experience as a workhouse master and as an attendant in an asylum associated with work therapy may have familiarised him with both rationales.[59]

---

[55] CVIS, 29 March 1859.

[56] Halliday, cited in L.D. Smith, *Cure, Comfort and Safe Custody*, Leicester University Press, 1999, p. 236.

[57] Asylums at Wakefield 1815, Gloucester 1823 and Hanwell 1831 pioneered the use of patient labour. The first and last reflected the reforming regimes of William Ellis and John Conolly, but the value of work was universally extolled.

[58] CVIS, 5 Sept. 1846.

[59] Owen may have worked under Ellis and/or Conolly at Hanwell before and after 1838.

Between 40 and 45 male patients were working in the gardens or asylum buildings, as observed by William Corthe of Stafford in 1849. He commented:

> I have visited the Asylum at Belfast and the Retreat at York, usually considered model establishments for the insane; & think the Norfolk Asylum will not suffer from a comparison with either, in *any* points . . . in some – the various ways in which the talents or ingenuity of the patients are trained into useful employment – it manfully excels them.[60]

Such praise was welcome, but the purchase of 30 acres of farmland in 1853 was critical. This was the minimum specified by the commissioners for asylums with 300 patients, though it had rarely been achieved elsewhere. It provided the NLA medical staff with a genuine opportunity as they believed that links between physical and mental illness could be countered by 'hygienic and medico-moral therapy', involving outdoor exercise and work which 'accords with . . . previous occupations'.[61] They considered good diet and a range of employment essential, since 'the more varied and extensive the occupations of the patients, the more fully will be the development of their individual capacities'.[62]

Work therapy supposedly stopped short of risk to patients' health, comfort or happiness and motives of 'any mistaken economy'.[63] In practice, it corresponded closely with institutional needs for food supplies and maintenance of the physical fabric. In 1854 a minimum of 34 male inmates worked in the gardens and on the farm, with 10 others as painters, carpenters, tailors, upholsterers and shoemakers. One tradesman was employed to direct and supervise patients in shoemaking and repairs, with another worker responsible for farmwork.[64] Similar arrangements for tailoring were introduced and additional workshops prepared to cover carpentry, plumbing, upholstery, glazing and glassware, smithery and engineering. Substantial revisions to the asylum in 1857 incorporated plans for 'carrying on industrial occupations to the extent deemed by the Committee to be desirable . . . The enlargement of those offices, apart from the call of accommodation . . . was therefore a matter of urgent necessity'.[65] Revising the assertions made in

---

[60] Visitors, 11 Sept. 1849. In the decade 1844–53 166 visitors, excluding lunacy commissioners, included clerics, army staff and poor law officials and doctors from France, Berlin, Ceylon and Ireland. Some were involved in post-mortem procedures: 28 of the 36 deaths in 1854 were investigated.

[61] AR, 1853, MO, p. 25.

[62] ibid., p. 21.

[63] ibid., p. 26.

[64] AR, 1854, MO, p. 29; Wages Book, Sept. 1854. Robert Watts was paid £11.14s. 0d for the quarter as shoemaker, Henry Bailey, paid £9.15s. 0d, was the other employee.

[65] AR, 1857, Supt, p. 1.

1853, the 1857 annual report acknowledged some work therapy as cheap labour. Although 'suitable work is provided for all the patients, male and female, who are in a fit state . . . the less skilful of the men have been set occupied in removing the earth thrown up in the formation of roads, and preparation of the ground for the new buildings'.[66]

By 1860 over half of the 152 men and three-quarters of the 188 women patients were working. Women performed all too familiar indoor tasks in the laundry and kitchens, or as ward helpers or cleaners. Steam-powered washing and wringing machines and drying rooms were introduced, however, partly because 'the labour of the patients in connection with washing . . . is not regarded a desirable occupation for them'.[67] Fifteen women were occupied in knitting, with roughly 70 others in workrooms. These provided a combination of entertainment and therapy, offering drawing, paperwork, the making of decorations, bric-a-brac, bonnets and prints for bazaars, with the definite purpose of fund-raising, for decorating wards and later for musical instruments, entertainment and excursions.[68] Rather oddly, given the importance of bread and beer in the diet and as expenditure items, baking and brewing were still not seen as suitable employment for patients.[69]

Although individual patient care remained an objective, the growth of the asylum and of work therapy meant that patients were increasingly regulated by the requirements of the asylum as a managed estate. A contribution to the political economy and greater self-sufficiency of the institution meant more signs of 'batch living' among patients, in wards geared to particular work tasks and the practicalities of washing or eating.[70] The asylum day began at 6.00 a.m. as the attendants prepared fires and day rooms. Sleeping rooms and dormitories were unlocked at 6.30 a.m. and able patients were expected to dress, with washing 'enforced or encouraged in those that are averse to cleanliness and performed for those unable to attend to themselves'.[71] An 8.00 a.m. breakfast was followed, on three days in the week, by a religious service in the chapel, which could now accommodate 420 persons. Work lasted from 9.00 a.m. until 12.30 p.m., with a mid-morning feeding break, and on fine days those unable to work but not infirm had outdoor exercise. After a brief return to the wards and dinner at 1.00 p.m. work for men resumed from

---

[66] ibid., pp. 2–3.

[67] AR, 1860, Supt, pp. 2–3. The remaining laundry workers were to be accommodated in a new ward and day room.

[68] Workroom and bazaar accounts, SAH 483, 1853–98.

[69] CVIS, 24 May 1861.

[70] Goffman's expression implies the loss of the patient's individuality and of face-to-face relationships, although such experiences were not unknown in contemporary farm or factory work; E. Goffman, *Asylums*, Penguin, Harmondsworth, 1961.

[71] AR, 1859, Supt, pp. 3–4. Lunacy commissioners had requested that attendants instruct patients in the use of these facilities, shave patients more frequently and ensure that body linen was changed more than once a week.

2.00 p.m. until 4.00 p.m. before further refreshments, but other patients were then normally in the grounds on suitable days until 4.00 p.m. in winter and 5.00 p.m. in summer. Supper was provided in day rooms at 6.00 p.m., usually followed by reading, music, cards or games until bed at 7.00 p.m. in winter and 8.00 p.m. in summer.

Early improvements to the airing courts had included the provision of raised mounds, enabling patients to see over walls and across the river valley, with shrubs and plants, followed by the opening of gardens, initially for female patients. More attention was soon paid to regular exercise and especially drilling, seen as essential to the promotion of patients' health, self-respect and self-control, with the practical advantage that 'the task of taking a vast number to a distance from the Asylum for air and exercise becomes comparatively easy'.[72] In 1853 land was hired for cricket matches, involving about 50 male patients altogether, and they levelled part of the asylum's own ground for the purpose in 1854, playing occasional matches against neighbouring clubs. A bowling green was also laid out but this was for staff only: male patients had to be content with an area for skittles. In the gardens a summer house was added and mixed picnics for 2–300 patients on the field just beyond the asylum walls, accompanied by brass band entertainment, became a regular feature.

A more ambitious railway excursion to Yarmouth for 130 patients in 1856 was repeated with 160 patients in 1857 and 247 patients went to Lowestoft in 1859. River trips were also introduced and convalescent women were allowed out with attendants to take tea at the homes of those who offered invitations. Such highlights complemented the fortnightly dances and occasional magic lantern shows in the late 1850s. A few patients could 'continue their own apparel where it is thought that a change will have a prejudicial effect' and others were allowed to avoid 'studied uniformity' or to recognise 'season and suitability' in their clothing.[73] By now the commissioners noted the cheerfulness of rooms aided by paintings, looking glasses, 'masses of ornaments' and 'entertaining periodicals' which, 'together with the aviaries, vivarium, plants and flowers contribute to the enjoyment of the patients and afford a relief and variety which they appear to appreciate'.[74] Many of these features may have been idealised – it is not clear who among the patients was asked for an opinion – and some represented particular treats rather than regular provision. Nevertheless they compared favourably with workhouse conditions and amenities available to the poorest outside the workhouses.[75] If they replicated and possibly reinforced the values of Victorian society, what values was a pauper asylum of the 1840s and 1850s supposed to reflect?

---

[72] AR, 1853, MO, p. 27.

[73] ibid., p. 19.

[74] CiL, 20 April 1861.

[75] K. Jones, 'The culture of the mental hospital' in G.E. Berrios and H. Freeman (eds), *150 Years of British Psychiatry*, Gaskell, London, pp. 17–28.

Patients and treatments

Even with a limited medical contribution to its overall direction, the asylum exhibited a cautiously optimistic outlook in the treatment and discharge of patients and publicly presented itself as a reforming institution.

Although the trend is understated in the averages presented in Table 3.2, annual admissions rose during the 1840s and constituted a higher proportion of the inpatient totals. As the equivalent of 44 per cent of new admissions was discharged, roughly the same as in the 1830s, this meant that a slightly higher proportion of all patients was leaving the asylum. The previous gender imbalance among discharged patients was also reduced. Admissions and existing patient numbers increased more rapidly in the 1850s and the proportion of those now classed as 'recovered' was only slightly below previous figures for all those discharged (see Table 3.3). Increasing numbers of probationary and other patients were discharged and patient readmissions then amounted to roughly one-fifth of all admissions. This suggests, if not a successful therapeutic regime, then one which sought to treat, discharge and, if necessary, readmit patients. By no means all those entering the NLA were expected to remain there: there was a considerable dynamic or throughput of patients. Nor was death the only way out of the asylum, for mortality rates fell in the 1840s and 1850s, as did the earlier surfeit of male over female patient deaths (see Table 3.2).

Table 3.2 Patients resident, admissions and mortality rates: annual averages, 1830–59

| | Average no. resident | | | Admissions | | | Mortality % | | |
	Total	M	F	Total	M	F	Total	M	F
1830–39	159	72	87	52	26	26	17.0	20.7	13.8
1840–49	185	86	99	72	33	39	16.7	16.5	16.9
1850–59	291	132	159	90	40	50	11.7	11.7	11.6

Notes: Residents and admission averages to nearest whole number. Discharge rates are presented in Table 3.3.

Medical officers' reports in the early 1840s still referred to patients 'in fits', in 'feeble condition' or 'sinking', although there were occasions when 'there is no man in bed or out of health', even if individuals were still reported as 'restless', or 'excited'.[76] On their admission several patients were categorised, somewhat dismissively, as in a 'low stupid state', though greater efforts were

[76] Physician's Report Book, 1843–5, SAH 150, 31 Oct. 1843.

made with others, such as 'June A— 31 of Docking, religiously insane and in great terror of eternal damnation'.[77] Younger patients, possibly admitted because their families could no longer cope with them, included George M— aged 20, 'a dangerous idiot', Robert P— aged 14, 'very violent', and John B— aged 20, 'incoherent and very violent'.[78] Little comment was made when elderly, bed-ridden or general paralysis patients died, but explanations were offered concerning others, such as Susan M—, aged 26, 'desponding for the last three years' or Sophia R—, aged 30, 'subject to diarrheea [sic] and sinking for a long time previous'.[79] James W—, Edward M— and Peter H— were among those who succumbed to repeated epileptic fits in 1844 and the prognosis for James M—, 'erysipelas in leg', and Robert P—, 'jaundice', was not good.[80]

Other patients continued to recover, or were discharged. Those monitored included Richard J—, 'admitted a month back, did not all that time exhibit any signs of insanity and . . . has been quite rational and well behaved', and Catherine B—, 'in a calm state and apparently rational and has been well since her admission'.[81] Similarly, William T—, 'who was under personal restraint at my last visit, is at work today'.[82] Physician's reports for 1844 show at least ten patients readmitted or discharged for a second time. Either a more flexible approach to treatment was being adopted or the doctors were responding to the pressures of overcrowding. There were occasions when, 'the day being very wet, the rooms on the women's side are crowded and several of the patients are much excited.'[83] Among those discharged in February 1844 was 'Mary Anne Elizabeth S— who is about 7 months gone with child . . . desirous of going home. She is much improved and may safely be managed at home.' Evidently she was readmitted, for in June it was 'recommended that the infant of MAE S— be detained in the asylum for the present'.[84] Simultaneously, patient Judith S—, 'expecting to be confined at end July' was also discharged, 'as it appears to the medical officers that she may be confined with her friends'.[85]

As the resident and visiting medical officers were both surgeons, they were always likely to focus upon the physical health of patients. However, Richard Foote MD, formerly assistant medical officer at the Wiltshire County asylum,

---

[77] ibid., 9 Nov. 1843. Sarah B—, 25, was also admitted 'religiously insane' on 25 Aug. 1844.

[78] ibid., 13 April, 11 July and 29 July 1844.

[79] ibid., 17 May and 12 Dec. 1844.

[80] ibid., 27 March 1844. J.W. was 30 years old when he died, E.M. died 24 Dec. 1844, aged 23.

[81] ibid., 4 Aug. 1844.

[82] ibid., 22 Nov. 1844.

[83] ibid., 17 May 1844.

[84] ibid., 14 Feb. and 21 June 1844.

[85] ibid., 21 June 1844.

became resident medical officer in 1852. The first published medical officers' report in 1853 was a revealing and optimistic document. It suggested that 'scarcely any insane person is entirely free from physical ailment' but saw the combination of good diet, exercise and medico-moral remedy as the basis of a curative regime.[86] Directing their remarks at poor law authorities, the doctors emphasised the dangers inherent in delay, for 'the "first few days" may produce such organic change in the brain of the lunatic as to render him incurable, a permanent tax on his parish and a permanent sorrow to his friends'. With immediate referral to asylum, however, it was felt that 'the percentage of cures may be increased to between 70 and 80 per cent'.[87] As convalescent care and help was deemed essential in avoiding the recurrence of illness, so opportunities should be provided for the 'convalescent and fit to follow their ordinary employment'.[88] Meanwhile, over 46 per cent of new admissions were discharged as 'recovered'. This represented a good performance according to a contemporary survey of county asylums, which suggested that 'less than 40 per cent may be regarded as a low proportion [of recoveries] and one much exceeding 45 per cent as a high proportion'.[89]

How were such results obtained? The medical staff elaborated on overall intentions and procedures and those specifics which they preferred to avoid, rather than upon particular treatments. Their first and otherwise detailed 31-page report concluded, rather abruptly, 'we must defer allusion to the pharmaceutical measures adopted on grounds of space'.[90] Admissons procedure now involved observation by attendants at night, 'to be especially reported on in the morning', with Foote making occasional visits or summoned in response to any sudden change in the patient's condition or behaviour, followed by daily reports. Attention was given to the class of persons with which the patient was placed, to appropriate occupations and amusements and the administration of any necessary medicines prior to further assessment. Patients were allowed visitors, though these were not encouraged in the first month and the medical staff could and sometimes did refuse access. The doctors also expressed the hope that alternative provision could be made for middle-class patients, as 'cases of this kind are not fit for a county pauper asylum'.[91] Such procedures asked a great deal of the asylum staff, who may have been irked by Foote's zealous approach, particularly as all were supposedly under Owen's superintendence. As will be seen, medical

---

[86] AR, 1853, MO, pp. 28, 25.

[87] ibid., p. 8.

[88] ibid., p. 10.

[89] ibid., p. 10. Foote probably had access to this information as the compiler, Dr Thuram, was his former medical superintendent at the Wiltshire County asylum. Thuram had worked at the York Retreat.

[90] ibid., p. 31.

[91] ibid., p. 30.

concerns for better off patients may have been interpreted differently by those concerned with asylum finances.

Reporting to the Commissioners in Lunacy in 1854 on his experience at the Wiltshire and Norfolk asylums, Foote stated, 'I have never seen mechanical restraint produce any beneficial effect . . . but have seen many cases greatly relieved by the removal of restraint'.[92] He believed that patients generally benefited from association under supervision but that a few required seclusion measures. At the NLA restraint measures were used on four occasions that year, three times to keep patients' dressings applied and once to restrain a suicidal patient. The use of a cold shower bath as means of medical treatment 'in cases of maniacal excitement' was first noted in 1856 and repeated on seventeen occasions in 1857, though not on those aged over 50 years. Evidently 'the warm bath, with cold douches to the head at the same time' was also 'materially useful', as were unspecified 'sedatives, tonics and stimulants'. In contrast, the doctors reported their 'resort almost never to depletion [of food and] very seldom to nauseant and depressing remedies', though aperients were used.[93] As all were regarded as standard procedures by contemporaries, the avoidance of more extreme measures was a benefit but the soothing tone adopted was less than reassuring. Treatments generally were said to be:

> rather moral than medical – rather hygienic than therapeutic: the moral control and discipline of a well ordered asylum – its amusements of various kinds and especially its light and voluntary labour, with . . . judicious adaptation to various cases and temperaments . . . are some of the means of cure, of relief, or of solace, upon which we depend.'[94]

Deaths were often casually attributed to old age, general decay, general paralysis, or 'exhaustion after mania'. Of those who died in 1853, '13 of the patients were upwards of 70 years of age' and others died from 'exhaustion', though the medical staff felt that diarrhoea and low fever among women patients were 'to be ascribed . . . to the crowded state of this department'.[95] How such explanations connected with the post-mortem examinations carried out on 28 of the 36 patients who died in 1854 is unclear but Foote may have opted for more rigorous investigation after concern was expressed by the commissioners. Although new buildings were added by 1860, 'as in the last three years the constant excess of female lunatics over the male has been considerably increased', suggesting that the prospect of overcrowding was not that remote.[96] Visiting commissioners approved of the placement of a female

---

[92] CiL, 1854, Appendix G, Treatment, restraint, seclusion etc., p. 134, section 21.

[93] AR, 1856, MO, p. 6; 1857, p. 7

[94] ibid., p. 6.

[95] CiL, 10 May 1853; AR, 1853, MO, p. 11.

[96] AR, 1860, Cttee, p. 3.

nurse in the male infirmary ward, but the infirmary was under particular pressure from the 20 or so patients taking medicines, those suffering from general paralysis and the elderly and feeble, a majority of whom were women. However, over one-third of deaths in 1860 occurred among newly admitted infirm patients and, with some feeling, the NLA staff exonerated themselves and criticised poor law medical officers for their delay.

> Debility from age or illness of insane persons imposes upon them some responsibility in ordering their removal . . . especially the occurrence of maniacal delirium toward the close of life, from phthisis or other exhausting disease, since it is obvious that no treatment can avail in such cases.[97]

This assessment pointed to a further role for the asylum, effectively as a hospice and provider of geriatric care, which required appropriate medical management and nursing and which was to become increasingly important. It also contradicted previous reminders from commissioners and justices that medical officers should 'at all times and more especial when the asylum was entirely or nearly full, promote the exchange of harmless chronic patients for patients whose case may be recent and supposed to be curable, or who shall be reported as dangerous'.[98] This confirmed a continuing, uneasy relationship between the asylum, as a place of cure, containment or relief for the dying, and the workhouse or poor law outdoor relief, still seen as suitable for the 'harmless chronic'. However, it also indicated that asylum medical officers were seeking to extend their management over the latter category of patients.

The 1853 medical report suggests that efforts were concentrated upon 88 new admissions, one-fifth of them readmissions, who were felt to have the greatest chances of recovery. Some 300 patients remained at the year end, one half of them affected by mania, one quarter by dementia, with one-sixth suffering from melancholia and almost one-twelfth from congenital idiocy or imbecility. Refining this broad classification, 30 of the patients were epileptic, 20 were affected by general paralysis and 10 were described as suicidal.[99] By 1860 the number of admissions had risen to 123, one quarter of whom were readmissions, confirming the turnover of patients at the asylum. The classification of illnesses was much the same, suggesting hard lives and additional stresses placed upon women. Poverty and debility were cited in one-third of cases and fever, old age, uterine disorders, 'change of life' and loss of friends were frequently mentioned, along with hereditary or congenital defect and intemperance. Most men were labourers or unemployed, with a few shoemakers and smiths; the women were largely described as the wives,

---

[97] ibid., p. 4.
[98] AR, 1855, Cttee, p. 3.
[99] AR, 1854, MO, p. 13.

widows or daughters of labourers, or as servants, seamstresses, housekeepers and charwomen.[100] Nearly half the new admissions could read and write, with a further 30 per cent able to read, and three-quarters of those 'with no education' were women.[101] Just over two-thirds of the 340 asylum patients at the close of 1860 had been there for more than two years and 99 of these for more than a decade.

Probation and discharge

Subject to some change in the gender balance, the proportion of newly admitted patients who were discharged was maintained during the 1830s and 1840s (see Table 3.3) and each year roughly one NLA patient in six was being released alive.

Table 3.3 'Getting out of the asylum', 1830–60

	Admissions			% discharged		
	Total	M	F	Total	M	F
1830–39	52	26	26	45	40	50
1840–49	72	33	39	44	45	42
1850–59	90	40	50	41.5*	41.3*	41.6*

Note: Asterisked numbers in the 1850s refer to patients discharged 'recovered'.

In 1850 the asylum was among the first to differentiate between 'recovered' and 'discharged' patients. This distinction was always problematic and subject to readmissions, but it usually signified a judgement made by the medical staff. It assumed increasing importance after legislation in 1853 amended the 1845 Act to allow the probationary discharge of patients.[102] It is noticeable that, with the asylum experiencing some overcrowding, its new resident medical officer, Dr Edward Casson, responded so positively. He discharged the equivalent of 60 per cent of new admissions in 1854, these including probationary patients, eleven of whom recovered, as well as thirteen others 'relieved' and two 'not improved'.

---

[100] These descriptions covered more than 75 per cent of new admissions. AR, 1860, Supt., p. 9.

[101] ibid., p. 9. Forty-eight new patients were single, 59 married and 16 were widowed women.

[102] The Lunatic Asylums Act, 1853, 16 & 17 Vict. c. 97 stipulated greater attention to medical presentation and reporting of the factors indicating insanity and clauses 16 and 17 dealt with probation.

The local justices approved of probation and saw virtues 'in the self control imposed upon the patient by the knowledge that he may at any time be compelled to return'.[103] They supported the experiment with an allowance, 'more liberal than the parochial, which the Committee of Visitors have ordered for a few weeks where it was deemed expedient'.[104] This was seen as a progressive measure, 'of essential service by diminishing, at a time most important to the mental health of the patient, the pressure of poverty ... allowing a gradual return to dependence upon his labour'.[105] Despite the focus upon work, grants were later provided for probationers whose poor bodily health 'prevents them undertaking any hard work'.[106] Initial results appeared successful, with eight of the first probationers recorded as 'cured' the following year, but numbers then fell off. Although five to eight probationers were discharged annually in the late 1850s, eighteen in total were readmitted, suggesting only qualified success.[107] Similarly with the provision of care: the justices were cautioned 'by consideration of the unfitness of most union houses ... for the reception of patients' and fears that some relatives could not provide 'sufficient means of surveillance and protection'.[108]

However, probation and discharge were still considered, despite problems with local poor law authorities. In Elizabeth P—'s case,

the overseer ... stated that he could only convey her to the Union house, and the Committee being of the opinion that it would be better for her to be with her friends a short time, discharged her upon probation for 5 weeks with a weekly allowance of 5 shillings and an enquiry to be made whether the Friends would receive her upon these terms'.[109]

James D— was discharged to the Erpingham Union on 30 August but was returned on 3 September, the Guardians protesting over their costs incurred and the 'want of judgement' shown at the asylum. Its medical officers responded that D— had not recently displayed signs of mental excitement, though there was always the possibility of relapse, and that 'he has regularly been at shoemaking since his return to the Asylum and is quite harmless and tractable'.[110] Either his discharge was premature, or unsettling, but he evidently did not wish to leave. In contrast, William G—, the overseer for Mutford and Lothingland Union, had his son returned from the NLA as the

---

[103] AR, 1854, Cttee, p. 2.

[104] ibid., p. 2.

[105] AR, 1856, Cttee, p. 4. Grants were given equally to men and women.

[106] Superintendent's Journal, 27 Aug. 1861. Owen made the request on behalf of two probationers; three others were 'fit to remain at large'.

[107] AR, 1859, MO, p. 6.

[108] AR, 1860, Cttee, p. 4.

[109] CVIS, 27 Dec. 1859.

[110] ibid., 27 Sept. 1859.

boy 'is more imbecile than dangerous' and his father 'undertook that he should come to no harm'.[111] However, no one wanted responsibility for Harriet K—, a convict discharged on probation as 'sane' to the Litcham overseer who, armed with medical certification, promptly demanded that she was re-committed.[112] The uncertainties surrounding mental illness and patient discharge were of little consequence to the Depwade Union guardians, who had books to keep and accounts to balance. They simply requested a list of chargeable patients and a clear statement in each case 'whether the malady is likely to be permanent'.[113]

Nevertheless, the continuing discharge of patients confirms that the asylum was more than an accumulator of inmates, 'warehousing the mad', and individual cases indicate the importance of caring relatives and some sensitivity on the part of the justices. In October 1859, for example, Eliza D— was discharged, John S— was to be 'delivered to the care of his wife' and Susannah B—'s father was asked 'to come and fetch her'.[114] Similarly with Sarah K—, 'quiet and of feeble mind, discharged on the application of her husband', although Mary F—'s husband was informed that she was not fit to be discharged at present. The condition of Anne C—, who had a baby in November 1859, caused the matron some concern, though the medical officer 'did not consider it desirable to remove the child from the mother's charge . . . for the present, every caution being taken to prevent danger'.[115] However, her discharge 'which has commonly been found admissible in like cases' was not allowed.[116] One further feature concerned the role of the commissioners in encouraging and identifying suitable individuals for release, as in 1861 when 'Mr Casson accompanied us . . . and we pointed out to him . . . such patients as appeared to us to be improving, and in which there is reasonable hope of early discharge'.[117]

From the early 1850s increased attention was paid to nutrition and the liberal use of spirits as tonics. This complemented work therapy, but also views that the insane required a better than 'normal' diet to combat asthenia, the diminution of vital power and bodily function. 'Depletion', the withholding of some food as punishment, was now officially frowned upon. Moreover, the medical officers pronounced: 'we entirely object to the idea that persons who vegetate in the wards should have only just enough food to

[111]   ibid., 19 March 1862.
[112]   ibid., 23 July 1860.
[113]   Cited in CVIS, 19 March 1862. The committee replied that NLA medical officers decided upon individual patients 'as and when the question of release or recovery arises'.
[114]   ibid., 25 Oct. 1859.
[115]   ibid., 29 Nov. 1859.
[116]   AR, 1860, Cttee, p. 4. In this case the baby stayed with its mother at NLA until it could be weaned.
[117]   CiL, 20 April 1861.

keep themselves alive.'[118] Officially, allowance was made for the individual needs of patients, but how this was achieved in asylum conditions was not explained. Much depended upon the asylum staff, though previous difficulties in ensuring that patients received their share of available food (noted in Chapter 2) were not encouraging.

A revised dietary, compiled by the medical officers in response to requests from the commissioners and Dr Foote, increased the patients' meat allowance by one-third.[119] Male patients breakfasted upon a substantial if monotonous 1.5 pints of oatmeal milk broth, half of which was new milk, and 6oz of bread. Women had 5oz of bread with butter and three-quarters of a pint of tea. Supper consisted of 6oz bread and 2oz of cheese with a half-pint of beer for men, but women were restricted to tea, bread and butter. Some limited variety came with the midday meal, the same for all patients. On three days this was based upon 4oz of meat and 12oz vegetables, wholly or mainly potatoes, with bread and a half-pint of beer. On the remaining days 10.5oz of meat pie or meat dumplings was served with 12oz of vegetables, the quantity of meat specified as 2.5oz without bone. Additional bread, cheese and beer were provided at breaks for outdoor workers, artisan and laundry patients. Main meals were supplemented by 'a considerable variety of vegetables introduced' from 1859, reflecting the successes of the asylum farm and requests by the medical officers.[120] Although its variety may have been exaggerated, the four shillings allowed for food per patient per week was double that reckoned to be available to Norfolk farm labourers and their families.[121]

Responses, improvements and crises

Through the years of Owen's superintendence the local justices were usually responsive and often positive in their relations with external authorities. As spending on patients and weekly charges rose to national average levels, the justices no longer sought to justify the asylum in terms of cheapness. They generally took the commissioners' criticisms to heart, though remedial measures were sometimes delayed, and tactfully maintained the position of the asylum against the economy-minded approach of poor law guardians,

---

[118] AR, 1853, MO, p. 22. Very occasionally some patients had food withdrawn, in James Arthur Scott's case, 'for being fat and short-necked'. Case Notes, SAH 261, July 1856.

[119] The asylum was supplied with 2,214 stones of butcher's meat in 1852 and 3,410 stones in 1853, according to G. Foote, cited in 'Misgovernment at the Norfolk County Asylum', *The Asylum Journal*, 7, 15 Aug. 1854, pp. 99–102, 101.

[120] AR, 1854, 'Dietary for patients'; AR, 1859, MO, p. 4. 'Meat' was usually mutton or beef, without bone. The recipe for asylum tea, was 1oz tea, 4oz sugar, 0.75 pint milk and 5.25 pints water.

[121] Digby, *Pauper Palaces*, p. 23.

even though some justices were themselves guardians. The outstanding area of criticism, by the *Asylum Journal*, concerned the asylum's alleged neglect of medical viewpoints and, in particular, the absence of a qualified medical superintendent, although this issue was also resolved by the end of 1861.

Was the NLA so badly out of step with professional views and did this have dire consequences for its patients? Medical explanations of madness in terms of stress, imbalances and overindulgence, which were often applied to wealthy patients, were applied much less frequently to the pauper inmates of county asylums and workhouses. The asylum regimen, the treatment of physical symptoms, links between physical and mental illness and a medical contribution in moral management, often using work therapy, were all emphasised by doctors nationally in justification of their own role. Such arguments were made by the NLA visiting doctors and resident surgeons well before Dr Foote secured his appointment in 1852. His optimistic assessment of the chances of therapy and cure, predicated upon earlier admissions, a reforming regime and full scope for his proposals, was not atypical. Sedation was used, but other invasive measures, such as nauseants and cold shower baths, were not routine and the claimed recovery rates at the NLA exceeded those nationally.[122] When faced with rising patient numbers and the implausibility of generalised cure, asylum doctors offered explanations which focused upon hereditary, helpless or infirm cases and then claimed their medical management as the best option in the most appropriate environment.[123] These arguments were also heard at the NLA before 1861. However, the *Asylum Journal*, while claiming to act 'in no spirit of partizanship', linked the asylum's alleged failings to the absence of a medical superintendent, even though its improvements were acknowledged.[124]

One issue concerned the resignation of Dr Foote in 1854. He was a zealous reformer at a pace too rapid for the local justices. He also believed that his medical qualifications entitled him to be disdainful towards Owen, the superintendent, and the matron and he had antagonised some of the asylum staff. A crisis over the control of patients, notably in the women's infirmary, resulted in allegations and counter-allegations of irregularity and improper behaviour and led the justices to request Foote's resignation.[125] A greater

---

[122] For medications, see Chapter 4.

[123] J. Andrews, 'Notes on mental health care and prophylaxis in late 19th century Britain' in J. Andrews, H. Bartlett and J. Stewart, *Health Care Discussion Papers*, 1, Oxford Brookes University, 1998, p. 18.

[124] The *Asylum Journal*, 15 Aug. 1854, p. 101. It explained the appointment of a medical superintendent at Bedford: (the justices) 'have reconsidered the conditions of this appointment. They advertised for candidates, offering the paltry sum of £100 per annum. They have elected a gentleman at a salary of £300 per annum, with board, etc.'. ibid., p. 102.

[125] Foote's account appeared in the *Asylum Journal*, 7, 15 Aug. 1854, pp. 103–4. The Journal endorsed Foote, though he was 'overzealous', and blamed Norfolk justices for their failure to appoint a medical superintendent.

crisis concerned the conduct of Dr Edward Casson, his replacement as medical officer. Casson was viewed as a suitable appointment and, after five satisfactory years, his salary was raised from £125 to £150 in 1860.[126] Meanwhile, Owen became subject to recurring illness and retired with superannuation of two-thirds salary in May 1861, Mrs Owen remaining as matron. The justices finally adopted the national practice of appointing a medical superintendent and Casson, then aged 33, was offered the post at an annual salary of £400 minus £150 for board and lodging, with Dr George Mackenzie Bacon appointed as his assistant.

Yet there was to be no Casson regime. On 27 July Casson was requested to resign, 'having shown himself unfit to fulfil the duties of the office', and he complied three days later.[127] Whatever had occasioned this crisis – there are no details or even hints in minute books or published reports – it represented a personal catastrophe for Casson. He committed suicide, taking prussic acid on 4 August, the coroner recording that he 'destroyed himself . . . being of unsound mind at the time'.[128] The justices decided that further comment was 'unnecessary as it would be painful to make any observations on the lamentable circumstances attending the death of the late Mr Casson'.[129] Mackenzie Bacon briefly acted as medical superintendent while the post was advertised in *The Times*, *Medical Times* and the local press. He was one of five shortlisted candidates from 26 applicants but only one of the nine justices supported him. The remainder plumped for William C. Hills, resident medical officer at the Kent County asylum for the past seven years.[130] An additional medical officer was appointed as junior assistant to Hills and Mackenzie Bacon, with visiting surgeon G.W. Firth retained in a consulting capacity once Hills took up his post in November 1861.

By then new buildings and conversion work had considerably improved the asylum environment. All wards were now self-contained for day and night, with water closets and lavatories, baths and washrooms. The older buildings featured enlarged windows and improved access to the airing courts, wooden floors replaced stone flags in 'nearly all' dormitories and the new rooms and corridors were 'light, airy and perfectly dry'.[131] With the new laundry, bedding and clothing could be washed, dried and made available within a few hours, enabling more frequent changes to be made. There had been some improvement in the patients' diet and a new dining hall for all patients 'in health' was first used on Christmas Day 1859.

[126] Visiting surgeon G.W. Firth requested an increased honorarium in February 1860, paid until the medical superintendent was in post in November 1861.

[127] CVIS, 27 July 1861.

[128] ibid., 10 Aug. 1861.

[129] ibid., 24 Sept. 1861.

[130] ibid., 27 Aug. 1861. Bacon became Assistant RMO at £100 per annum.

[131] AR, 1859, Supt, p. 2.

The asylum more closely resembled a managed estate, with a multiplicity of functions which reflected the diversity of its patients and their perceived needs, moves toward greater self-sufficiency and relations with external authorities. Inmates who were deemed capable of work were expected to do so: work therapy was a broad and expandable concept, embracing political economy and stretching towards self-sufficiency. It reduced staffing and maintenance costs and was inequitably rewarded with the minor comforts or treats which enhanced a dull institutional life. Yet for many patients work was a link with the past, an element of 'normality' in a greatly changed existence which, for a few, pointed to another future beyond the asylum. If asylum life was hard and controlled, the outside world offered few agreeable alternatives to work for the poor and fewer still for the insane, dependent, or unmanageable poor.

A therapeutic regime focused mainly upon newly admitted patients, with sufficient numbers regarded as recovered or placed on probation to suggest more returns from the asylum than is conventionally acknowledged.[132] Some patients were discharged 'not improved', if they could be supported by family or friends or managed elsewhere, and workhouses were not always considered a suitable environment. Readmissions indicate that these measures were not necessarily successful, but the effort does not suggest a wholly repressive regime. Many patients remained because they could not look after themselves physically or in socially acceptable ways and no other care was available. These included the aged, infirm and debilitated, those suffering from forms of breakdown or with congenital defects, as well as those considered potentially dangerous. Their steadily accumulating numbers suggest the asylum as a place of last resort or hospice not simply of custody or containment. Asylum doctors saw them as grist to the professional mill but, certainly at the NLA, medical staff could not impose this agenda, given the role of commissioners, justices and poor law authorities.

Responding to the commissioners' promptings, the justices were advised by medical staff. Some were also poor law guardians and collectively the committee still operated with an eye to poor law authorities and in awareness of the relative costs of poor law and asylum provision.[133] But they determined the timing and extent of change within the asylum and, as magistrates, they

---

[132] J. Walton, 'Casting out and bringing back in Victorian England: pauper lunatics 1840–70' in W.F. Bynum, R. Porter and M. Shepherd (eds), *The Anatomy of Madness*, Vol. 2, Tavistock, London, 1985, pp. 132–46. Concerning 'bringing back'; 'there was very little of it . . . a disastrous failure for the moral treatment system', p. 142.

[133] Compare with Scull's view that the lunacy commissioners eroded local regulation: the justices still had to consider the guardians and ratepayers and central regulation had further to go. B. Forsythe, J. Melling and R. Adair, 'Politics of lunacy: central state regulation and the Devon Pauper Lunatic Asylum 1845–1914' in J. Melling and B. Forsythe (eds) *Insanity, Institutions and Society 1800–1914*, Routledge, London, 1999, pp. 68–92.

were also committed to maintaining order outside it. They readily embraced reforms such as work therapy, discharge 'not improved' and probation for reasons of their own. The part-reclamation of patients through work or probation had moral dimensions, strongly endorsed by the established political elite and poor law guardians, and economic significance: support from families or friends was critical to maintaining discharged patients at reduced cost. An early enthusiasm for probation coincided with considerable overcrowding and calculations that cash allowances for probationers were less than charges for patients, particularly outcounty 'boarders', may have featured. Any spare capacity after the asylum was extended was viewed similarly: offers were already being made to other authorities responsible for the insane and it may be more than coincidental that asylum capacity by 1860 matched exactly estimates made for the total Norfolk county insane in the early 1840s. Nevertheless, the amount of patient mobility through discharge procedures and, if necessary, readmission suggests more to the asylum regime than incarceration and physical control.[134]

The inspection and regulation of asylums also offers one illustration of relations between central and local authorities in a supposed age of laissez-faire. Variations in the stance taken by the lunacy commissioners might reflect the seriousness of a problem or the vigour of a particular individual. Commissioners disapproved and regretted defects, they exhorted and cajoled over improvements, which were then publicly endorsed or praised, but they could not enforce changes except by invoking the Secretary of State.[135] Their first visits left the local justices in little doubt on non-restraint or the need of a resident medical officer, which became a legal requirement in 1845. With these objectives attained, the commissioners then focused upon staffing levels, the patients' bedding and effects in the early 1850s. Whether they could always 'examine every patient' is questionable: at times their reports were bland and, on one occasion, over-congratulatory. Within months of Hills' appointment, the commissioners praised 'the excellent condition and management of this Asylum which, under the management of Dr Hills, has evidently improved in many respects and is now in a state of great efficiency'.[136] This verdict reflected real progress but overstated the case; it diminished the achievements of the Owen regime and understated continued shortcomings, even as Hills began to identify and address these.

---

[134] Scull understates 'bringing back' but Wright possibly overstates it, not allowing sufficiently for temporary probation, readmission and the possible recycling of certain patients (e.g. with drink-related illnesses).

[135] Eighth Report of the Commissioners in Lunacy to the Lord Chancellor, 1854, recorded that the Norwich Corporation had been reported since 'they persist in neglecting to make fit provision for their Pauper Lunatics', pp. 21–3.

[136] AR, 1862, CiL, p. 6.

4

A medical superintendent, expansion and reform, 1861–87

William Hills was 33 years old when he became medical superintendent at Norfolk Lunatic Asylum on 17 October 1861 and he completed his working life there, retiring early in 1887. He had obtained his M.D. at Aberdeen and held membership of the Royal College of Surgeons and the Association of Asylum Medical Officers. Given the context of his appointment, the temptation to associate Hills' regime with reform and 'medicalisation' at the asylum is strong. Evidence might include: a greater emphasis upon treatments, drugs and medicines; the public presentation of medical explanations of recovery, sickness or death; a more caring and therapeutic approach to patients by attendants and nurses; and revised concepts of management and of the political economy of the institution. Such changes can be exaggerated. Although Hills made an active beginning, the lunacy commissioners probably overstated improvements in their endorsement of his appointment. Between 1861 and 1887 patient numbers doubled, from 370 to over 730, pressuring the asylum fabric and facilities. Increasing acceptance of the asylum as an appropriate place of care, sometimes in the absence of suitable alternatives, also reflected further medical claims made on behalf of asylum therapies. Yet a sense of lost momentum later surrounded Hills' retirement when, in turn, high hopes were transferred to his successor.

Meanwhile, continuity was provided in the stable membership of the committee of visiting justices. It still met monthly, though the variable timing of weekly visits, suiting the justices' personal convenience, made inspections less predictable. The committee also retained formal control over the discharge of patients, and much routine continuity was embodied in long-serving members of staff, not least the clerk to the justices, William Girling. More pertinently, the challenge of medicalisation to conventions and to contemporary authority may be questioned. Hills also brought to the NLA a heightened sense of economy, expressed in the desire to save costs and utilise patients' skills. This was confirmed in his interpretation of work therapy, changes to the patients' dietary and promotion of an auxiliary asylum as an efficiency aid. He linked the use of probation for patients with a proactive stance on the admission of boarders, acknowledging openly systems of cross-subsidy and savings to Norfolk ratepayers. Though Hills shared with the lunacy commissioners hopes of further improvements, notably in the care of 'idiots' and in nursing standards, he did not press the committee on such matters.

Hills' first proposals concerned hygiene and overcrowding and he faced immediate difficulties with escape attempts and a smallpox outbreak. In October 1861 the asylum contained over 390 patients and he informed the justices: 'the crowded state of the Asylum generally requires the urgent consideration of the Committee . . . to meet the emergency I am compelled to have beds made up on the floor of the associated rooms.'[1] A month later he produced a revised laundry list for the asylum, 'the present plan being very unsatisfactory', having also dismissed one 'inefficient' laundress. His thoroughness was indicated in letters to the matron at Colney Hatch asylum concerning Smith's 'cleansing powder' and 'washing powder' as replacements for soda and soap.[2] This hygiene campaign soon refocused upon the formidable combination of wooden beds, straw mattresses and fleas in the crowded male ward 4. Gas lighting was to be extended, beginning with bathrooms and stairways. Following an escape attempt, Hills ensured that the responsible attendant 'should pay a portion of the expenses incurred . . . in the hope that it may act as a wholesome check to him and others'.[3] Music was to feature more prominently and Hills planned an attendants' band to offer 'treats to patients' more economically than outside entertainers.

Overcrowding and new accommodation

Hills also requested new isolation rooms for infectious disease cases or 'excitable' patients who required seclusion. Temporary expedients sufficed until buildings flanking the main entrance and incorporating six rooms for patients and supervisory accommodation were added in 1862.[4] In a portentous experiment, he reserved a detached cottage for nine women patients, in the charge of an ex-workhouse inmate, previously 'quite unmanageable in the Union'.[5] A steady refurbishment programme introduced smaller ceramic baths and finally enabled each woman patient to have a 'fresh' bath. All rooms were papered or painted and blinds or shades fitted by 1865, with wooden flooring laid in all day rooms and dormitories by 1877. The lunacy commissioners generally found the wards 'clean, well-ventilated and cheerful' and were mostly satisfied with the patients' bedding, sets of clothing, means

---

[1] Medical Superintendent's Journal (MS Journal), 1861–78, SAH 131, 29 Oct. 1861.
[2] ibid., 23 May 1862.
[3] ibid., 26 Nov. 1861. Two patients escaped in Sept. 1861. One was returned by the police, the other climbed the wall, 'descended into the road . . . and soon met with the Reverend Cole who, with his usual politeness, offered the runaway a seat in his jig and speedily conducted him back to the asylum'. MS Journal, 24 Sept. 1861.
[4] Designed by the new County Surveyor, R.M. Phipson. Plans are at Drayton Old Lodge.
[5] Annual Reports (AR) SAH 28, 1844–76, 1865, Medical Superintendent (MS), p. 6. As provision for women patients improved, the cottage was later used by four male patients.

for daily washing and 'the supply of brushes and combs'.[6] Safety arrangements benefited from police patrols 'on duty nightly outside the building, to give an alarm, in event of fire' and the addition of a surrounding water main, with hydrants 'placed at intervals outside the Asylum, so that water can be thrown on every part of it'.[7] Each ward later had one window cut down to floor level for use as an emergency exit.

Until the 1860s the asylum fabric was roughly symmetrical, with equal numbers of male and female wards, but bed shortages were exacerbated by the low ceilings of many older wards, and insufficient cubic space per patient. Lunacy commissioners in 1868 'noticed hardly a dormitory today on the female side that had not too many beds . . . even the wards built for infectious cases . . . were filled with ordinary patients'.[8] With room for 230 women patients there were 227 residents on average, even after transfers to Norwich city asylum. Hills again acknowledged, 'we have been reluctantly compelled to make beds intended for one case accommodate two, whilst others have slept on the floor of an associated room'.[9] New wards for 52 patients, built on the pavilion plan and connected to the women's wing by a single corridor, were completed in September 1869 for roughly £4,000. They offered a day room, bathrooms and dressing room, fifteen single bedrooms, dormitories and attendants rooms. Furniture was 'of polished birch . . . of a superior kind' and, as elsewhere in the women's wing, there were white counterpanes and curtains, with coloured paintwork and wallpaper and 'homely domestic' fittings, all of which the lunacy commissioners found 'difficult to praise too highly'.[10]

Yet women patients were again temporarily placed with the Ipswich Borough and Northampton asylums in 1871 and 1874. Hills wanted more wards, facilities and space not least because 'air for 100 cannot any more than food be made to serve a larger number'. He proposed additional buildings for quiet and chronic patients, thereby 'leaving the existing building for the more recent and excitable cases'.[11] The lunacy commissioners declared that fifty more beds were 'absolutely necessary' but insisted on no further additions on the asylum site.[12] Another complication arose from legislation that they had instigated in 1874. This promoted the care of insane paupers in county asylums by offering grants of four shillings per person per week, thereby subsidising asylum accommodation. It duly encouraged the transfer of

---

[6] AR, 1863, MS, p. 7; 1869, MS, p. 10; 1877, CiL, 15 Feb. 1877, p. 8.
[7] AR, 1874, CiL, 9 July 1874. In 1886 Justice R.B. Longe designed a mobile ladder to evacuate first-floor wards.
[8] AR, 1868, CiL 23 Oct., p. 8.
[9] AR, 1868, MS, p. 6.
[10] R.M. Phipson's plans for ward 5 are at Drayton Old Lodge. See also AR, 1870, CiL, p. 6.
[11] AR, 1872, MS, pp. 6–7.
[12] Reports of Commissioners in Lunacy (CiL) 1844–1925, SAH 141, 24 March 1873.

suitable patients to asylums, but disadvantaged recovering asylum patients or candidates for probation. As the commissioners acknowledged, 'since the capitation grant now allowed for the maintenance of patients in Asylums, the Guardians generally decline to receive them back, however harmless.'[13]

Given this additional contribution to overcrowding at the NLA, the commissioners offered a compromise, encouraging local justices to provide a 'neighbourhood workhouse' for 200 imbecile and chronic patients, to be run as a second county asylum, if sufficient space for airing courts was available. The justices purchased 15 acres of land, allowing Hills to demonstrate his theory that, for such patients, 'moral treatment, supervision, and general care and attention . . . can nowhere be so well carried out as in Institutions specially adapted for the Insane.'[14]

Plans for the annexe, a separate auxiliary asylum several hundred yards to the north of the main buildings on the site of a cricket field, were announced in 1876. The buildings were to be of 'somewhat plain, simple and comparatively cheap construction', later described as 'a sort of go-between the Asylum and the Workhouse'.[15] Designed by the architects Cornish and Gaymer, they were modelled on Metropolitan Asylums Board institutions at Leavesden and Caterham. They comprised a two-storey 'H' shape with large and rather barn-like male and female wards linked, or rather separated, by an administrative cross-section, behind which lay a single storey complex of kitchens and staff rooms. Costing £33,920, virtually the same as the 'main' buildings of 1814, they accommodated 250 patients, two and a half times the original capacity. 'Chronic lunatics, imbeciles and idiots' were placed under the care of Hills' assistant, who became resident medical officer, a head female attendant and a relatively modest staff of attendants and nurses. Some £3,000 was allocated for new furnishings and building funds were raised through a special quarterly rate.[16] Construction, delayed in the hard winter of 1878–9, took three years, during which ten women patients were transferred to the Ipswich Borough Asylum and 23 men were temporarily accommodated in the NLA's former craft shops.[17] Eighty beds were available by March 1879 and 155 patients were already resident in the 'partly furnished' auxiliary buildings a year later.

Clearly, the justices hoped not simply to address overcrowding but to rehouse some asylum patients and attract new ones from workhouses at reduced cost and on price-competitive terms. The comparatively cheap

[13] ibid., 14 July 1876.

[14] AR, 1875, MS, p. 4.

[15] D. Thomson, 'Norfolk County Asylum', *Eastern Daily Press*, 18 June 1903 (see Chapter 5).

[16] This levy produced £13,950 from 1879–82: outstanding amounts and Local Government Board support are unclear.

[17] Annual Reports 1877–86, SAH 29, 1879, MS, p. 4.

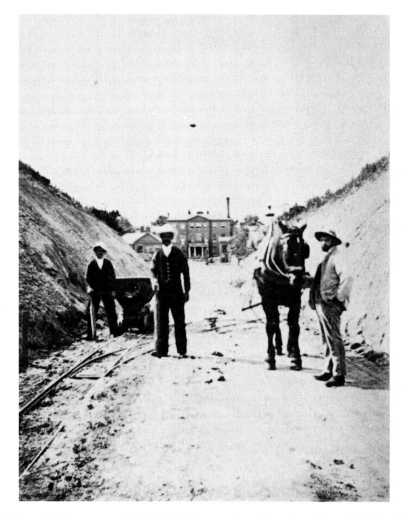

Figure 4.1 Annexe road c. 1876, looking south to the main asylum (Middleton)

standards of accommodation, less intensive nursing, a 'reduced (though sufficient) dietary', and the importance of state subsidies were openly acknowledged. Thus,

> we do not expect that the Guardians will . . . take any steps towards maintaining the lunatic paupers of the quiet and harmless class out of the Asylum as long as they can get them cared for at 4s 2d per head per week, which is the cost at present when the 4s weekly allowance is taken into account.[18]

---

[18] ibid., 1880, CiL, p. 7. P. Bartlett, *The Poor Law of Lunacy*, Leicester University Press,

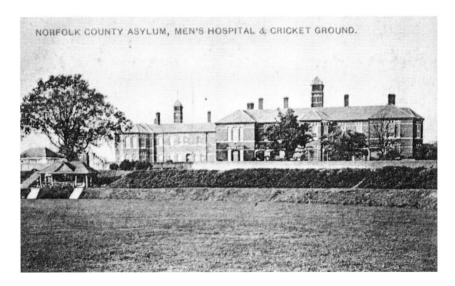

NORFOLK COUNTY ASYLUM, MEN'S HOSPITAL & CRICKET GROUND.

Figure 4.2 Men's asylum c. 1901: 1880 buildings and new wards on left (Roberts)

Moreover, the delineation of auxiliary asylum facilities suggests a very early provincial and proto-public sector form of the 'Idiot Asylums', few of which had yet been constructed.[19] NLA admissions increased, from an 1875–9 annual average of 144 to 182 for the period 1880–5. Consequently, the auxiliary asylum already contained 261 patients on 1 November 1884 and, with additional beds, its capacity was quickly raised to 280. Whether standards of care could be improved so readily is questionable: official ratios of one male attendant for every 25 male patients and one nurse for every 20 female patients deteriorated and these made no allowances for staff time off, absences or holidays.[20]

Patients and treatments

Hills' arrival at the asylum coincided with the beginning of an era of 'therapeutic pessimism'. Nationally, 'ideas about evolution, inheritance and natural selection invaded medical thought . . . and fuelled continuous debate about the relative importance of heredity and environment, mind and body; but . . . they did little to explain and much to obscure the nature of many

1999, does not cover the importance of this subsidy of asylum accommodation in discussion on the placing of pauper lunatics.
[19] see M. Jackson, *The Borderland of Imbecility*, Manchester University Press, 2000, p. 23 and M. Thomson, *The Problem of Mental Deficiency*, Clarendon, Oxford, 1998.
[20] ibid., 1884, CiL, 1 Nov., p. 7.

illnesses'.[21] His first report as medical superintendent, unlike those of earlier medical officers, was pessimistic in tone. It reflected doubts, most influentially expressed by Dr Henry Maudsley, concerning the treatment of insanity and mental deficiency.[22] Hills noted that almost one quarter of new NLA patients were aged over 60 years and he indicated that just 22 of those currently under treatment might recover. Thus:

> so large a proportion either from age or the nature of their disorder offer little if any prospect of recovery; and this increase of incurable patients must, of course, diminish the number of dismissals and tend gradually to a stagnation of the institution.[23]

Given this analysis, the further undermining of the asylum's therapeutic role by the admission of chronic or 'hopeless' cases became a recurring theme in Hills' reports. Medical superintendent or not, he had no control over the admissions process and, failing to stem the flow of 'inappropriate' cases, he later offered such patients reasonable standards of care, nursing and facilities in his proposal of the auxiliary asylum. Hills soon identified those patients whose 'only malady was age and its attendant feebleness of intellect' or those at the asylum because they were 'unmanageable at home or in the workhouse' as problem groups.[24] In his fifth year as medical superintendent he noted: 'as usual, many patients were brought to us in a state which precluded all hopes of their surviving more than a few months; and there were many aged persons as heretofore.' A decade later, 'the admissions, I am sorry to say, still consist of hopeless cases of dementia, imbecility and senility &c, &c, which occupy space and entail an outlay that might be more profitably employed'.[25]

Hills' concern was for the public reputation as well as the therapeutic record of the asylum. He stated publicly, after twelve patients had died within one month of their admission, 'how little care and discrimination were exercised on the part of the medical men who sent them . . . such carelessness tends to raise our death rate above its normal percentage and to bring undeserved discredit on the Asylum'.[26] Some patient transfers were truly scandalous: poor James P— died hours after his transfer from the Aylsham workhouse, emaciated, covered in bed sores and with a broken rib. The coroner, recording death from softening of the brain and exhaustion, added

[21] J. Harris, *Private Lives, Public Spirit: Britain 1870–1914*, Penguin, Harmondsworth, 1993, p. 57.

[22] Henry Maudsley (1835–1918) was an early exponent of hereditary features in 'degeneration' in the 1860s, adding a susceptibility to criminal influences to the many weaknesses of the 'defective'.

[23] AR, 1844–76, SAH 28, 1862, MS, p. 4.

[24] AR, 1863, MS, p. 3.

[25] AR, 1865, MS, p. 3; 1874, MS, p. 3.

[26] AR, 1879, MS, p. 4.

that 'a great error in judgement was committed in removing [the] deceased in an open cart and that he ought to have had some extra diet before the journey'.[27]

Diagnostic problems and an absence of alternative facilities featured in other 'inappropriate' NLA admissions. Hills remarked that some patients 'suffering from ordinary brain disease, pure and simple [were] fit objects for an Infirmary . . . many such cases are to be found in the hospitals of London and other large cities'.[28] Increasing numbers of 'idiot' children and juveniles were referred over the 1870s, probably in consequence of the growth of state education and growing professional interest in the 'weak-minded'.[29] In May 1877 Hills noted that 'two idiot boys, possessing a fair amount of intelligence, were admitted; these were certainly not cases for us, as they were capable of being educated to some extent and of being taught in time a trade'.[30] Two others, aged 7 and 10 years, arrived 'from Birmingham' in 1879 and the lunacy commissioners commented upon the presence of 'a large number of idiot lads who are not fitted for the wards of a lunatic asylum' in 1881.[31] Hills urged a combined effort from Norfolk and adjoining counties to provide 'special establishments', though this particular solution lay fifty years in the future (see Chapter 6). These evident sympathies were not extended to anyone who drank excessively or whose referral to the NLA arose more from 'the trouble he gives at a workhouse, or in his own house, than upon any other consideration'. It was fundamentally 'not right that such criminal patients should enjoy the benefit of an Asylum; and associate with inmates, who deserve our commiseration; their detention is a great mistake'.[32]

'On reviewing the so-called causes of insanity' in 1868, Hills concluded that; 'most common are intemperance, poverty, bodily disorders, family broils, and disease of the brain &c.'[33] His early reports emphasised links between debility and insanity; the possibility of successful outcomes, given early and proper treatment; the importance of work therapy; and problems associated with the recurrence of illness and readmission. Thus 'the malady almost invariably arises from debility' and he noted 'the general impression . . . that Insanity is incurable, as the disease frequently relapses'. A recovered and discharged patient could be subjected to 'a fresh attack of insanity by

[27] MS Journal, 1878–88, SAH 132, 5 April 1880.

[28] AR, 1878, MS, pp. 4–5.

[29] Over the late-nineteenth century 'idiocy' was increasingly differentiated from imbecility (congenital defects) and milder forms of 'weak-mindedness'. J. Saunders, 'Quarantining the weak-minded: psychiatric definitions of degeneracy and the late-Victorian asylum', in W.F. Bynum, R. Porter and M. Shepherd (eds), *The Anatomy of Madness*, Routledge, London, 1988, Vol. 3, pp. 273–95, 274.

[30] AR, 1877, MS, p. 6.

[31] MS Journal, 26 Oct. 1879; AR, 1881, CiL, p. 9.

[32] AR, 1868, MS, p. 4.

[33] ibid., p. 4.

exposure to its causes and become again an inmate of an Asylum'.[34] Under these circumstances readmission did not demonstrate the asylum's failure to cure: if general hospitals could be credited with 'curing' the same patient several times after bouts of bronchitis, why should asylums be condemned for achieving comparable results?

This reasoning was plausible but, in explaining positive outcomes, Hills revealed a preference for physical exercise and a work ethic as therapeutic measures and as templates for 'normal' behaviour. Thus, in 1866:

> the recoveries have been unusually numerous, viz. 56.93 per cent of those admitted! This . . . is a fresh demonstration of the importance and advantage of early treatment, and of the folly of delay . . . whereby their chance of recovery is lessened . . . the mental faculties become blunted through disease and the want of salutary exercise and excitement which occupation, wages and self-maintenance afford.[35]

Yet more than 22 per cent of admissions during the 1860s and 1870s were readmissions, suggesting that former patients experienced problems in obtaining a living, coping or complying with life outside the asylum. It also implied that some, for example men prone to major bouts of drinking, experienced the asylum as a slowly revolving door. Each time 'recovery' was acknowledged, rather in the manner of bronchitis cases in general hospitals. Explanations of this kind seem more convincing than Hills' assertion (not substantiated by asylum statistics, see Table 4.1) that greater recoveries among men were due 'partly to the great recuperative powers of the male sex'.[36]

A comparison of asylum admissions in two sample years, 1870–1 and 1885, suggests a much younger and more varied age profile than Hills' was apt to describe. Over one-third of new patients were aged 20–40 years and a similar proportion were aged 40–60 years. Less than one-third were more than 60 years old.[37] In almost one-third of the 1870–1 cases no prime cause of insanity was indicated but, among the remainder, there were two 'physical' for each 'moral' cause. Debility, epilepsy, senile decay, hereditary factors, male intemperance and 'puerperal' features affecting women were present in roughly equal proportions and there were two rape victims. Poverty, adverse domestic circumstances, or the death of a close relative were cited as the main 'moral' causes, with several instances of religious fervour, 'disappointment in love' and 'immorality'. Large proportions of the 1885 admissions were still triggered by 'unknown' features or were readmissions but almost one-fifth of

[34] AR, 1864, MS, pp. 3–4.

[35] AR, 1866, MS, p. 4.

[36] AR, 1871, MS, p. 4.

[37] Does this suggest general problems, for example agricultural unemployment or breakdown of a rural micro-economy (Scull's thesis) rather than the inability of families to deal with particular members, notably juveniles or aged relations?

those examined were now identified with hereditary or congenital defects, suggesting a new medical interest and possibly a convenient label.[38] Using those other great labels of insanity, over 70 patients suffered from forms of mania, 35 from melancholia and 10 from dementia. Whatever the changed medical conditions implied in this classification, the social backgrounds were familiar: half the men admitted were farm labourers and nearly two-thirds of the women were housewives, domestic servants or housekeepers.[39]

Hills' explanations of asylum mortality centred upon patients 'worn down by age and long standing cerebral disease' or arguments that 'the aged and feeble' were vulnerable 'to the most trifling disorder'.[40] One quarter of those who died in 1867 were aged 70 years or over, yet all bar four of the 29 patients who died in 1870 were less than 60 years old. Nor were their disorders 'trifling'. Shortly after Hills arrived at the NLA there was a smallpox outbreak. Five patients were isolated with two nurses 'specially obtained from Norwich' in hastily converted rooms in the boilerhouse. The three patients previously vaccinated survived their 'modified' infection but Augustine C— and Esther W— died.[41] Hills reported that all patients had been examined and monitored, 'and in every case where vaccination had been neglected and the patients willing, they were vaccinated, the same . . . with regard to the servants generally'.[42] The experience convinced Hills of the need for reception rooms as a precaution against infectious disease, though this approach was not developed during his period of office into the provision of admission centres for the wider observation of new patients.

In 1865 Hills reported an abnormally high number of 43 deaths with a brief public comment concerning his suspicion of typhoid fever. He did not refer to an earlier, private record:

> during a portion of the time the reservoir has been under repair we have experienced great inconvenience in being compelled to use the river water unfiltered, the impure state of the river during the hot weather made it very objectionable to drink.[43]

Although the quality of spring and well water was good, river water was still used for washing and the lunacy commissioners were not convinced that

---

[38] The 1871 Annual Report covered 154 admissions over 15 months, 1870–1: there were 135 admissions in 1885.

[39] AR, 1885, Classification of disorders, p. 17. Other males included several tradesmen, two farmers, a solicitor, a teacher and a vet. In addition to widows, a separate group of 'wives' had been married to a farmer, parson, publican or miller.

[40] AR, 1864, MS, p. 5; 1865, MS, p. 5.

[41] MS Journal 1861–78, SAH 131, 8 Jan.–22 Feb. 1862.

[42] ibid., 23 April 1862. Note the suggestion of choice in vaccination: Hills may have been sensitive to the strong anti-vaccination movement in Norwich.

[43] ibid., 14 July 1864.

separately marked taps represented a risk-free solution. Another typhoid outbreak in 1880, ascribed to sewer gas and the inadequate trapping of old drains during building work on the auxiliary asylum, may have had a simpler explanation.[44] Outbreaks of influenza or pneumonia, as in 1864, 1865, 1877 or 1883, were generally accompanied by comments that 'the weather was cold and damp and the invalids already depressed by diseases of the nervous system consequently fell an easy prey'.[45] Similarly, 'twelve deaths occurred from phthisis, a disease so frequently associated with insanity, and not an unfrequent cause of the mental disorder'.[46] Tuberculosis, the major killer disease of the nineteenth century, accounted for perhaps one-fifth of deaths at the asylum, where overcrowding and deficient cubic space per patient in older wards still featured. Outbreaks of erysipelas in both wings of the building were reported in 1875 and 1879 but various forms of 'paralysis', 'exhaustion/convulsions' and 'inflammation of the brain' ranked among the remaining frequent causes of death.

Although drugs featured in asylum treatments, evidence concerning their use or dosages is limited and the underlying rationale was often short-term control over the patient. Croton oil, a powerful purgative, was used to calm or distract excited patients, who were then given warm baths. Hills also reported that, in cases of mania, veratine (veratrum viride) was 'of great efficacy . . . in lowering temperature and pulse without producing any untoward or unpleasant symptoms'.[47] Curare was administered as a muscle relaxant in certain conditions of paralysis, though overdosing caused muscle paralysis. From 1870 chloral hydrate was given to those affected by 'nervous insomnia' or hysteria, sometimes combined with valerian, a sedative used also for 'neurotic conditions'. Henbane derivatives lowered the heart rate of otherwise violent or unmanageable patients, and hyoscyamine was also used for temporary pain relief. Digitalis, considered a heart tonic, also featured in treatments of diseases of the central nervous system, including general paralysis, delirium tremens and epilepsy. MacKenzie Bacon believed that 'the influence of the sexual organs . . . [was] . . . the great point to be considered' and expressed disappointment with results from bromide of potassium, 'though I have given the drug largely to all sorts of cases'.[48] Bromides of ammonium or sodium were also used for their analgesic properties, however,

---

[44] CiL, 15 Feb. 1877. Following the typhoid outbreak, the original drains were closed and trapped. AR 1881, MS p. 9. Lunacy commissioners specified taller ventilation pipes in the auxiliary asylum and filter plants replaced subsidence tanks to reduce problems with sewer gas. AR 1885, MS, p. 10.

[45] AR, 1877, MS, p. 4. The 1883 outbreak killed eight patients, several dogs and a cat, one indication of the asylum's pet population. AR, 1883, MS, p. 5.

[46] AR, 1877, MS, p. 4.

[47] AR, 1873, MS, p. 6.

[48] G. MacKenzie Bacon, 'On the treatment of epileptic insanity', *Practitioner*, 1869, 2, pp. 334–346, 337.

and Hills felt that bromide had produced 'a marked improvement in the temper and demeanour of the patients . . . the wards are quieter'.[49]

In the contemporary medical literature Henry Maudsley noted that 'opium undoubtedly occupies the foremost place' but warned against the use of drugs in cases where bodily disease was likely to be the cause of mental disorder.[50] Hills, emphasising the value of exercise and work therapy, may have followed the published advice of another early psychiatrist, G.H. Savage, and sedated patients 'as a means of controlling with the hope that, quiet being established, cure would follow.'[51] Too frequent or excessive sedation could prove disastrous; 'you have to deal with a tottering edifice, and severe measures may be rapidly destructive . . . I have seen excitement and violence . . . relieved more effectually by rum and milk than by morphine'.[52] Side-effects were also recognised: opium shared with chloral nitrate the limits of temporary relief and the dangers of addiction and loss of appetite, although cannabis tincture was prescribed at the NLA and 'its value is well known to asylum physicians'.[53]

Ellen B—, aged 19 years and 'low in spirits', was given iron tablets because she was not menstruating. When these caused headaches and diarrhoea, she was given opium, which was then associated with her mood swings and 'dietary disturbances'.[54] Jane S—, who suffered from bouts of mania associated with each menstruation was 'in this respect . . . now better in consequence of her taking t. Cannabis Ind.'[55] Cannabis was also used to treat headaches and to reduce 'restlessness' or shock among those who had been bereaved. It was also used for stomach ulcers, though bismuth was more frequently mentioned in their treatment and for ulcerative colitis. Zinc ointment was considered effective for a range of skin conditions, rather optimistically in cases of erysipelas. Spirits were seen as tonics and expenditure on them in 1860 dwarfed the £37 spent on all other drugs and medicines. Dispensary costs doubled by 1870 and had quadrupled by 1885 but this represented a fraction over one penny per patient per week in 1877, compared with 1.5 pence for wines and spirits.

Modest numbers of patients went on probation. Maria F— was released with a temporary weekly allowance of four shillings in November 1861. She was readmitted, but Hills later engaged her 'as a housemaid on a month's trial,

[49] AR, 1867, MS, p. 8.

[50] H. Maudsley, 'On opium in the treatment of insanity', *Practitioner*, 1869, 2, pp. 1–8, 7–8.

[51] G.H. Savage, 'The use of sedatives in insanity', *Practitioner*, 1886, 37, pp. 181–5, 181.

[52] ibid., pp. 182–3. Savage was then medical superintendent at the Bethel, London.

[53] Cannabis tincture was used as a relaxant. S. MacKenzie, 'The value of Indian hemp' in *British Medical Journal* 15 Jan. 1887, pp. 97–8; 'Indian hemp', ibid., 4 July 1891, p. 12.

[54] Case Books, 1861–5, SAH 263; E.B., 1861–6.

[55] ibid., J.S., 1862–72.

she is one of the patients who will be discharged today'.[56] The conduct of probationers was monitored: in the case of Mary A—, Hills 'received a very unfavourable report . . . consequently I deemed it necessary to send for her'.[57] Mary B— was still less fortunate: her discharge was cancelled after the asylum received information 'respecting her home, which is now much impoverished by the recent drunken habits of her husband'. There were also occasions, as in November 1884, when the discharge of a patient recommended by Hills and his staff was overruled as 'premature' by the lunacy commissioners.[58]

A brief review of patient case notes indicates the range of their experiences and treatments or measures adopted in the asylum. Margaret C—, affected by 'religious mania', sold the contents of the family home to raise money for the Free Church. Over four years her delusion that she was 'empowered to save the nation' turned to belief that she was 'sent here to undergo persecution for Christ's sake'. Her husband visited but 'she would not recognise him' and, in the belief that 'she was too wicked to live' she stabbed herself, refused food and had to be force fed. Soon afterwards she showed signs of TB and died at the age of 36. The 'eccentric' sisters Harriet and Margaret J— also pawned their furniture but equated their reduced circumstances with demonic possession and asked the local vicar to 'pray out' their cottage. In the asylum they were kept together in a double bedroom but reacted violently, believing the devil to be present, and refused food, thinking it was poisoned. When Margaret collapsed she was put on extra diet and porter: she gradually recovered and became 'industrious' and was discharged after one year. Harriet, meanwhile, 'pretends to be weak for the slightest exertion and feigns hysterics when interfered with; the could douche is now administered'. With better nourishment and her sister's recovery, however, she also improved, expressed a desire to leave and was discharged two months after Margaret.[59]

George C— was an unemployed shoemaker, deaf, drunk and debilitated, who came to the asylum via the police station and workhouse after attempting suicide 'by cramming food down his throat and by strangling'. Within a week he was working in the shoemaker's shop and a month later his 'depression has quite passed away giving place to cheerfulness and jollity'. Food and a working environment where his skills were valued were evidently all that he required and he was discharged 'recovered' after four months. William D—, an 18-year-old labourer, was more troublesome. 'A source of great annoyance to his neighbours on account of his drunken habits', he had become violent and was readmitted to the asylum. He settled and was 'anxious for his discharge' but when this was refused he became 'very excited and mischievous'. For a month he had spells in the padded room or was

---

[56] MS Journal, 26 Nov. 1861; 24 June 1862.
[57] ibid., 11 Jan. 1863.
[58] ibid., 31 July 1879; AR, 1884, CiL, 1 Nov., p. 10.
[59] Case Books, 1870–4, SAH 265; M.C., 1870–4, H.J. and M.J., 1870–1.

'packed' in tight sheets and he was variously given chloroform, bromide and hyoscyamus, measures discontinued as his excitement lessened. Having 'settled down again' he remained 'industrious' and 'rational' for five months, and was then discharged.[60]

Susannah P— was also successfully treated in a traditional manner. She was married with two children but had twice previously been admitted and was regarded as having hereditary predisposition. When one child died she was 'low-spirited', then violent and destructive. For two weeks after her admission in April 1870 she was repeatedly packed, as 'the efforts of three nurses are required to restrain her'. Morphia and then 30 grains of chloral daily were ineffective so she was twice blistered on the back. Whether this diversion or the passage of time was effective, medical staff felt that 'since the application of the blister her natural state of mind has returned. She now converses rationally and is free from all excitement, she sleeps well . . . and is clean in habits' and pronounced her recovery. Poor Sarah W— derived little benefit after she began to 'wander away from home' when she was 19 years old. Diagnosed 'manic', she constantly covered her face, cowered under tables and said only 'I want to go home'. Within two weeks she was 'in a semi-hysterical condition . . . placed in wet sheets [packed] but without any benefit'. She was then given the shower bath 'but instead of acting beneficially it terrified her . . . the treatment was discontinued; she now begs we will not kill her'. 'Owing to the earnest solicitations of her parents', she was discharged to their care after five months in the asylum and one month's probation.[61]

Other patients settled to an institutional life. John P—, aged 50, already had a brother in the NLA and a sister said to be deranged and was regarded as having hereditary predisposition to insanity. He underwent no treatments but was 'manageable and industrious' and 'of great service in attending to the wants of the feeble and paralytic'. Whenever his return home was suggested he responded, 'What have I done that I should be sent away?' After four years he was transferred to the chronic case book and acted as a ward helper in 'the private department'. Edward J— had spells in prisons and workhouses and was regarded as a 'congenital imbecile' on his admission in 1861. Dr MacKenzie Bacon, still much taken by phrenology, noted 'narrow head: his look sufficiently betokens his mental capacity'. Edward J— worked in the dining hall and as a ward helper, 'well and willingly so long as he is well-supplied with tobacco'. George F—, transferred with Edward J— from Docking workhouse, also had 'a badly shaped head' but was employed in the laundry and with the bricklayers for ten years, before he died from phthisis. William B—, 'of average size, with a large head', spent his adult life in the asylum, working on the farm and periodically being 'ordered to bed on a low

---

[60] ibid., G.C., 1870; W.D., 1870.
[61] ibid., S.P., 1870–1; S.W., 1870.

diet' for 'very disgusting habits'. He received very little medication until his transfer to the infirmary shortly before he died from heart disease in 1903.[62]

In contrast, Aaron D—, a 34-year-old 'idiot' whose mother could no longer care for him, had little time left. He soon 'improved, as he can be kept clean, he appears quite happy . . . gives very little trouble', but he developed a cough, deteriorated rapidly and he died within six months from phthisis. Like Margaret C—, he may have contracted his fatal illness within the asylum.[63] William G— was a particularly tragic figure. A 34-year-old carpenter, he was 'a large powerful man' but disappointed in love and in a state of 'acute melancholia'. His first eighteen months in the asylum were highlighted by escapes, recapture and conflicts with attendants but he also attempted suicide by throwing himself on to a fire, down stone staircases and hanging himself. Doctors admitted that 'he has suffered . . . at the hands of those who wish for his welfare, in the shape of physic, [cold] baths, black-eyes, broken ribs and a fractured lower jaw. He has survived all these . . . but is not much better for anything'. Over the next three years he literally wasted away, succumbing to pneumonia and tuberculosis according to his post-mortem report.[64]

For all Hills' faith in diet, rest, exercise and supervised work, immediate measures were often required. Long-sleeved dress was used to prevent 'serious self-injury' and padded and seclusion rooms were improved.[65] Thus Stephen B—, who was biting himself and had tried to tear his mouth, was 'confined in a long-sleeved dress by order of Dr Hills'.[66] Detailed reports were required but unofficial recourse to such facilities was always possible. Patients could lodge complaints but, as one lunacy commissioners' report stated, 'No restraint is recorded. Every patient in residence had the opportunity of making known to us any complaint, but we had none, not of an insane character'.[67] Typical observations were that:

> the medical books shew that two men have worn the leather-locked gloves since the last visit; one for six weeks, by day, to prevent self-injury, and the other, similarly for three weeks, in consequence of a surgical operation. The seclusion has been limited to 7 females, who have been secluded altogether for a total of only sixteen hours.[68]

---

[62] Case Books, SAH 263, E.J., 1861-??; G.F., 1861–71; W.B., 1861–1903. SAH 265, G.P., 1870–4.
[63] ibid., A.D., 1870.
[64] Case Books, SAH 263; W.G., 1861–5.
[65] MS Journal, 24 Oct. 1861, 27 Jan. and 26 June 1862.
[66] Case Books, SAH 263; S.B. (1861) was given opium and, later, porter and beef tea. He had warm baths and supervised exercise, improved, worked on the farm and was discharged within two months.
[67] AR, 1885, CiL, p. 5.
[68] AR, 1871, CiL, 10 June, p. 12.

Self-injury was not the only consideration, however, for maniacal excitement, destructiveness and indecent behaviour led to ten patients being secluded for a total of 61 hours in 1884. Hills also reported that 'faradization was employed in some cases of dementia, with favourable results' but, even with the best of intentions, galvanism like force-feeding represented a further imposition upon patients.[69]

Roughly 60 epileptic and 20 suicidal patients were dispersed through the asylum in the 1860s and their supervision posed difficulties, particularly at night. Attendants and occasionally outsiders were engaged as night watchers before a regular night staff was appointed. All were to 'visit all the epileptics every hour, or oftener; if any seizures are anticipated, and . . . sit within hearing distance of most epileptic patients', but deaths from epileptic seizure were sometimes reported 'during the absence of the attendant on his rounds'.[70] Responding to the lunacy commissioners, the justices agreed on 'special night wards, for Suicidal and Epileptic; under the constant supervision of an attendant, whose whole time and energies shall be devoted to them'. These reduced the risks faced by 90 or more epileptic patients in the mid-1880s.

Suicidal patients could be wholly unpredictable, as when E.P. attacked 'helpless paralytic' patient C—, thinking that 'he ran needles in his eyes and had destroyed the sight of several women whom he knew'.[71] They were probably heavily sedated, as staff resources were stretched but very few suicides occurred. Hills considered as his 'worst suicidal case' a woman who cut her throat and made repeated attempts, 'thrusting her head through a pane of glass etc', over an eight-month period in 1879. Using special care measures 'together with frequent doses of sedative medicine, every variety of which was used . . . we were able at last to thwart her efforts'.[72] One patient drowned himself in 1885, the first such incident for fifteen years, but two others, 'trusted' for five and sixteen years respectively, hanged themselves in separate incidents away from the asylum buildings in 1886. Precautionary measures were rarely wholly effective.

Sudden, puzzling or suspicious deaths attracted coroners' inquests, but only one-third of deaths led to post-mortem investigations. Hills wished to increase these but faced 'strong prejudice generally entertained by relatives against investigations which are otherwise so desirable', as recognised by the lunacy commissioners.[73] Considering himself a man of science, he was alternately frustrated and bemused by such opposition. He encouraged visitors to counter:

[69] AR, 1884, CiL, 1 Nov., p. 8; AR 1874, MS, p. 6.

[70] AR, 1873, MS, p. 4.

[71] MS Journal, 25 June 1862. According to the coroner's inquest C— was 'seized with convulsions (similar to former attacks prior to the accident)' and died on 30 July.

[72] AR, 1879, MS, p. 5. Eight months later 'she died somewhat suddenly from syncope'.

[73] AR, 1871, MS, p. 4; 1880, CiL, 19 Aug.

absurd ideas as to the behaviour of lunatics and our treatment of them . . . in the minds of many of the Norfolk rustics . . . I have been requested, on several occasions, to show them 'as a favour', the room in which we smother the more violent lunatics!![74]

The NLA was among pioneers in weighing and photographing patients 'before and after', on their admission and discharge, an exemplary practice according to the lunacy commissioners.[75] There were also moments when Hills' surgical background enabled him to cope with the unexpected: in 1863 a patient's child was 'born with an imperforate anus, for which she was operated upon with satisfactory results. The infant remained in the Asylum a month, and since her transference to the Union (to which she is chargeable) I have learnt she is doing well.'[76]

Published records of treatment are summarised in Table 4.1. Increasing patient numbers reflected not only admissions but also reduced mortality among the residents. There were increasingly more female than male patients, although imbalances were slightly less obvious among admissions (54–57.5 per cent) than in total numbers (55–60 per cent) in the period covered. Contrary to Hills' views on male resilience, women had lower mortality and higher recovery rates, although male mortality rates fell from the 1870s. Proportionate to the average number of residents, new admissions

Table 4.1 Average patient admissions, recoveries and mortality by decade, 1850–89

	Average no. resident			Admissions			% admitted recovered			Mortality %		
	Total	M	F	Total	M	F	Total	M	F	Total	M	F
1850–59	291	132	159	90	40	50	41.5* (12.8)	41.3* (12.5)	41.6* (13.0)	11.7	11.7	11.6
1860–69	382	172	210	122	56	66	45.3 (14.6)	41.7 (13.4)	49.3 (15.6)	11.5	13.0	9.9
1870–79	495	199	296	139	59	80	42.4 (11.7)	40.0 (13.2)	44.0 (9.6)	11.1	13.2	9.6
1880–89	692	291	401	170	76	94	42.3 (10.4)	38.2 (10.0)	45.7 (10.7)	9.9	11.2	9.0

Notes: From 1850 the patient numbers asterisked refer to those classed as 'recovered', not simply discharged. Figures in parentheses are for the proportion of all patients discharged.

[74] AR, 1874, MS, pp. 6–7.
[75] AR, 1881, CiL, 8 June. This practice was under way from 1873 at least and probably reflected the photographic interests of assistant M.O. Seymour and Cannell, the asylum engineer.
[76] MS Journal, 11 Jan. 1863.

declined from over three-tenths in the 1850s and 1860s to less than one quarter in the 1880s.

An increase in the number of long-term patients occurred even though NLA recovery rates were comparatively high and probationary procedures were maintained. This reflected the opening of the auxiliary asylum, after which overall recovery rates were an inappropriate indicator of the multiple dimensions to the asylum's value and work. Some patients recovered, with or without therapy or medication, others received medically managed forms of care. Asylum accommodation remained largely custodial, but was increasingly offered to patients who had no suitable alternatives. In 1885, for example, half of the 61 patients who recovered did so within six months of their admission and two-thirds of the remainder recovered in the next six months. Mortality patterns were more even. Some patients, very weak or seriously ill on admission, died within their first month in the NLA but most deaths occurred among longer-term patients, in two cases residents for over forty years.[77]

Medical staff and attendants

Hills was assisted by a succession of younger resident medical officers who tended to move elsewhere to secure promotion. The first of these, George MacKenzie Bacon, was forced to resign in July 1863 after the night watch discovered him with a nurse in ward 1 nurse's room but he later became medical superintendent at Fulbourn Hospital, Cambridge.[78] Drs Charles White and Frederick Sutton served one year each but William Tayton stayed until 1875. T. Seymour was then appointed, becoming head of the auxiliary hospital and senior assistant medical officer from 1880, with T.J. Compton appointed as Hills' junior assistant in the main asylum. When Seymour resigned because of ill-health in 1882, Compton was promoted and a new succession of junior assistants, Drs McWilliam, Cocks, Creasy and Little, followed until 1887.

One feature in this high turnover of junior staff was the poor salary. Hills received £400 less board and lodging in 1862, increasing to £475 in 1869, £500 by 1878 and £600 by 1885. However, his assistant was paid just £80 in the 1860s and £100 in the early 1870s and, as senior assistant with sole responsibility for the auxiliary asylum, Compton received a salary of £180 in

---

[77] AR, 1885, p. 12.
[78] MS Journal, 19 July 1863. Nurse Mary H— was dismissed too. MacKenzie Bacon, appointed at Fulbourn in 1866, was described as a Guy's graduate, a bachelor with independent means 'at that time travelling on the continent perfecting his French and Italian and visiting foreign asylums'. D.H. Clark, *The Story of a Mental Hospital, Fulbourn 1858–1963*, Process, London, 1996, p. 13.

1885.[79] Although Mrs Owen continued as matron after Hills arrived, she resigned in ill-health on 26 August 1862. Emulating early nineteenth-century practices, Mrs Hills then became matron, at a salary of £150 less board and lodging. When she died prematurely in 1868 Hills retained a housekeeper, but Miss Nati was appointed head female attendant in lieu of matron and James Ramsey became the head male attendant from 1870. Bertha Waters, aged 33, later replaced Miss Nati in the main asylum, her deputy being based in the auxiliary hospital.[80]

Until 1880, each ward typically had two attendants, with additions as required for difficult duties. Regular night attendants replaced the previous casual, rotation-based system in 1862, but just one was initially appointed for each side of the asylum, rising to a complement of two men and three women in 1885. To their credit, the medical staff protested at the early discrepancy in night staff salaries, which commenced at £21 for the male but was fixed at £12 for the female attendant, 'although her duties on her side are more onerous'.[81] An indication of workloads comes from Hills' request in 1862 for an additional attendant on the new women's ward 4, where one attendant 'has to make 48 beds and clean three large dormitories, these duties take her too long from the day room, where her presence is imperatively needed'.[82] Six years later four attendants on this ward remained fully occupied by more than forty patients requiring special supervision or in 'helpless' condition. In addition to their own work, the two laundry maids had responsibility for 22 working patients and on male 'working class' wards one attendant took out the farm-work or gardening parties, the other remaining with non-working patients.[83]

Although the number of attendants increased during the 1860s and 1870s, ratios of male staff to patients were barely maintained and those for females deteriorated. Improvement in the main asylum by 1885 largely reflected patient transfers to the auxiliary and those remaining probably required more intensive nursing.[84] Corresponding figures for the auxiliary asylum had deteriorated rather than improved by 1884. On three occasions in the five

---

[79] Based on Annual Reports. Mr C. Williams was the consulting surgeon after G. Firth died in October 1879.

[80] Harriet Waters, matron until December 1898, may have been Bertha's sister or the same person.

[81] MS Journal, 23 April 1862. This was partly corrected in October 1864 and night attendants received £5 minimum quarterly in 1865.

[82] ibid., 27 Dec. 1862

[83] AR, 1869, CiL, p. 10.

[84] A snapshot in 1884 suggests five men's wards with two attendants and 21–32 patients. At least two were working wards. Ward 6 had 14 patients and one attendant, and the infirmary ward 18 patients and one nurse. There were nine women's wards. Four wards and two working wards each had 23–30 patients and two nurses, but ward 9 had 56 patients and four nurses. The laundry ward had 29 patients and three staff, including two laundresses, and the infirmary ward had 18 patients and one nurse.

Table 4.2 Attendant numbers and ratios to patients at the Norfolk Lunatic Asylum, 1862–85

| | Attendants | | Ratio of attendants to patients | |
	M	F	M	F
1862	11	15	1:15.2	1:13.3
1869	12	17	1:15.5	1:14.0
1876	14	20	1:14.5	1:15.6
1880	16	23	1:15.3	1:15.2
1885 main	12	22	1:14.1	1:13.9
auxiliary	5	7	1:25.0	1:19.4

Source: Based on annual reports and excluding matron/head attendants and night attendants.

years after 1880 lunacy commissioners remarked that staffing levels were inadequate in larger wards and that 'nowhere does the staff appear too strong'.[85]

Under Hills' superintendence the asylum wages bill almost trebled, reaching £1,720 in 1885. There were more nursing staff but also craftsmen, a cellarman/butcher, storekeeper, farm bailiff, two cooks and a kitchen maid, three laundresses and three house servants by 1880. Pay was tightly controlled and geared to incremental rises rather than broad additions to basic rates. In 1864, as in 1854, a new male attendant earned roughly eight shillings weekly and few experienced men cleared ten shillings. Most female attendants were paid less than five shillings, although some received six.[86] By 1874 experienced male attendants were paid twelve shillings, the standard wage by 1885, when senior staff earned 17 shillings. Perhaps in recognition of the successes of the asylum farm the wages of G. Breeze, the farm supervisor, were raised by 25 per cent to 22 shillings in September 1876. He and the head attendant were the top wage earners, on 24s 9d per week by 1886. Female attendants commenced on 5s 2d per week in 1874 although two-thirds earned just over six shillings. Rates were essentially the same in 1885 but a successful agitation in 1878 enabled women to cash in their beer allowance, reckoned at an extra shilling per week.[87] Only one of the 21 male staff had taken the same option by 1885.

[85] AR, 1885, CiL, 1 Nov., MS, p. 5.

[86] Based on wages books. In 1865 quarterly pay was: males £4 12s 0d basic, average £5, senior and night attendants £6; females, basic £3, most £3 2s 6d, senior £4–£5, assistant matron £5. Others included laundresses up to £4, cook £5 10s 0d, kitchen maid £3 10s 0d, housemaids £2–£2 5s 0d. Total wages were £640.

[87] MS Journal, SAH 132, 27 April 1878. Quarterly pay in 1875 was; experienced male attendants £7 16s 0d; females, basic £3 7s 6d, most £4, assistant matron £10, laundresses £5–£5 10s 0d, cook £6 5s 0d, kitchenmaid £4, housemaids £2–£2 10s 0d. Total wages were £1,140. Wage rates were substantially the same in 1886, but wages totalled £1,720.

If NLA attendants were poorly paid they probably made local rather than national comparisons. An experienced male attendant earned the same or less than a Norfolk farm labourer before 1870, but had the significant additions of beer and board. Each worked long hours but the attendant worked all year round, with few days off and was expected to cover for colleagues: a working week of at least 84 hours was standard even in 1910. Few late nineteenth-century Norfolk farm-workers were assured of twelve shillings regularly in the contracting labour market and Norwich wages were routinely the lowest or equal lowest among the 44 towns surveyed by the Board of Trade. Nevertheless, the attendant's basic pay was matched by strike money doled out to shoe-workers by their union in 1890 and a Norwich navvy, then paid 3.5d–4d per hour and working a 60-hour week, earned at least the seventeen shillings paid to senior asylum attendants.[88]

NLA wages books dating from 1854 indicate some 30 waged asylum staff with 75 arrivals or departures by 1870, excluding unsuccessful probationers. Asylum working conditions were not particularly attractive. Staff were recruited on the basis of character references for a probationary period, but had no formal training.[89] Hills' emphasis upon music and exercise established a tradition that male attendants should play an instrument or a sport, particularly cricket, which lasted well into the twentieth century. Any additional stresses, incurred for example during infectious disease outbreaks, were likely to prove too much for some. Thus the resignation of four attendants and a housemaid within a nine-day period during the 1862 smallpox outbreak was understandable, if not particularly worthy.[90] There could be harsh discipline and many restrictions. Hills insisted that attendants held responsible for escapes should suffer financial penalties or worse, yet he acknowledged publicly that some patients would escape, 'due to . . . cunning and to the very desperate attempts . . . marked craftiness and determination. In these days of non-restraint, with many facilities at hand . . . we are occasionally outwitted'.[91] Bad episodes, as when 'Edward D—, an epileptic, fell on the fire in a fit, his head is rather badly burnt' or when a patient secreted the key to a ward medicine cupboard and killed herself using chloral hydrate, also affected staff.[92]

Poor safety arrangements and staff shortages were endemic but some staff were culpable. During the winter of 1861–2 patient William G—, 'a constant source of anxiety from his cunning and determined attempts to destroy

---

[88] Digby, *Pauper Palaces*, p. 23; S. Cherry, *Doing Different? Politics and the Labour Movement in Norwich 1880–1914*, CEAS, Norwich, 1989, pp. 30–33.

[89] See P. Nolan, *A History of Mental Health Nursing*, Chapman & Hall, London, 1993, p. 54 and Chapter 5 below.

[90] MS Journal 2, 13 Feb. 1862.

[91] AR, 1877, MS., pp. 4–5.

[92] MS Journal, 22 Dec. 1861; AR, 1871, MS, p. 5. Fireguards completely enclosing open fires were then fitted; the 1871 suicide was reportedly the first of its kind.

himself', suffered broken ribs and a broken jaw on separate occasions whilst being undressed by two attendants. Hills blamed no one for the first incident but an attendant admitted that 'his hand had come unintentionally into contact with G—'s chin' in the second. Only the fact that he was 'normally kind and attentive' saved him from the consequences of this 'injudicious behaviour' and Hills promptly revised the rules of conduct for attendants.[93] So when Mary R— complained that probationary attendant Jane B— 'had slapped her face . . . such treatment being highly reprehensible, I discharged her immediately'.[94] This reduced but did not prevent examples of staff violence, such as when John N— 'blundered' down a patient and broke his collar bone. Gross neglect of duty, for example, when a patient under special observation died during an epileptic seizure, or when another was scalded in an untested bath, was still occurring and led to staff dismissals in 1880.[95]

Hills was particularly uncompromising on questions of habit or character. 'Charles W—, night attendant, returned from half-day leave in a state of inebriation' and was promptly discharged. Attendant J.B—, who had allegedly beaten a woman in Thorpe village, was also dismissed, even though Hills 'had an excellent character (reference) with this servant, he had been 21 years in the army, was a sergeant and in possession of three good conduct badges!!'[96] As Dr MacKenzie Bacon found, 'improper' sexual activity was not tolerated and even indirect evidence of it among attendants was sufficient cause for dismissal. Elizabeth F— was discharged when she took a patient on leave, went to public houses, had beer and brandy 'and returned in a fly with two men'. Mary P—, dismissed because of 'grave suspicions of immorality . . . was extremely impertinent'. Farm bailiff S.L. and attendant Phedora F— were discharged after 'carrying on a clandestine courtship . . . this foolish lovemaking had been going on for about five months, and almost entirely by correspondence.'[97] Cases of theft were vigorously pursued by the justices and superintendent, presumably to deter others. One attendant received six weeks' hard labour for stealing a flannel jacket, 'the property of the Inhabitants of the County', and the asylum shoemaker, prosecuted for taking home one pair of leather soles, value 8d, was acquitted but nevertheless dismissed and his family were evicted from their asylum cottage.[98]

Several women attendants resigned because they were about to marry, which was not allowed in most contemporary nursing and, with insufficient family accommodation, asylum work did not suit married men. Typically,

---

[93] MS Journal, 23 Dec. 1861 and 24 March 1862. G— recovered from his injuries, made further suicide attempts but died from other causes on 31 Jan. 1863.
[94] ibid., 16 May 1862.
[95] AR, 1880, MS, p. 4.
[96] MS Journal, 26 May 1862 and 5 March 1864.
[97] ibid., 2 Dec. 1863, 16 June and 7 Dec. 1864.
[98] Clerk and Steward's Report Books, 1861–72, SAH 143, 22 March 1865, 20 Sept. 1865.

Hills commented that 'several experienced hands left, either to be married or to accept the more tempting offer of higher wages'. However, the loss of eleven nurses in 1887, nine of whom went into private nursing or to other asylums, suggests poor working conditions at the NLA.[99] Ironically, these departures possibly reflected the introduction of ambulance first aid training by medical officers the previous year. Asylum staff were clearly employable elsewhere and their pay, conditions and pensions needed further attention.

Work therapy, entertainment and exercise

Hills' efforts to maintain the proportion of working patients as overall numbers doubled confirm the medical superintendent's role as an administrator focused upon economy and self-sufficiency, as much as a doctor espousing the therapeutic value of work or crafts. When Norwich City Asylum patients, temporarily accommodated at the NLA, were painting the men's wards, Hills noted 'one of the men is a painter by trade and I regret to add that we shall lose him when the city patients are removed'.[100] Patient labour soon featured prominently in ward redecoration. As the asylum's straw mattresses encouraged fleas, Hills thought it 'a wise economy on the part of the Committee at once to replace', suggesting coconut fibre and other materials which were sampled before he chose a softer 'German wool'.[101] Silk flock pillows were also examined but were more expensive than horsehair substitutes. These samples stimulated in-house industry rather than extensive product orders. In 1865 Hills reported that 'all who evince the least capacity are taught tailoring or shoe or mattress making' and, four years later, that two inmates, engaged solely on producing hair mattresses, had almost completed their task.[102]

A recurrent theme, hardly indicative of 'medicalisation' in work therapy, was 'that we get so few artisans, whose labour would be remunerative; our patients are for the most part of the agricultural class'.[103] In January 1863 Hills noted proudly: 'the gas having been laid on in the several [work]shops our tradesmen work ten hours today for the first time.'[104] Under supervision, patients soon produced and repaired all the boots required by the establishment and similar results were anticipated from tailoring. The clerk and steward further suggested that 'some of the furniture should be manufactured on the premises. At the present time we have a very good

---

[99] AR, 1877, MS p. 5; 1887, MS, p. 11.
[100] MS Journal, 23 April 1862.
[101] ibid., 26 Nov. 1861 and 23 Feb. 1862.
[102] AR, 1865, MS, p. 7; 1869, MS, p. 10. Sixty patients were still in 'straw beds' early in 1868.
[103] AR, 1870, MS, p. 4.
[104] MS Journal, 14 Jan. 1863.

carpenter as a patient and . . . a turner . . . some of the more important articles needed might be made in an advantageous manner'.[105]

More farmland was also required because the asylum possessed 'an abundance of labour and the application of our patients to agricultural pursuits would vastly promote their chances of recovery' and because Hills would not condone 'patients idle in the wards who would otherwise advantageously be employed'.[106] Extensions to asylum buildings and recreational space absorbed land acquisitions until 1877, when 52 more acres were purchased. The proportion of male working patients rose from 40 to 45 per cent, depending upon seasonal activity, to 45–50 per cent by 1880. Until then, outdoor workers, farming or gardening, had barely exceeded those in the kitchens, ward helpers or cleaners. At least 55 per cent of women patients worked indoors, 125 as cleaners, ward, kitchen or laundry helpers in 1885, with a similar number doing needlework. These patients contributed to the fabric, furnishings and general upkeep of the asylum and to its image as a hive of industry as well as a hospital and therapeutic community.[107]

Hills' commitment to the work ethic, endorsed by the justices, included reward and deprivation. Noting that Thomas J—, probably a private patient, 'whose assistance in the office is very valuable, expresses a great desire to see the Exhibition' , Hills requested several days' leave for him to attend with Mr Girling, the house steward, as with patient Robert C—.[108] Working parties of between ten and thirty patients were occasionally accompanied to Norwich for more modest treats, for example, the pantomime in the winter of 1862–3 and Tombland fair the following April. Yet a few months later Hills abolished the ward helpers' afternoon allowance of beer, cheese and bread, 'the men not doing anything to entitle them to it', and Boxing Day 1863 saw him preoccupied with wage deductions for three women attendants who had been off sick.[109]

Wider entertainments were conducted with economy in mind. Shortly before Hills arrived the justices replaced annual excursions to Yarmouth or Lowestoft with an 'annual frolic'. A picnic on the asylum cricket field, where patients were 'regaled with an ample supply of good things', was followed by sports and games and then singing and dancing in the dining hall until 10. p.m.[110] Hills summarised the following year's event as a 'merry day . . . much more feasible and economical than taking so large a number of patients

---

[105] Steward's Report, 28 July 1863.
[106] MS Journal, 24 Sept. 1863, AR, 1863, MS, p. 5.
[107] AR, 1885, CiL, p. 5. In 1877 the patients produced 260 pairs of boots and repaired 800 pairs, 150 sets of trousers, waistcoats and jackets plus repairs, more than 500 dresses and chemises and 300 skirts. In addition to sheets, bedding and pillows for the asylum, women patients made mats, scarves, bonnets, baby clothes etc., sold at the asylum bazaar.
[108] MS Journal, 25 July and 15 Oct. 1862.
[109] ibid., 24 Oct. and 26 Dec. 1863.
[110] ibid., 24 Sept. 1861.

far from home'.[111] Other entertainment included shows with slides, dissolving views and ventriloquists but the great standby through the winter months was the fortnightly asylum ball, attended by up to 300 patients. As the asylum band had made 'great progress', it performed on these occasions and thereby saved £10 per year on visiting musicians, as Hills carefully noted.[112] Boat trips continued for smaller groups of patients and a horse and van were purchased in 1865 to provide outings for elderly patients, who could also sit in the new summer house, constructed from disused wrought iron fireguards. From 1871 these activities were enhanced by William Johnson's bequest of £2,000, an unusual benefit for a county asylum, the interest providing trips, recreation and small advances to assist convalescent patients.

Otherwise, exercise was the thing. Hills reported in 1863 that 'all the patients capable of appreciating the enjoyment of walking beyond the wall, do so three times a week'. The proportion later diminished with the ageing of the asylum population and the infirmity of those in the auxiliary hospital but staff shortages also featured. When the lunacy commissioners complained that 350 patients, almost half the asylum population, received no exercise beyond the airing courts in 1880, a reduction to 250 within twelve months indicated previous shortcomings in the asylum regime rather than in its patients.[113] The cricket field served as a major social space and, occasionally, as the site for escape attempts or secret rendezvous, but cricket was promoted as a healthy, orderly team game for male patients to play and females to watch. The patients' team was 'vanquished' by boys and fathers from Thorpe Grammar School in a 'well-contested game' in 1863 but a repeat match 'terminated in our favour . . . the weather was propitious'.[114] After the cricket pitch was required as building land for the auxiliary asylum, no able-bodied patient's effort was spared to clear and level ground for a new one.

More patients derived their spiritual comfort from religious services. Church attendance was recorded by the asylum chaplain and monitored by the justices and lunacy commissioners but it is to be hoped that the services were more uplifting than these records. Three-quarters of patients were expected to attend and a nave was added to the church in 1881 to accommodate growing numbers whilst maintaining sexual segregation. Unlike his predecessors, J.D. Paulett developed the chaplain's journal, recording his ward visits and efforts to improve the asylum library. In 1872 he considered just 35 of the 210 available books suitable for retention, prior to restocking with religious works. He established a lending library for patients and attendants with some success, but acknowledged shortages of 'light

---

[111] ibid., 8 Aug. 1862.

[112] ibid., 25 May and 22 Nov. 1863.

[113] AR, 1882, CiL 1882, p. 8. This improvement was confirmed in their inspection in 1885.

[114] MS Journal, 19 July and 9 Sept. 1863; 6 May 1864.

literature'. A reforming spirit can be detected in his requests for 'slates and copy books' for the younger patients and campaign against the segregated burial of asylum patients, which had caused 'much distress' to their relatives. Whether Paulett became frustrated or had overstepped the mark, a new chaplain was appointed in 1875 and the dour recording of church attendance and burials recommenced.[115]

Although the asylum dietary was largely unchanged, weekly patient costs were pared from roughly six shillings in 1861 to 4s 8d by 1885. Hills' first effort was distinctly personal: asylum tea was 'very well for the general use of the Establishment, but I beg to ask that some of better quality may be allowed for the officers'.[116] He substituted tea or milk and water for beer for all infirm patients in 1871, 'without any detriment to health . . . some appear more quiet and cleanly for it'. Beer was stopped for all excepting outdoor male working patients in December 1879, Hills concluding that 'the patients now eat more than formerly; there is less waste and also less excitement and turmoil after dinner'.[117] Women patients ate little other than bread at breakfast and supper whereas men still had an oatmeal breakfast with broth served on two evenings in the week. The other dietary innovations were that 'Australian meat has been used, cold, for dinner on Sundays' from 1871 and soup and bread replaced meat and vegetables on two other days in the auxiliary asylum from 1880.[118] These economies failed to impress the lunacy commissioners, who criticised the lack of fresh fruit and vegetables in the dietary, even noting occasions when 'the meat pie given today was rejected by several patients'.[119] Whether NLA patients had a poorer diet than contemporary Norfolk farm labourers, costed at just two shillings per family member, is arguable but some deterioration probably had occurred.[120]

Political economy

Hills' appointment had little effect on the governance of the asylum and possibly increased attention to the institution as an economic entity. The Reverend Thomas Blofield, chairman of the justices for eleven years prior to Hills' arrival, retained the post for five more years, subsequently remaining on

---

[115] Chaplain's Report Book, 1 Jan. 1860–31 Oct. 1862, SAH 152; 25 Oct. 1872 (library), 27 May 1873 (books), 23 June 1873 and 22 July 1874 (burial ground).

[116] MS Journal, 23 June 1863.

[117] AR, 1872, MS, p. 5; 1879, MS, p. 6.

[118] ibid., 1872, MS, p. 5; 1881, MS, p. 6. Refrigerated meat became a cheap substitute in many institutions and was probably of dubious quality, particularly in early years.

[119] Farm output and bonuses ('Mr W. Birkbeck's annual gift of oranges . . . much appreciated and . . . "expected" by the patients', MS Journal, 1 Jan. 1879) were insufficient for the lunacy commissioners, e.g. in 1882 and 1885.

[120] Digby, *Pauper Palaces*, p. 23.

the committee. He was succeeded by other clergymen justices from land-owning families, Jeremiah Burroughs (1867–72) and R.G. Lucas (1873–83), each with long committee membership. Before the Local Government Act of 1888 the domination of landowners, clergy and armed forces of the justices and hence the NLA committee was assured. William Girling, clerk to the justices from 1850 until 1888, embodied this continuity in daily routine. He was responsible for inventories and purchases, general upkeep and operations, including the farm and use of patient labour. His report books show that Girling provided much of the impetus for work therapy, for example suggesting that furniture-making should begin in 1863. Hills' approval of shoe-making and pride in the self-sufficiency of the asylum in this respect stemmed from Girling's detailed cost comparisons, which involved direct purchases and making up from part finished materials, leading to conclusions that, 'after allowing for the value of patients' labour, there results a saving of at least 9d a pair'.[121]

Even before its expansion in 1877 the asylum farm provided food supplies and modest cash surpluses. Crop and stock sales were roughly one-third higher over the following decade, averaging £960 annually, which was more than double the expenditure on livestock, feed etc. Healthy balances were not greatly diminished by rent or other costs and they occasioned periodic transfers as 'expenditure' from the farm account to the asylum maintenance account, for example £300 in 1886.[122] Some cash allowances were possibly made for patients' farm labour, as with shoemaking, for annual surpluses averaging £100 were itemised as 'labour', possibly for carting asylum coals and goods. Girling was responsible for some very fine-tuning of livestock accounts. Armed with one-year forecasts of asylum food requirements and stores, he sold any surpluses. Asylum farm produce was costed against that of other suppliers so that, if the value of asylum farm pigs fell below current pork prices, they were slaughtered and butchered for immediate use; if not, they were retained for more profitable sales.[123]

Cost considerations determined patient numbers' totals and even their location. Hills reported considerable overcrowding in 1862 but observed that an excess of deaths over admissions and the discharge of five patients in December made it 'unnecessary to send any of the patients to their respective unions'.[124] This adjustment of patient numbers under medical criteria was not simply in response to overcrowding but intended to maintain and indeed

---

[121] Steward's Report, 26 May 1863. Asylum boots and shoes 'were of superior quality to those bought from Norwich tradesmen'.

[122] AR, 1877–86, Farm Accounts. Annual sales averaged £960 and costs, excluding rent, £475. With additional farm surpluses on labour, stock adjustment and cash in hand, there were probably transfers to asylum general accounts in the guise of rent on asylum-owned land and other charges. Annual farm balances averaged £446.

[123] Steward's Report, 25 Oct. 1862 and 24 Feb. 1863.

[124] MS Journal, 30 Dec. 1862.

maximise asylum income. As new wards were added in 1869 the asylum's spare capacity was quickly and productively used. Some 22 women patients were accepted from Ipswich on a weekly charge of 14 shillings compared with the standard 8s 6d. When the NLA again became overcrowded in the late 1870s such opportunities were lost. Hills contacted other asylums seeking the most economical placement for NLA patients before suggesting that a reduced number of women patients be sent to Ipswich Borough asylum, where the weekly maintenance charge was 16 shillings.[125]

With the NLA reorganisation of 1880 new opportunities arose. By 1882 the asylum had an average of 715 patients, almost 50 of them on probation or 'out', generally on weekly allowances of three to four shillings. Each of these represented a net saving to the asylum of up to five shillings on standard costs, excluding some allowance for capital costs. These annual savings amounted to £800, some of which was used to trim standard weekly charges from 8s 10d to 8s 7d, with a remaining balance of £350 carried forward. It was additionally reckoned that the 46 outcounty and 20 private patients provided an income £900 greater than their maintenance costs, a sum also used to subsidise the standard 'Norfolk' charge by a further six pence per week.[126]

Individual case notes also confirm the importance of financial issues. A magistrate signing committal papers for a non-pauper patient was promptly billed for his care, his refusal to pay prompting a general ban on such 'informal admissions'. Norfolk patients found to be non-paupers, in one case a farmer's son, were charged at the higher outcounty rate and individuals found to have private means were set appropriate fees or sent to private institutions. These issues often arose when the asylum received additional information, sometimes from patients who were less confused than formerly or from their relatives. Occasionally asylum authorities felt that others were deliberately taking advantage. Hills was genuinely shocked to discover that patient Fanny F—, married to a house carpenter in service to the Duke of Sutherland, had been returned to Norfolk and the asylum 'as a pauper!!'[127]

Table 4.3 indicates the determined efforts to control costs in a situation where total income increased in line with, or less rapidly than, overall patient numbers. A modest but growing proportion of income was derived from outcounty or private patients, rather than from Norfolk ratepayers, and thus to their advantage. Expenditure on food dominated maintenance accounts, even with the asylum farm and reducing dietary costs per patient. Hills'

---

[125] ibid., 27 April, 20 June 1878.

[126] Based on Annual Reports 1880–3. Average weekly patient costs were 8s 9d, but Norfolk unions were charged 8s 3d per patient. 'Outcounty' charges were 14 shillings and 14–21 shillings for private patients. This convenient situation deteriorated from 1885 as Suffolk County Asylum patients were returned.

[127] Respectively in MS Journal, 20 May 1863, 20 Feb. 1879, 6 Feb. 1880 and 22 March 1879.

Table 4.3 Income and major items of expenditure at the Norfolk Lunatic Asylum 1860–85

	1860	1870	1880	1885
Net annual income	£7,723	£9,685	£15,236	£17,031
'Norfolk' (%)	93.7	87.3	97.9	88.2
'Outcounty, etc.' (%)	6.3	12.7	2.1	11.8
% Expenditure on:				
Officers' salaries	9.2	8.8	7.1	7.9
Attendants/wages	7.1	7.3	9.1	10.1
Food	50.3	50.3	53.5	50.3
Beer, spirits	9.1	8.4	4.6	3.4
Fuel	8.0	8.4	8.7	9.3
Clothing, bedding	9.7	9.0	10.8	11.7
Drugs, surgery	0.5	0.6	0.8	0.9
Sundries	3.6	3.7	4.1	4.0
Balance at beginning of year	£1,582	£1,897	£2,167	£2,742
Balance at year end		£1,035	£2,448	£2,825
(Repairs, etc. on capital account)	£1,516	£2,086		£5,723

Notes: Net annual income excludes beginning and end of year balances. The 1870 financial year was officially 9 months, Jan.–Sept., but Oct.–Dec. income has been added.

restrictions on beer and the reduction of spirits consumption had a visible effect on spending after 1870, with that on fuel tightly controlled, even as the use of gas lighting was extended. Increasing items of expenditure included attendants' and nurses' salaries, a function of greater numbers rather than generous payments, and the patients' clothing and bedding.

As the NLA's first medical superintendent William Hills was expected to enhance its therapeutic role and to manage a micro-economy efficiently. He had to satisfy the committee and, indirectly, local ratepayers and also the lunacy commissioners, as the external authority notionally concerned with safeguarding patients' interests. A man who could develop much-needed musical resources but remain focused on the £10 thus saved and who had an employer's eye for patients' talents probably sensed little in the way of tensions in these roles. Hills' strong sense of the work ethic and financial prudence in work therapy and even in patients' treats would not have been out of place in a justice of the peace or a poor law guardian. And on his retirement the lunacy commissioners recalled they had 'at all times found him ready to support their suggestions . . . and undoubtedly great improvement has been effected during his term of office'.[128]

---

[128] AR, 1886, CiL, 24 Nov. Hills spent his retirement in Thorpe and died in 1902.

These were appropriate remarks for the occasion, but the commissioners' tone soon changed. They criticised staffing levels, the patient dietary, lack of brightness and objects of interest in the main buildings, notably in some 'very shabby and dilapidated' rooms on the men's side. Similarly, 'the day rooms, in their dull, bare appearance present a striking contrast to those in most county asylums of the present day'.[129] Either Hills' reforming enthusiasm or his powers of persuasion with the justices had diminished and their shared sense of economy had not put the asylum in good standing for the longer term. His major innovation was the auxiliary asylum, the embodiment of medical claims to manage and care for, rather than to cure, those seen essentially as infirm or senile. Though he recognised the asylum as inappropriate for its youngest patients, Hills could not prevail upon the justices to produce a tolerable alternative. Lunacy commissioners 'were sorry to see idiot children in the wards with the adult lunatics, but fear there is no more prospect of any alteration than . . . more than four years ago'.[130] Despite these deficiencies the NLA sustained official patient recovery rates slightly ahead of national asylum averages. And, even if many were readmitted, the concept of the asylum as a revolving door for some was more optimistic than many patients or their relatives expected, and more than some latter-day historians have allowed.

---

[129] Annual Reports 1887–96, SAH 30: CiL, *viz.*, 19 Nov. 1887, p. 17; 21 July 1891, p. 16; 11 March 1893, p. 17.
[130] AR, 1885 CiL, p. 6.

5

'Successful conversion': a managed community, 1887–1915

David Thomson, born and educated in Edinburgh, received his M.D. and studied in Dresden before he became medical officer at the Derby County and then Camberwell asylums. He was senior medical officer at Surrey County Asylum and only 30 years old when appointed medical superintendent at Norfolk County Asylum on Boxing Day 1886. Yet he was already 'favourably known' to the lunacy commissioners, who had 'some confidence that, under his charge, this Asylum will not fall back'.[1] Thomson took up his position on 12 February 1887 and remained there until 1 May 1922, well beyond his due retirement date, because of emergencies created by the Great War. In that time he was mainly responsible for the extensive reorganisation of the asylum and its modernisation to standards considered comparable with best contemporary practice. He also supervised the asylum's conversion to a military hospital, the subject of the next chapter, and its eventual reinstatement and renaming as a mental hospital.

Thomson's arrival coincided with changes in the regulation of county asylums and a determined effort by the lunacy commissioners to secure improvements. Under the 1888 Local Government Act Norfolk County Council became responsible for maintenance of the asylum, from April 1889 renamed the Norfolk County Asylum and run by a committee of seventeen visitors appointed from the elected councillors. Four members of the new committee had been members of its predecessor, providing an element rather than any guarantee of continuity in its management. The 1890 Lunacy Law Amendment Act altered procedures for the certification of patients, requiring the approval of a qualified medical practitioner and the formal consent of a judge or justice of the peace, rather than a clergyman or poor law relieving officer. It also required the annual recertification of existing asylum patients by their medical superintendent. A further clause restricted any cash surpluses generated from private patient care to asylum building accounts but, as will be seen, the indirect and medium-term subsidy of certain asylum patients and ratepayers continued.

Initially, Thomson complained that legislative requirements consumed medical superintendents' time and that 'the treatment of patients . . . cannot

---

[1] Annual Reports (AR), 1887–97, SAH 30, 1887, Commissioners in Lunacy (CiL), 19 Nov., p. 13.

help being in a greater measure delegated to their less experienced colleagues'.[2] Although he remained accountable to the committee of visitors, he grasped the reform opportunities offered, initiated relevant policy-making and effectively assumed personal control of the asylum. Ultimately his efforts to improve asylum sanitation strained relations with Norwich Corporation and the Norfolk county surveyor and his determination to modernise the asylum fabric impinged on other personnel, notably the engineer and clerk of works. Attendants and nurses also found that Thomson had decided views concerning training, ward practice and working conditions. Late nineteenth-century asylum growth was a national phenomenon and NCA annual admissions and patient numbers rose by 50 per cent between 1887 and1914. Thomson managed this increase and reorganised patient care within new or refurbished facilities on sexually segregated lines. Although his therapeutic approach was much less innovative, this secured his reputation as a moderniser and improved the asylum's professional and public image. The NCA's dramatic conversion as a military hospital in 1915 thus disrupted longer-term changes, recognised in the reopened and renamed Norfolk Mental Hospital in 1920.

Improving the physical environment

A succession of lunacy commissioners' reports suggested that the asylum had slipped behind contemporary practices, though Thomson was not held responsible and was indeed said to be overworked. Immediate action to reduce fire risks and improve emergency procedures was requested, with further use of river water restricted to fire control purposes. Auxiliary asylum patients were to receive the full dietary and a more sympathetic redecoration of the asylum, with better heating and lighting, was urged. Extended farm-working and a more varied diet necessitated further land purchases and other improvements in patient amenities, exercise and recreation required the resolution of staff shortages, improvements in staff training and off-duty facilities.[3] These recommendations determined Thomson's first steps, immediately supported by the new committee. Within one year two-thirds of all patients were working, notably on the redecoration and part-refurbishment of the asylum, its grounds and cricket field, with a greater proportion taken on walks beyond the asylum estate. Ambulance training was extended and a trained fireman was appointed.[4] Additional staff, a new mess room for nurses and the restoration of full dietary in the auxiliary asylum were also noted approvingly in the 1890 lunacy commissioners' report.[5]

---

[2] AR, 1891, Medical Superintendent (MS), p. 13.
[3] AR, CiL, 19 Nov. 1887, 21 July 1891, 11 March 1893.
[4] AR, 1889, MS, p. 11.
[5] AR, 1890, CiL, 22 March, p. 17.

However, there were other problems to confront. Dysentery and typhoid fever between 1890 and 1893 were linked to contamination by sewer gas and defective inspection facilities in the main asylum. River water was no longer used but water quality analysis, whilst exonerating the asylum's wells and spring, confirmed that vegetables were washed in contaminated water on the asylum farms. New pumps were ordered to increase the water supply and Thomson, having personally checked all drains and covers, then devised and supervised the installation of an improved water heating and drainage system.[6] He blamed Norwich City Corporation and its Whitlingham sewerage works for the 'disagreeable effluvia . . . arising from the sewerage farm and river' and for continuing problems at the asylum, an outburst which had political repercussions.[7] In the 1894 diphtheria outbreak Thomson isolated suspected cases and introduced antiseptic gargling on the affected wards, leaving the management of cases and tracheotomies to his assistant Dr Spence Law and an assistant matron experienced in fever nursing.

Even the more critical of commissioners' reports acknowledged ward improvements and refurbishment. Although 'the bedding of the Asylum was exceedingly neat and clean everywhere' the laundry facilities, formerly suitable for 350 patients, were forty years old.[8] Three staff and at least 30 working patients were fully occupied 60 hours each week by the requirements of 900 patients and staff. Thomson, matron Hamer and the county surveyor visited five modern steam laundries in London before revised plans for a new laundry block with residential accommodation for 40 working patients were approved by Norfolk County Council in January 1896. After excavation work by patients to limit costs, the laundry block opened in July 1897. Costing £6,000, it featured washing machines with alternating offset drums and a continuous drying room capable of handling 20,000 items per week. Seven staff and 60 patients were employed but efficiency gains and the release of main building accommodation for outcounty patients were intended to offset running and capital costs respectively.[9] Along with improvements to main kitchens, the new laundry represented the first phase of modernisation and expansion of the asylum fabric.

---

[6] This utilised white glazed half-channel pipes, sunk into the tiled floors of bathrooms, washrooms etc., leading to external open traps and preventing the introduction of sewer gas. Thomson specified a bath at 100 degrees Fahrenheit to be drawn in 40 seconds and emptied in 30. Work was completed with the rebuilding of the auxiliary asylum in 1903. AR, 1903, MS, p. 15.

[7] AR, 1899, MS, p. 8. The asylum committee held similar views, see C. Mackie, *The Norfolk Annals*, Norwich, 1901, Vol. 2. 1851–1900, 3 July 1879.

[8] AR, 1894, CiL, 8 May, p. 17.

[9] AR, 1895, MS Special Report. E.F. Cannell, 'The progress of a century; Norfolk County Mental Hospital Engineering Department', 1914, SAH 325 contains illustrations of the new washing machines.

In 1899 the lunacy commissioners issued 'a very satisfactory report on the state of the wards, which were bright and clean . . . the dormitories were in excellent order . . . the dress of the patients good, that of the women being very bright and varied'.[10] Yet there were signs of renewed overcrowding at the asylum. Patient admissions exceeded 200 for the first time in 1894 and the average number resident climbed beyond 850, compared with roughly 700 on Thomson's arrival. On three occasions in the 1890s more than 30 patients were discharged 'not improved', mainly to local workhouses, confirming the offloading of quieter patients to make room for more serious cases. After the commissioners commented upon insufficient male facilities, particularly for epileptic patients, Thomson responded at the visitors' committee in March 1899. Some 200 beds in the main and 140 in the auxiliary asylums were insufficient for male patients but he was unwilling to discharge patients to workhouses, given the prospects of readmission and poorer standards there. Transfers to other asylums were unacceptably expensive but the use of diminishing spare accommodation on the female side would incur conversion costs and any discharge of outcounty women patients would mean lost income. The laundry block and the conversion of an attendants' dormitory had provided the only new beds since 1880 but qualitative improvement was also required, since 'our accommodation for the sick, infirm, paralysed and the epileptics has not been increased in due proportion, and is inadequate on both sides of the main building'.[11]

Thomson's proposals reshaped the asylum's physical environment and provided its twentieth-century template. He recommended the building of a new male infirmary and attendant block as part of an asylum reorganisation featuring complete sexual segregation. The former auxiliary asylum would be converted for males only and 150 women patients would transfer to those main buildings previously occupied by 200 men. Existing large auxiliary wards would house working and 'quiet' patients, with new infirmary, epileptic patient and attendant blocks constructed to enhance site facilities, providing 390 beds and some spare capacity. In the refurbished former main building 560 beds were more than sufficient for current Norfolk and outcounty women patients.[12] Accepting these proposals in May 1899, the committee appointed the London architect A.J. Wood, 'a specialist in asylum work'.[13] With modifications the male asylum was costed at £22,886 and an additional

---

[10] Minutes of the Committee of Visitors (CVIS), July 1898–Sept. 1906, SAH 13, 12 May 1899.

[11] ibid., 5 Jan. 1899.

[12] ibid., 20 March 1899.

[13] ibid., 4 May and 12 Aug. 1899. Woods was to receive 5 per cent commission on the costs of all work, viz. infirmary £7,222, epileptic block £5,984, attendant block £4,041 and new workshops £1,620. Auxiliary ward modifications, improved day rooms, dining areas and side wards cost £1,816.

£9,021 was earmarked for new power plant to provide heat and electric lighting to both asylums. Having undertaken responsibility for Postwick chapel in March 1899, the committee obtained exclusive control of road access to the asylum's cottages and prepared for further improvements to the women's asylum.

At this point major obstacles were encountered. The national commissioners in lunacy felt they had been inadequately consulted and insisted that more land to the north-west side was necessary to provide 'an adequate area around any additional buildings'. This land belonged to Lord Rosebery and much persuasion, involving the lunacy commissioners and the Secretary of State, was required before an additional 13 acres could be purchased.[14] With more spacious siting of the new buildings, modified plans, involving improved boiler capacity for greater quantities of hot water, were agreed by the asylum committee in April 1900. Wood's recommendation of suitable specialist contractors caused some concern but the competitive tendering for general building work was delayed until June 1901 by a dispute throughout the Norwich building industry.[15] Soon afterwards, the asylum committee corresponded with the Local Government Board over allegations by Thorpe St Andrew's Parish Council that the asylum burial ground was full and that 'three people are actually being buried in each grave'.[16] Within three months an acre of land to the north east of the asylum site was purchased as burial ground and plans for a small chapel announced to minimise adverse publicity or complications with the Local Government Board.

Instead, a different problem emerged. Some £65,908 was needed for the asylum projects and Norfolk County Council attempted to borrow £70,000 from the Local Government Board, planning to release agreed sums to the asylum building account, from which contractors would be paid. However, a Local Government Board investigation initially led to refusal of the full loan in January 1901. Sanitary arrangements for the enlarged asylum were considered inadequate, land purchases were not allowed under the loan application and full details concerning £3,000 expenditure on furnishings were required.[17] These latter points could be resolved but Thomson's long-standing complaints concerning the Norwich Corporation sewerage works and river pollution stirred political issues. The asylum always objected that expansion plans at Whitlingham 'were continuing instead of abolishing the

---

[14] ibid., 31 Oct. and 7 Dec. 1899; 1 Feb. and 2 April 1901.

[15] ibid., 5 May and 6 June 1901. Contracts were with W. King and Son of London (£52,353 for buildings) and Norwich firms Laurence & Scott (£2,456 for electrical plant) and G.W. Mann (£3,485 for piping and wiring). Architect's fees, furnishings and contingency funding were a further £7,614, making a total cost of £65,908.

[16] ibid., 20 Dec. 1901 (re. letter received 5 Dec.) and 6 March 1902. Plans were approved by the LGB in June 1902 and the chapel and ground consecrated by the Bishop of Norwich on 26 March 1903.

[17] ibid., 5 Dec. 1901 and 17 Jan. 1902.

existing nuisance' but it was, as Norfolk County Council acknowledged, itself a polluter. Thomson's argument, that a system of peat and coke filters and ditches produced waste water 'at least as pure as the water into which it flows', was counterproductive. Improvements 'without delay' were demanded in January 1902 as relations between Thomson and T.H. Heslop, the county surveyor, deteriorated. By November the asylum accepted that further argument meant only 'great inconvenience, and prevents arrangements as to [the] loan . . . the County Council are also pressing the Committee to proceed'.[18] Work finally began on a new sewage disposal system in June 1903, three months after the new asylum buildings were completed and two months after the last male patients moved from the main asylum. Costing £2,350 it met Local Government Board specifications for automatic electric pumps, accumulation and stormwater tanks, thereby facilitating the full release of loan funds.

Considerable disruption arose from building work and patient transfers. A major feature of construction work was the excavation of a new 300-yard tunnel and road link between the two asylums using patient labour (see Figure 4.1). This took more than three years and involved a 15-feet deep cutting and the extraction of at least 10,000 cubic yards of earth. Building works were extensive and Thomson stated: 'I long for the time when the last of the hundreds of outside workmen employed here shall have left and we can resume the ordinary life of the institution.'[19] The cost-saving virtues of work therapy were again demonstrated in clearing-up operations and the laying out of grounds after the contractors had left.

In their revised form the twin asylums occupied 150 acres and provided 1,012 beds, roughly 130 of which represented spare capacity. They were first lit by electric lighting on 26 February 1903, providing results described by Thomson as 'beyond all praise'.[20] The male asylum became fully operational from 4 April. Its central administration block, added to the former auxiliary asylum, contained medical offices and living quarters for the second assistant medical officer, the dispensary and pathology laboratory. Located behind were the kitchen, stores and bakery, servants' quarters (and billiards room for medical officers!), with separate post-mortem room and mortuary. All the new ward blocks were self-contained. Those extending to the north east comprised visiting rooms and a ground floor ward A for acute and recent patients, with the 'excited and troublesome' accommodated on the first floor ward B. The south-west side included a separate infirmary and special nursing block for the

---

[18] ibid., 12 June 1901 (asylum objection), 25 Jan. 1902. The asylum consulted F. Wallis Stoddart, a Bristol sanitary engineer, and proposed the 'Stoddart continuous filter system'. The LGB rejected it, insisting upon arrangements to prevent stormwater from causing overflows of sewage. 3 April, 4 Sept. and 6 Nov. 1902.

[19] AR, 1897–1905, SAH 31, 1902, MS, p. 16.

[20] AR, 1903, MS, p. 10.

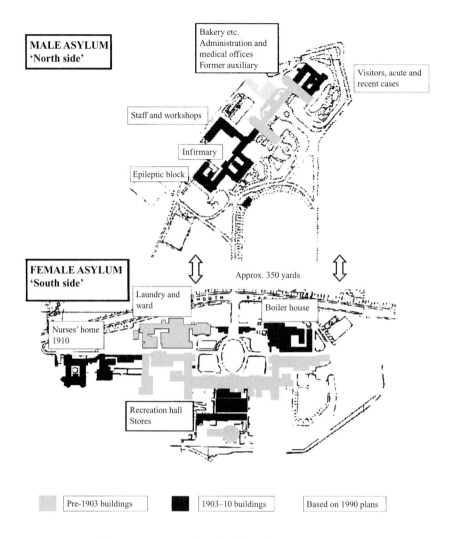

Figure 5.1 1903 plan of male and female asylums

physically sick and reception patients, respectively wards D and E, each with 33 beds. Both wards had a higher proportion of bedrooms and a generous spatial allowance. In the new epileptic block, wards F and G were arranged on two floors and provided for 70 patients. Behind the infirmary were the attendants' mess, games and recreation rooms, leading off to various workshops and the photographic studio. Lastly, the wards on two floors of the former annexe were extended and refurbished for use by working patients as ward C.[21]

---

[21] 'Norfolk County Asylum', *Eastern Daily Press*, 18 Sept. 1903. Reorganisation in 1907

Immediately south of the Norwich to Great Yarmouth road lay the power plant, workshops and stables. The engineers' department included a redesigned central boiler house which heated both asylums, using a 260-yard steam main to the new male asylum buildings, and the pump house. Electricity was generated by compound steam engines and used for lighting, the laundry, bakery and pumps, with accumulator rooms providing a silent source of energy for nightlights.[22] Building maintenance workshops were separated from the boiler house and a fire station was established. Wards were equipped with alarm bells and telephones and emergency iron staircases, repeatedly requested by the lunacy commissioners, were installed.[23] Defunct heating pipes were used to provide ring water mains, equipped with hydrants and pumps able to throw jets of water above roof level at either asylum. A brigade of twelve trained attendants operated them and other staff were instructed in the use of indoor hoses and emergency procedures. In the old 'main' buildings, now the women's asylum, the former male wards 3 and 4 were converted at a cost of £1,170 as female epileptic wards 11 and 12, each with 40 beds. This asylum now comprised 14 wards, each combining dormitories, single bedrooms, day rooms, kitchen and stores, and sanitary arrangements, providing 560 beds in total. Wards 1 and 10 were set aside for the infirm, with ward 2 for the physically sick. Recent and acute cases were placed respectively in wards 3 and 4, with the 'turbulent' and 'excitable' in wards 5 and 6. Quiet and chronic patients occupied wards 9, 13 and 14 with convalescent patients in wards 7 and 8.

Rounding off the pre-war modernisation, work on a separate nurses' home began in 1909 and was followed by a recreation hall and central stores in 1910. Standing in a two-acre site west of the women's asylum, the nurses' home was built to rectangular design around a court and was fronted by a verandah and bay windows, with a balcony on the first floor. A hall, dining, reading and general rooms led to single rooms off corridors along each side of the court, with double rooms and a conservatory at the rear. Fifty nurses were accommodated in 28 single and 11 double rooms at a total cost of £6,376.[24] Meanwhile, the use of former nurses' rooms allowed 60 more beds to be placed throughout the women's asylum. The hall and stores cost £9,173 and were located between the central administration block and the chapel. A mechanical stoking and underfeed system was also introduced in 1910 to

---

created three farmworkers' wards (A, B, C). Wards D–G were unaffected and H was for convalescents.

[22] The new boilers cost £11,124. The old ones, sold to 'Norwich City Hospital', Hellesdon, were used until 1939, according to Cannell. Other items included engineer's house (£425), phones and alarms (£796) and mortuary chapel (£420). Wood's commission was 'approx. £3,000'.

[23] AR, 1899, CiL, 7 March and 12 May; 1901, CiL, 11 June.

[24] AR, 1910, MS, p. 10. This included a photograph and plans. Building costs were £5,625; furnishings £876 and alarms, phones etc. £235.

improve fuel economy, while water softening plant and tanks were added to assist the maintenance and efficiency of the laundry.

Visiting lunacy commissioners observed that 'the asylum throughout is in excellent order' and concluded, perhaps too readily, that 'the many improvements . . . have brought up the Institution to a high standard as regards the comfort and well-being of the patients'.[25] The completion of new buildings at a cost of £73,000 to the public purse led to an inspection by county councillors, to which poor law guardians, representatives from local hospitals and the medical profession were also invited. Yet an asylum was still an asylum to many of those who purported professional or political interest and the local press reported that 'the responses were not so numerous as might have been expected'.[26] Historically, the physical fabric and mechanical functioning of the asylum were probably at their best between 1903 and 1914. This positive contribution to the quality of patients' lives and the working environment of staff was not the sole feature to be considered, however.

Staff, nursing standards and working conditions

For most of the 1880s the lunacy commissioners considered that there were insufficient nurses at the NCA and in 1893 they recommended an additional medical officer.[27] However, a pressing problem was the retention of current medical staff, as a procession of junior officers including Drs Hartman Brown and Ryan came and went. When Maxwell Little, the senior medical officer, left after five years' service in 1891, Dr Wreford was promoted and his replacement, John Spence Law, settled to take charge of the women's asylum in 1903. Thomson could not obtain suitable junior officers in the 1890s, although his Edinburgh connections secured a succession of graduate locums until Dr Duff, seven years above the conventional age limit, arrived in 1902.[28]

A qualified dispenser was appointed the next year, taking responsibility for photographic work and acting as clerk to the medical officers. This post suggests the growing importance of drug therapy but it certainly relieved the medical staff. Thomson's reluctance to undertake annual recertification was well known. Referring to a patient who thought that he was made of brass, Thomson wrote:

> he has this delusion and will never lose it. I see him nearly every day . . . a member of the committee sees him once a week, his case has already been fully described

[25] AR, 1905, CiL, 8 May, p. 14.
[26] *Eastern Daily Press*, 18 Sept. 1903. The open day was held on 17 Sept. 1903.
[27] AR, 1893, CiL, 11 March, p. 17; 1896, CiL, 11 April.
[28] CVIS, 5 June 1902.

in various statutory books. I have no interest in his detention . . . and yet once a year he has to be brought to my office, half an hour has to be wasted over useless formalities and a report sent up to Whitehall, and so on, with the other 7 or 8 hundred cases.[29]

A subsequent deterioration in patient records, criticised by the lunacy commissioners, was belatedly addressed by the dispenser and admissions and current case books were improved, although many long-established case histories 'should be at once written up to date'.[30]

In 1903 salaries for senior and junior medical officers rose by one quarter, to £250 and £160 per annum respectively, and these had further increased to £414 and £200 by 1914. Evidently this was insufficient for the junior staff: after Dr Duff, Dr Gavin left in awkward circumstances in 1909 (see below), to be followed by Dr Chambers, who took up a senior appointment in Dumfries in 1911, and then Dr Flynn.[31] Nor did it augur well for Thomson's hopes that, with the introduction of a postgraduate diploma in mental medicine in 1910, the asylum might attract and retain 'the more distinguished type of young medical graduate'.[32] Meanwhile, he successfully pressed his own case by referring to his increasing workload and the salaries of medical superintendents at comparable asylums in Northampton, Somerset and Wiltshire. A substantial medical superintendent's house was completed in 1892 and, with board, stable allowance and pay awards, the value of Thomson's salary rose to £925 in 1898, £1,100 in 1903 and £1,418 from 1910, a real increase even in inflationary times.

Until the late 1880s there were few signs of improvement in staff to patient ratios, (1:13 for nurses and 1:15 for attendants), or in the training of staff beyond first aid measures.[33] Thomson's attempts to improve standards began with more general use of the epithet 'nurse', though vestiges of male terminology continued in the new nurses' 'mess room'. He persuaded the committee to re-establish the position of matron and to abolish those of asylum housekeeper and chief nurse. Thus, 'the dual female control is unsatisfactory and, in the same way as a medical superintendent should have complete control and authority in the asylum, so ought there to be one female officer'.[34] Mary Hamer, chief nurse for the previous five years, became matron and Miss Parry, the asylum housekeeper, left to become matron of the Beccles workhouse. James Ramsey retired after eighteen years as head male attendant in 1888, but sergeant Fairbanks from the army hospital corps completed just one year in the post and his successor, James Hulse, had to

[29] AR, 1891, MS, pp. 12–13.
[30] AR, 1905, CiL, 8 May.
[31] Wages Book, 1911–1920, SAH 99, 1911.
[32] AR, 1906–15, SAH 32, 1910, MS, p. 14.
[33] AR, 1887, CiL, 18 Nov.
[34] AR, 1891, MS, p. 14.

resign, 'having shown signs of intemperate habits'.[35] Charles Fox, previously the charge attendant for ten years, then became head attendant through to the War Hospital period.

Attendants and nurses at the NCA, as elsewhere, had little formal training before the 1890s. They were expected to work long hours and could be almost permanently on call in periods of crisis for poor fixed rates of pay. Their responsibilities were considerable and many possessed valuable skills. Male staff experienced in farm work or gardening were useful to the asylum economy, 'artisan' attendants made prized contributions towards institutional self-sufficiency and work therapy, and ex-servicemen were considered good for order and 'character' in male wards. If instances of abusive behaviour towards patients occurred, close contact and common interests between staff and patients also implied engagement, persuasion and even role models. Among asylum reformers, John Conolly had recognised in 1830 that 'the influence of a healthy person's mind becomes the chief therapy in mental disease, and the mental nurse its most important agent'.[36] A national study has concluded that late nineteenth-century asylums in areas such as Norfolk were serviced by local communities and family networks. These provided recruits but also informal training and realistic expectations concerning the work involved as 'the attendants were, over the years, building up a fund of knowledge about caring . . . which was often passed from one generation to the next as children followed their parents into asylum work'.[37]

Nevertheless their status was low and, if family men were encouraged, married women were not. Consequently the turnover of women nurses was particularly high, averaging 45 per cent at the NLA in 1887 and 1888. Some failed to complete their probation period, some left to marry, but others moved into more lucrative or less stressful nursing work. Thomson hoped to retain staff with additional pay increments and to raise standards through personally controlled and systematised training, enhanced status and a pensions scheme. He felt that 'young women of more education, culture and possessing more musical and other accomplishments than formerly' could be attracted by 'fair remuneration, comfortable quarters, liberal board . . . and amusements and recreation . . . and properly teaching and training them how to perform their duties'.[38] When provision for asylum staff pensions was specified under the 1890 Lunacy Law Amendment Act, Thomson quickly produced a model for NCA staff. This offered superannuation of up to two-thirds pay from the age of 60 and was based upon a maximum starting age of

---

[35] AR, 1892, MS, p. 10.

[36] J. Conolly, *An Inquiry Concerning the Indications of Insanity with Suggestions for the Better Protection and Care of the Insane*, Taylor, London, 1830, p. 31. Conolly was then medical superintendent at Hanwell Asylum, Middlesex.

[37] P. Nolan, *A History of Mental Health Nursing*, Chapman & Hall, London, 1993, p. 48.

[38] AR, 1894, MS, p. 10; 1895 MS, p. 10.

35 years and pro-rata payments for a minimum of fifteen years' satisfactory service. But dismissal meant disqualification and, revising the staff rules, Thomson assumed powers 'to suspend without warning for any acts of unkindness, harshness or insolence, violence towards patients, disobedience of orders, transgression of rules or negligence; also for intemperance or immorality, whether occurring within or without the hospital boundaries'.[39]

When the philanthropic Miss Whaley established a club room for all Norwich nurses in 1895, Thomson encouraged asylum nurses to attend, also offering reciprocal visits to the NCA. An outdoor uniform, symbolic of new standards, was also introduced. The completion of the medical superintendent's house between the main and auxiliary asylums in August 1892 allowed a reshuffle of accommodation, which benefited the assistant medical officers, matron and head attendant. Married male attendants were further encouraged by the building of six more cottages on the asylum estate. Using the 1885 Medico Psychological Association *Attendants Handbook*, staff training was introduced in combination with practical ward sessions. This became compulsory for new recruits from 1895 and seven of the first ten attendants and nurses entered obtained the MPA certificate of proficiency in 1896.

Thomson now pressed for staff pay increases and contemplated asylum-based contract nursing as a source of fee income, emulating the more prestigious voluntary general teaching hospitals.[40] From 1899 nurses' annual salaries commenced at £18 and rose incrementally to £25. Male attendants mostly earned 16 shillings weekly, with board, lodging and uniform, but there were bonuses for MPA certificate holders, night staff and senior or long-serving staff. At least two-thirds of male attendants held the MPA certificate by 1900, a proportion roughly double the national average.[41] Better pay helped to reduce staff turnover and there were 25 asylum cottages available to married men, but facilities for single men were poor and 'not much is done to make their mess room a comfortable resting place when the day's work is over'.[42] All male attendants were allowed one full day's leave every eight days and with alternate evenings off subject to emergency cover, these arrangements being extended to nurses in 1900.

A day staff of 33 attendants and 33 nurses provided one nurse or attendant per eleven patients by 1900.[43] Yet one-third of nurses still left annually, a

---

[39] Rules, 1895, p. 3. Mrs V. Roberts of Thorpe St Andrew kindly allowed me to examine a hand-copied version of these rules.

[40] AR, 1895, MS, p. 10.

[41] Roughly 7,500 out of 20,000 nurses and attendants nationally held the MPA certificate in 1906, with slightly more women than men. L. Massie, 'The role of women in mental health care in 19th century England', *International History of Nursing Journal*, 1, 2, 1995, pp. 39–51, p. 47.

[42] CVIS, 6 July 1899; AR, 1900, CiL, 12 May 1899.

[43] AR, 1900, CiL, 22 March. Plus matron, 2 assistant matrons, head male attendant, 3

feature which Thomson linked increasingly with the competitive upsurge of poor law and local government board nursing.[44] Reliable nurses were promoted through the ranks and efforts made to retain them. Matron Hamer, employed as a nurse from 1886, had a salary of £100 in 1910. Her assistants, Laura Shulver and Rebecca Wheatley, had similarly commenced in 1893 and 1894 and now had annual salaries of £52.[45] All charge attendants and half of the charge nurses held the MPA certificate by 1907, but nearly half of new qualifiers left that year and overall staff turnover was almost 30 per cent. An improved working environment in the new and refurbished asylums was a modest bonus and deliberate efforts were made to provide a contrasting setting when the new nurses' home was constructed. This utilised different building materials and furnishings and included a tennis court and cycle shed to encourage outdoor pastimes. Accommodation was sufficient for all except the night staff and the 14 required for emergencies. Thomson's rationale, at a time when less than one-third of county asylums possessed such accommodation, was interesting. 'Nurses are most unsuitably housed; they are never free, day or night, from association with the insane and the attendant turmoil and strain, and at night, or when off duty, have not the opportunity for rest and recreation their arduous occupation demands.'[46]

For all these efforts, the Edwardian era witnessed significant price inflation and rates of pay at the asylum, unchanged since 1899, became a source of considerable discontent. Thomson recognised that NCA salary and wage spending per patient was increasing but remained below national levels.[47] Industrial unrest at some asylums in Lancashire marked the formation of the National Asylum Workers' Union in September 1910 and the first campaigns for pay increases, a 70-hour working week and 'a fair trial by the visiting Committee of any member of the staff before dismissal'.[48] Within a year there were over 4,000 members, including a group at the NCA, which delegated G.E. Hopton to the first annual conference in Birmingham in July 1911. Some union demands were incorporated in the 1911 Superannuation Amendment Act and the NCA committee announced 'considerable additions to the pay and the hours off duty of the nurses, attendants and

---

night attendants and 4 night nurses, with an establishment of 47 in the laundry, stores, trades and maintenance etc.

[44] CVIS, 30 Dec. 1899. Of the 33 nurses who left in 1900, 1902, 10 married, 11 obtained other jobs or disliked asylum work, 6 were ill and 6 'unsuitable' or dismissed. Twenty-two probationers failed to complete their three-month term. Based on 1900, 1902 annual reports.

[45] Female staff wages book, 1910–14, SAH 88, 1910.

[46] CVIS, 3 Sept. 1908.

[47] Viz 2s 1d at the NCA (cf. national average of 2s 8d in 1897) and 2s 10d in 1906 (cf. 3s 2d) CVIS, 3 Nov. 1898; AR, 1906, MS, p. 11.

[48] *History of the Mental Hospital and Institutional Workers Union 1910–31*, Manchester, 1931, pp. 12–15.

house servants'.[49] Nurses now earned £20–£38 annually with board, working eight days followed by one and a half day's leave, which could be spent away from the asylum and supplemented with a 1s 9d allowance in lieu of board. Non-emergency 'free time' was granted between 8. p.m. and 10. p.m. and annual leave, linked to years of service, increased between 14 and 21 days. These improvements required more staff, with 57 day and 5 night attendants and 64 day and 8 night nurses in 1913, an average of one per 8.8 patients. Nearly half the NCA attendants and more than one quarter of nurses had been there for five years or more and annual turnover of nurses fell below 20 per cent and of attendants to just 7 per cent in 1914. It was just at this point, with many staff grievances apparently resolved, that practically half of the attendants were lost to war service.

Thomson's initial reforms and zealous approach had possibly curbed staff misbehaviour in the late 1880s and 1890s, those discharged ranging from probationers to the head attendant. Many 'routine' incidents may not have been recorded, but several later ones were detailed. In August 1900 a laundress was dismissed when 'certain articles belonging to the Asylum' were found at her home in Norwich. More seriously, when patient Frederick B— suffered a broken jaw the visitors committee accepted the testimony of four attendants that he was known for 'striking his head against the wall'. But ten months later Walter V— was dismissed for ill-treating a patient and the committee prosecuted him for assault.[50] After a visitor complained that patient Sarah H— had been poorly treated and suffered an injured hip, her daughters made no allegations against the nursing staff in the subsequent inquiry, but suggested that their mother was frequently cold.[51] These were portrayed as isolated incidents and, in a selective interpretation which tempted fate, Thomson even announced the extinction of 'the rough and often brutal "keeper", whose principal qualification for the work was physical strength'.[52]

Patients, illnesses and recoveries

In 1910 the number of patients at the NCA exceeded 1,000 for the first time and the 1910–14 annual average was roughly 350 greater than that for the 1880s, even though the population of rural Norfolk continued to decline. Nationally the expansion of the number and size of asylums has been linked with their reversion to holding and custodial roles, notably in response to 'hereditary taint' and 'degeneration' within the wider population. The experience of poisoning through harmful environment, poor nutrition, or

[49] AR, 1913, Cttee, p. 4.
[50] CVIS, 2 Aug. 1900, 5 Sept. 1901, 5 June 1902. Vincent was fined £2.
[51] ibid., 3 Dec. 1903.
[52] AR, 1906, MS, p. 10.

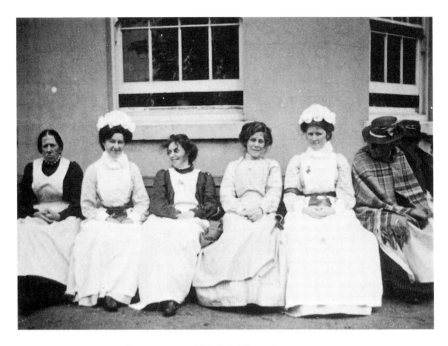

Figure 5.2 Nurses and patients c. 1900 (Middleton)

alcohol abuse was allegedly carried with increasing severity through successive generations, producing irremediable conditions among asylum inmates.[53] Certain family group characteristics were linked with perceived 'national degeneration' in a period of economic uncertainty and fears for imperial security.[54] Hysteria among women was also diagnosed on a much greater scale, providing a medical explanation of gender imbalances within asylums whilst contributing to them.[55] At the NCA Thomson detected hereditary taint in his patients and increasingly referred to it in explaining forms of mental disorder. In contrast, hysteria was rarely diagnosed and the proportion of women patients fell slightly, from a 60 per cent peak in the 1870s, to average 56 per cent from 1900 to 1914.[56]

---

[53] See R.C. Olby, 'Constitutional and hereditary disorders' in W.F. Bynum and R. Porter (eds), *Companion Encyclopedia of the History of Medicine*, Routledge, London, 1993, Vol. 1, pp. 412–37, and J. Goldenstein, 'Psychiatry', Vol. 2, pp. 1350–72.

[54] See G. Searle, *Eugenics and Politics in Britain 1900–14*, Science in History Series, Leyden, 1976; J. Harris, *Private Lives, Public Spirit: Britain 1870–1914*, Penguin, Harmondsworth, 1993, pp. 241–5.

[55] E. Showalter, *The Female Malady: Women, Madness and English Culture*, Virago, London, 1993.

[56] Cf. Showalter, but see J. Busfield, 'The female malady? Men, women and madness in nineteenth-century Britain' in *Sociology*, 28, 1994, pp. 259–77.

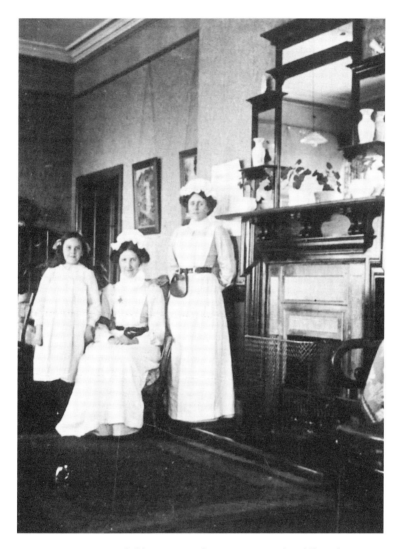

Figure 5.3 Child patient and nurses c. 1900 (Middleton)

Such features might be explained by the asylum's location and the social composition of its patients. For example, the 165 admissions in 1890 consisted of 81 men and 84 women whose age distribution was uniform, with almost as many aged 15–30 years (38) as aged over 60 years (41) and half aged 30–60 years (82). Almost all men had rural occupations, as farm or general labourer, shepherd, gardener, hawker or unemployed, with seven tradesmen and five farmers. Apart from four factory workers, the women were house-wives, had 'no occupation' or were engaged in domestic service. These women had limited access to medical practitioners and were probably

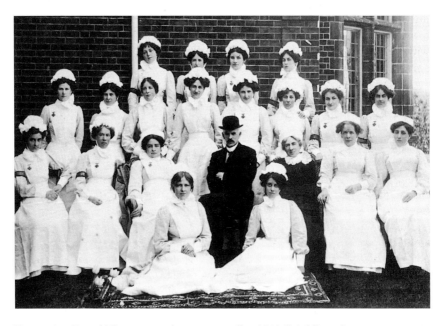

Figure 5.4 David Thomson with nursing staff c. 1910 (Middleton)

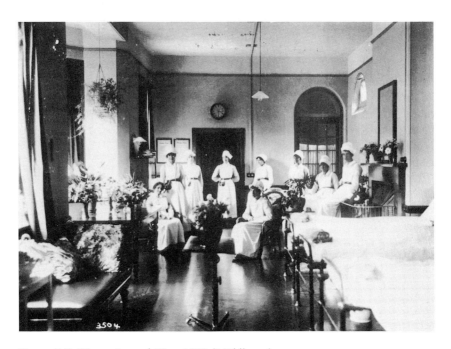

Figure 5.5 Women's ward 10, c. 1900 (Middleton)

unaware of psychiatric consultations. Some 43 per cent of patients were diagnosed with forms of mania, 28 per cent with melancholia and 10 per cent with dementia. Just 6 per cent had congenital defects, similarly with general paralysis cases and most of the remainder were epileptic.[57]

A predominance of 112 women within 188 admissions in 1900 partly reflected insufficient accommodation for male patients: it was less noticeable after new asylum buildings opened in 1903. Although the principal and associated causes of insanity were stated, the largest single category was still 'unknown', followed by 'hereditary' factors, 'other bodily disease' and old age. Other 'physical' causes included noticeably few examples of male intemperance and four cases of sunstroke, reflecting characteristics of rural working life in Norfolk. 'Moral' cases comprised the minority but a feminised one: women were referred to in nine-tenths of 'domestic' causes and exclusively under 'love affairs (including seduction)'.[58] The 236 patients admitted in 1910 came from similar social backgrounds to those of 1900 or 1890 and 55 per cent were female. Their disorders, grouped under similar headings, included proportionately fewer cases of epilepsy (4 per cent), general paralysis (4 per cent) or dementia (9 per cent). Under a reclassification of the causes of insanity the 'uncertain' category covered 25 per cent of admissions, as did 'heredity'. 'Stress' applied in 20 per cent of cases, alcoholism in 10 per cent, with senility, 'puerperal state' and 'climacteric' the remaining features affecting more than 4 per cent of admissions.[59]

This overview confirms the increasing importance attached to hereditary features by 1910 but also Norfolk's low levels of alcohol-related illness, general paralysis and epilepsy, each associated with the degeneration thesis. More women than men were admitted, but the disparity was not widening and new 'catch-all' terminology was not yet deployed. Great uncertainty concerning the causes of mental disorders remained and the extent to which admissions or discharges were determined on purely medical criteria is questionable. For example, NCA annual admissions averaged 181 in the years 1900-02 but leapt to 318 in 1903 as new asylum buildings opened. The number of men and women discharged 'not improved' averaged 9 and 14 respectively between 1900 and 1910 but the 1905 totals alone were 48 and 42. Variance in such figures suggests some element of restocking and clearing of the asylum, involving other county institutions and the physical transfer of patients. Concepts of insanity, the corresponding needs and location of the insane were also elasticated, a feature vividly demonstrated during the Great War but evidently applicable in non-emergency situations.

---

[57] AR, 1890, admissions tables, p. 25. Four people were diagnosed 'not insane'.

[58] AR, 1900, admissions, p. 26. The social composition of patients was largely unchanged but included 4 soldiers, 3 nurses, 2 bookmakers and a surgeon. Moral causes constituted one quarter of those attributed.

[59] AR, 1910, admissions, p. 24.

Although Thomson's annual reports focused upon the causes of insanity and their implications, the possibilities for asylum patients, and the comparatively good record of patient recoveries achieved, he took every opportunity to enhance the asylum's financial position. His approach to the apparently random causes of insanity was predicated upon underlying features which made some people more vulnerable than others. Thus, 'intemperance, childbirth, ill-health, domestic trouble and anxiety can only produce insanity in minds predisposed to it by hereditary taint, for surely these causes are rife around us without causing insanity'.[60] He also felt that poor physical health was responsible for perhaps one quarter of mental disorders and appears to have drawn upon humoural theory in linking liver and heart disease with depression, or over-stimulation with epilepsy. This may also explain his three-month experiment in 1891, in which he confined epileptic patients to a vegetarian diet, 'with no appreciable results'.[61] Predisposition and humoural elements were offered in explanation of why men were likely to have maniacal symptoms and, whereas 'half the women suffered from melancholia . . . in the men less than one-third suffered from this form of insanity'.[62]

Later Thomson looked to poisoning of the central nervous system by toxins from disordered nutrition (alcohol) or sexual excesses (syphilis), again in 'those predisposed by hereditary defect'. Alcohol featured in one-twelfth of NCA admissions, half the national average, and the incidence of general paralysis and epilepsy was comparatively low. Yet he insisted that hereditary taint was the great understated feature, though 'brain degeneration in old age' might account for 15 per cent of insanity.[63] By 1905 his analysis was shot through with eugenicist ideas and the most authoritarian of recommendations. 'Pending further research', he suggested that:

> half the amount of occurring insanity is due to hereditary defect and could be prevented by rendering infertile and incapable of producing tainted progeny anyone who became a person certified to be of unsound mind. Nature's methods of doing this are so slow . . . and we try to prevent them by preserving the unfit . . . perpetuating the vicious circle and adding to the already great burden of insanity borne by the race.[64]

There was little consideration of individual minds here and Thomson overtly opposed 'wasting any more time among the quagmires and pure will-o'-the-wisps of pure psychology'.[65] His prognosis that perhaps fifty of the remaining patients in 1887 were curable indicated a phlegmatic, traditional emphasis

---

[60] AR, 1889, MS, p. 10.
[61] AR, 1891, MS, p. 13.
[62] AR, 1889, MS, p. 10.
[63] AR, 1902, MS, p. 10.
[64] AR, 1905, MS, p. 9.
[65] AR, 1906, MS, p. 8.

upon the basics of care, work therapy, exercise and modest comforts for the others. He was also sceptical concerning the widespread use of drugs in treatments, as these 'merely modify a symptom and do not prevent the malady running its course'.[66] However, Thomson was less conventional in arguing that the aged and physically infirm should also be cared for within the asylum environment. Indeed,

> unlike most of my professional bretheren . . . I consider that the County Asylum is the only place where such cases can be properly dealt with . . . they tax all the special resources . . . of accommodation and skilled staff, and cannot . . . be treated in any kind of institution other than an Asylum.[67]

Patient case books for the period reveal sad and tragic lives and medical staff tendencies to associate observations with family histories. Even tenuous linkages produced classifications such as 'hereditary', 'congenital' or combinations such as 'hereditary; melancholia' or 'hereditary (menopause)', with little subsequent comment before 'transfer to chronic book'. Arthur G—, an 'idiot from birth' with a club foot, was 'troublesome and destructive' to his family and was admitted aged 6 years in 1878. Over 41 years his two entries were 'hobbles about wonderfully' and 'a slobbering idiotic creature, untidy & slovenly, is unemployable'. Mabel C—, 'hereditary (epileptic)' was 7 years old when admitted in 1908. She was 'inoffensive . . . simply chatters in an imbecile way . . . is a great favourite on the ward' and 'adds to cheeriness on the ward', but her repeated falls required stitching and no cause was given, apart from 'some pyrexia, temperature', for her death five years later. Caroline A—, aged 23 and suffering from depression, would not take care of herself and was force-fed. She subsequently improved but refused to work and was diagnosed 'chronic dementia'. Showing signs of tuberculosis, she was given extra diet and cod liver oil but died in May 1896, aged 35 years. Mary B— had threatened her husband and children and was five months pregnant when admitted but was diagnosed 'hereditary; melancholia'. She was reluctant to eat and was treated with sulphur for constipation, then given sedatives after her husband's visit made her 'restless'. She had a premature delivery and died four days later of 'exhaustion'.[68]

Christmas S—, aged 53 and a fisherman, had already experienced Yarmouth workhouse and Norwich gaol before he was admitted, diagnosed with 'dementia'. With delusions that 'he has been fighting all over the world, that he has a silver plate in his skull . . . that he has his coat covered in medals', he also fought patients, attendants and asylum hygiene. After his

[66] AR, 1891, MS, p. 12.
[67] AR, 1900, MS, p. 8.
[68] Case Books (from admission date); A.G. 1878–1915, SAH 268; M.C. 1908–13, SAH 296; C.A. 1884–96, SAH 271; M.B. 1887, SAH 285.

escape and recapture, Thomson 'ordered a low diet for punishment'. A year later S— had a stroke and was subsequently described as a general paralysis case, 'being roused only for a few minutes on the administration of a nutrient enema'. Little could be done for Noah L— or Alfred F—, middle-aged men suffering from dementia and general paralysis, who died within months of admission, or for Charles K— and William H—, both in such 'feeble health on arrival' that they died within days. The deaths of Susanna P— (56) and John C— (66) were associated with exhaustion from 'recurrent mania' and 'mania/ hereditary' respectively, whereas the 'acute mania' of farmer Robert G— (45) was associated with 'depression of business'.[69]

Ellen H—, just 15 years old and affected by amenorrhoea, was admitted and diagnosed, somewhat curiously, as 'mania/change of life' in January 1894 and died within four months. However, considerable efforts were made to save Ethel D—, aged 19 years and also a domestic servant suffering from amenorrhoea. Diagnosed 'hereditary (ill health)', she was provided with extra diet and special attention and given nightly chloral draughts to curb her restlessness. She developed scarlet fever and was nursed in the isolation block; her peeling skin condition was treated with olive oil and eucalyptus. After five months she was settled and eating better, 'rather simple in her manner but quite orderly and industrious' and was successfully discharged after a trial period in August 1908. In contrast, Alice G—, aged 28, received very little treatment before her discharge. With a previous history of depression, 'stays in bed till midday . . . fits of temper and swears', 'the prospect of getting married seemed to excite her and upset her mentally', hence the diagnosis 'previous attack (love affairs)'. A few months later she was working in the laundry and left after a successful trial period in June 1908.[70]

Two other case histories illustrate unpredictable exceptions to the idea of long-term confinement. The omens for Arthur B— were not good: he was born in a workhouse, suffered from epilepsy and was considered 'rebellious and violent'. Transferred to the asylum at the age of 20 in 1884 he was then given 'mixt. epilept' with some success, but his violent outbursts led to periods 'in seclusion on a low diet' and confinement in bed. A settled spell working as a painter ended in a drunken escape attempt on parole, but his selection for the asylum football team marked a rapid improvement. For several years he constantly requested discharge and appeals to the lunacy commissioners finally succeeded in 1899. B—'s regular medication, work and sports contrasted with Rosa C—'s asylum experience. After five months' treatment for 'melancholia and stupor', she was readmitted in 1907, still only 17 years old. She was given thyroid extract and worked for a time as a maid,

[69] ibid., C.S. 1884–8, SAH 271; N.L., A.F., C.K., W.H., R.G. and J.C. all 1894, SAH 273/1; S.P. 1894, SAH 288.
[70] ibid., E.H. 1894, SAH 288; E.D. and A.G. 1907–8, SAH 296.

but then became excited and noisy. Over the next five years, she had 'galvanism applied to hands for hysteria' on three occasions, respectively following a violent episode, escape and suicide attempts. She was regularly sedated, spent long periods confined to bed, was allowed home to visit her mother, and twice put in strong clothing in the padded room. By February 1912 she was 'very depressed . . . asked for battery but was refused as the last course did no good'. Having exhausted her options, Rosa either simply accepted work or saw this as her remaining strategy: she was 'much brighter and daily employed' in December and left 'recovered' in April 1913.[71]

NCA treatment books for the period are dominated by first aid for cut lips, septic fingers and bruised foreheads. Diagnosis of 'cancer of stomach', the reporting of suicide, or the calling in of the consultant surgeon to trepan a patient following an accident were rare events. Empty spaces within their standard page format confirm the small numbers of general paralysis or epileptic cases under continuous treatment compared with cramped, over-spilling entries for more recent or acute mania. Fractures, accidents, instances of erysipelas were highlighted, presumably for their compilation in annual reports, as with falls, whether accidental, during fits, 'struggle with patient X' or occasionally, 'struggle with nurses'. In the early 1900s there were five or six annual instances of an accident, fall or attack by a fellow patient resulting in broken limbs, with a similar number of escapes. Other regular specifics included maniacal excitement, epileptic seizure, 'loose bowels', debility, weak heart and TB, but Elizabeth C—'s 'hysteria' was rare and 'neurasthenia' was not reported.[72]

The 1890 Act (section 40) limited use of mechanical restraint to the prevention of self-injury or harm by a patient to others, under constant supervision and visits by a medical officer. In most years solitary entries were made, although particular individuals might be restrained on several occasions: in 1891 a woman patient with a cut throat was bandaged in tight sheets for 33 hours altogether.[73] These official records should be considered alongside the more regular use of seclusion, occasional accusations made by patients to lunacy commissioners, staff dismissals for misconduct and some doubtful electric 'treatments', exposed in 1909. However, Thomson did encourage visitors and poor law officials to the asylum and 'their' patients, with limited success.[74]

---

[71] ibid., A.B. 1884–99, SAH 271; R.C. 1907–13, SAH 296.

[72] Treatment Book, July 1908–April 1915, SAH 240. Only one suicide (5 March 1911) was recorded.

[73] Register of mechanical restraint, 1894–1915, SAH 202. Lunacy commissioners inspected and signed the register and referred to the lack of such restraint at the NCA (e.g. 22 March 1900).

[74] When Thomson arrived there were years where no Norfolk poor law union visited or inspected. In the early 1900s about one-third did so regularly and, by 1910, one half.

Table 5.1 Patient numbers resident, admissions, recoveries and mortality, 1880–1914

	Aver. no. resident			Admissions			% admitted recovered			Mortality %		
	Total	M	F	Total	M	F	Total	M	F	Total	M	F
1880–89	692	291	401	170	76	94	42.3	38.2	45.7	9.9	11.2	9.0
1890–99	778	327	451	191	82	109	36.9	35.7	38.3	10.3	12.1	9.0
1900–09	925	402	523	224	103	121	33.7	31.4	38.2	10.9	12.5	9.8
1910–14	1,035	453	582	225	103	122	31.5	28.1	34.4	11.2	11.4	11.0

Note: The percentage of admissions 'relieved' was 3.8 per cent 1890–99, 5.3 per cent 1900–09 and 5.6 per cent 1910–14.

A downward trend in the percentage of patient recoveries by 1914 was not offset by greater numbers discharged 'relieved'. Mortality levels were stationary and tended to increase from 1900. These features reflect an increasing proportion of longer-term patients, including transferees from Norfolk workhouses, and the 'outcounty' cases accepted as the NCA expanded. Improving recovery rates in the late 1880s varied between 46 and 52 per cent, ahead of the 40 per cent national asylum average. Thomson's claim that 'this maintains the reputation of this Asylum for a high recovery rate' was optimistic, as results possibly reflected the low proportion of general paralysis and epileptic cases at the NCA.[75] Over the whole period 1887–1914 between 75 and 90 per cent of those recovering did so within twelve months of admission, though 33 to 50 per cent of deaths were recorded among this group. This illustrates the multi-faceted asylum: as a hospital treating patients with acute forms of illness, some of whom were also physically very sick; and as a long-term residence for chronic patients whose bodily health also varied.

Like his predecessor, Thomson linked levels of recovery or death with a large proportion of 'manifestly incurable' patients and offered selective statistical commentaries, even allowing for annual fluctuations. Thus the 1901 figure of 49 per cent was indicative of 'our normally high recovery rate . . . 12% higher than the 1901 average rate in English county asylums', although it exceeded the NCA's own 1890–1900 average by almost as much (see Table 5.1).[76] Before the 1903 reorganisation deaths from bronchitis and pneumonia were associated with elderly patients and low temperatures on some wards and corridors. Typhoid fever and dysentery fatalities around 1890 also suggest serious sanitary problems then. Apart from particular outbreaks, for example influenza in 1890, diphtheria in 1894 and erysipelas in 1907, more post-mortem examinations confirmed tuberculosis and 'chest or lung

[75] AR, 1888, MS, p. 10; 1890, MS, p. 10.
[76] AR, 1902, MS, p. 10.

infections' as major killers. In 1910, for example, they caused one-third of the 117 deaths, with one-sixth from senile decay, one-tenth from heart disease and similarly from general paralysis.[77] The amount of long-term illness also helps to explain why improving standards in the modernised asylum had no immediate impact upon patient mortality.

Work and exercise, especially outdoors, were still seen as critical to improved health, better rest and tranquillity on the wards. Efforts to re-establish a cricket field and to extend boundary walks raised the proportion of working male patients to two-thirds in 1889. Up to three-quarters became involved when earthworks or clearing up was necessary, as with the new roadway in 1900 or the recreation hall and stores in 1910. Most of the 250 male working patients did these tasks, farming or gardening, but 50 were ward helpers and 20 or so were in the repair shops. By 1910 the latter employed over 30, with the upholsterers producing six hair mattresses per week and the shoe and tailoring shops also repairing footballs, 'football knickers', boots and cricket pads. Over 90 men were in farm gangs and three worked in the new bakery. Both sexes helped on their respective wards and kitchens but the laundry became an exclusively female zone after a woman patient became pregnant there in 1888. Her partner played no role, at least in Thomson's explanation, as 'the woman was of an erotic temperament, single and . . . had two illegitimate children'.[78] This early example of a 'dangerous woman' was marginalised and the three-quarters of women patients who worked were restricted to indoor ward help, cleaning, needlework, and the laundry or kitchens. Only the laundry patients were allowed the additional 'outdoor' bread and cheese and 'female' 9oz portions of pie or dumpling and 8oz of vegetables compared with the respective 'male' 10oz and 12oz amounts.[79]

References to patients' entertainment and activities focused upon highlights shared by relatively small numbers and the few initiatives undertaken before the new recreation hall opened hint at dull routine. Excursions to Cromer and Lowestoft were reinstated in 1889 and parties went to the circus and on river trips and picnics, the latter enjoyed by 200 annually in the early 1900s. Roughly one-third of patients regularly attended concerts, dances and film shows with coffee and cake. Gilbert and Sullivan nights, introduced in 1907 'with the help of some Norwich friends', reached larger audiences in the new hall, with weekly film shows and whist drives now standard features. Perhaps Thomson found food for thought after he was 'struck by the capacity of quite imbecile patients to learn and play whist'.[80] An outdoor asylum fair was added to sports day and, in well-organised

---

[77] AR, 1910, Deaths, p. 21.
[78] AR, 1888, MS, p. 11.
[79] AR, 1900, Dietary, p. 30. Extra soup on Saturday was possible part-compensation for such refinements.
[80] AR, 1907, MS, p. 10; 1910, MS, p. 15; 1913, MS, p. 10.

sporting fixtures, cricketers were more successful than footballers.[81] But male team games offered only spectator roles or inadvertent leisure for women, who were otherwise restricted to walking, ironically 'to make up for the want of out-door employment'.[82] 'Daily walks in and beyond the Asylum estate . . . in fairer weather' were taken by 400 patients by 1890 and still more had weekly walks beyond the enlarged post-1900 estate. Recreation in the grounds and gardens was the standby, although a consistent 15 per cent of able patients remained within the airing courts.[83]

The chapel harvest festival was usually the best-attended event as seating capacity here was ample. Patients' religious needs were met by two Sunday Anglican services and one for up to a hundred Nonconformists, held on a larger ward. However, 'there are so few Roman Catholic patients that no regular service is held . . . a priest visits the sick when required'.[84] Lunacy commissioners monitoring these events and patient attendance were concerned at shortages of 'an interesting kind of literature'. There was 'still the need of more amusing books . . . bibles, prayer books, hymn books are furnished in abundance . . . old theological treatises and some religious works form the bulk of the library'.[85]

Asylum finances

Thomson and the committee of visitors matched their predecessors' attention to asylum finances and self-sufficiency. Substantial capital investments were presented as county assets and justified as long-term efficiency gains quite as much as therapeutic advantage or patient comfort. Annual reports detailed the capabilities of the boiler house and laundry and the 1903 reorganisation was equated with modernisation, though it was much concerned with reshuffling the existing building stock and sexual segregation. Similarly with the nurses' home: Thomson's proposal began with the overcrowding on female wards and the need to maintain contracts for outcounty patients. Unlike ward blocks, a nurses' home would liberate beds throughout the women's asylum without the need for more staff. As a capital project, it could be financed 'from the profit made on the Yarmouth patients' and was, therefore, 'soundest both from a financial and administrative point

---

[81] Thirteen full cricket matches were played in 1888, 20 in 1889 and at least 20 in 1891. Football, organised from 1889, began with 10 games. In 1906 the asylum cricket team won 17 and drew 5 of 33 matches played, the football team winning 7 and drawing 3 of 28 games played. AR, 1906, MS, p. 10.

[82] AR, 1888, MS, p. 10.

[83] AR, 1900, CiL, 22 March p. 15; 1910, MS, p. 15.

[84] *Eastern Daily Press*, 18 Sept. 1903.

[85] CVIS (CiL inspection), 12 May 1899.

of view'.[86] Descriptions of the recreation hall and stores recognised patients' contributions and likely benefits, but 'work therapy' was increasingly replaced by overt discussion of patient labour, self-sufficiency, and contributions to earnings or savings in asylum budgets.[87] Thomson also obtained personal control over the functioning and administration of the NCA. Arguments that new plant required new skills signalled the replacement of Charles Cannell, the engineer for 36 years, by Robert Humes, nominated by and responsible to Thomson. Unsuccessful in merging the posts of engineer and clerk of works, Thomson still obtained control over staff, works and materials featured in building accounts, subject to formal consultation with the county surveyor.[88] He could therefore integrate the planning and working of the NCA, as an institution and an economic entity.

Table 5.2 indicates principal features and trends in maintenance accounts to 1914. Income tended to exceed expenditure, not least because of earnings from outcounty and private patients and, from 1900, a greater contribution from the asylum farm. Control over provisions may reflect the farm's success and the costing of farm-supplied food, at 7d per head in the 1900s compared to 3s 5d for other foodstuffs, suggests hidden subsidies.[89] Post-1900 reductions in clothing, furnishings and bedding were probably temporary and reflected building work, which included new furnishings and equipment charged to capital accounts. A growing staff of nurses and attendants employed at improving rates of pay clearly required more resources, as did the reduction in working hours in 1911. Medical officers' salaries featured less prominently, not least because the dispenser was substituted for a fourth doctor. Spending on 'necessaries' was also broadly contained: 'miscellaneous' items are difficult to account for but 'profit on private patients' featured in 'expenditure' because this was transferred from maintenance to building accounts.

The weekly cost per patient averaged 9 shillings in the decade to 1897 and 10 shillings over the next decade, reaching a peak of 11s 8d in 1903.[90] Charges to Norfolk poor law unions had partly been offset by direct subsidy from outcounty or private patient charges (see Chapter 4), but the 1890 Act prohibited the direct cross-subsidy of patients or county ratepayers. This had considerable implications for the NCA financial strategy, although longer-term subsidies could still be achieved via the supplementation of asylum building accounts. Outcounty admissions in 1891 included 20 Suffolk and 16

---

[86] ibid. (MS on overcrowding), 25 Aug. 1908.

[87] New Buildings Account 1876–1912, SAH 355. Minor repairs 1887–1900 averaged £1,150 annually, overwhelmingly on piecework payments to listed tradesmen. These may have included labourers' wages, or patient labour may have been provided.

[88] J.B. Poutney, the asylum bandleader, was Clerk of Works 1889–1912, and P. Hansell Clerk to Justices, CVIS 1875–1913. The county surveyor remained in a consulting authority but Thomson had secured control. CVIS, 29 July, 4 Sept. and 29 Nov. 1902.

[89] AR, 1906, table of costs, p. 59.

[90] ibid., MS, p. 11.

Table 5.2 Income and expenditure at the Norfolk County Asylum by principal items in maintenance accounts, 1890–1910

	1890	1900	1910	1914
Net annual income	£17,637	£23,637	£34,741	£34,789
(% from outcounty, private patients)	4.8	10.5	16.5	16.6
(% from farm*)	3.4	5.0	10.2	5.3
Expenditure items (%)	£17,980	£23,629	£28,880	£35,336
Provisions	47.9	37.2	36.7	37.3
(of which farm*)	(4.2)	(3.4)	(5.2)	(7.7)
Salaries – medical officers	7.9	7.2	8.5	7.7
– nursing	12.5	13.7	18.5	19.6
Necessaries (fuel, soap, etc.)	12.4	14.1	14.3	14.0
Clothing	7.0	7.0	4.6	3.3
Furnishing/bedding	4.7	4.7	3.3	3.6
Drugs, etc.	0.9	0.8	0.9	1.0
Profit on private patients	1.8	0.6	5.9	4.1
Miscellaneous	5.2	6.3	6.9	

Note: Income excludes any previous balance from the previous year and expenditure excludes any balance carried forward to the following year.

Source: Annual Reports.

* See discussion of farm contribution below.

London County Council patients, each charged at 14 shillings weekly or 4s 8d above the 9s 4d Norfolk charge. Temporary transfers also arose from building work or overcrowding at other asylums but the prospect of overcrowding within the NCA threatened these lucrative additions. This featured prominently in Thomson's efforts to reorganise the NCA and to maximise its patient capacity. In 1900 he stated plainly that the 37 Middlesex local county council women patients, resident at the NCA for five years, represented a surplus over costs of £3,307. In token exchange Norfolk had three boys at the 'special idiot department of Middlesex County Asylum, there being no suitable accommodation or educational training for such cases in this Asylum'. Similarly the return of 40 Hertfordshire County Asylum patients relieved NCA overcrowding but Thomson lamented, 'their three years residence . . . yielded a profit of £2,176/5/11d to this County'.[91]

Given previous expansion the inclusion of spare capacity in the 1903 rebuilding was a sensible planning decision, but the opportunity for additional revenues undoubtedly featured. Great Yarmouth county borough agreed in December 1902 to transfer its patients from Ipswich and to place

[91] AR, 1900, MS, p. 11.

new ones at the NCA. The net increase of 130 patients at the NCA between 1902 and 1904 reflected the addition of 142 outcounty patients, 60 from Middlesex and 82 from Yarmouth. When 20 male patients arrived 'under contract' from Essex in 1906, Thomson saw therapeutic benefits, since 'they occupy our vacant beds and yield us a substantial profit, and further the infusion of urban residents among our almost exclusively rural and agricultural residents has had an enlivening and brightening effect'.[92] As with his remarks upon the convenience of visiting patients, plausible for Yarmouth but not for Middlesex- or Essex-based relatives, he was being selective. Much depended upon the form of these patients' illnesses and the greater incidence of general paralysis and tuberculous 'urban' patients may also have featured in increased NCA mortality rates.

With strong poor law associations, the asylum rarely attracted private patients but examples like Emma M—, found to have private means in August 1902, or those with friends willing to pay were transferred to private status within the NCA. In 1910 16 such patients were charged between 14 shillings and 31s 6d weekly and 135 outcounty boarders at 14 shillings or 15 shillings. Combined, these fees exceeded £5,700, compared to the regular Norfolk income of £25,400 that year. Profits from them, averaging £1,700 in the period 1910–13, were transferred to the building account, where they represented over 26 per cent of spending on asylum repairs, money not required from Norfolk ratepayers.[93]

Another substantial contribution came from the asylum farm. Annual fluctuations between asylum and general market sales suggested continuing efforts to maximise farm earnings for the asylum and total sales almost doubled over the 1890s, exceeding £2,000 by 1900. Farm accounts now included livestock valuations and their adjustment affected annual balances but surpluses averaged £250.[94] Industrial quantities of vegetables were grown annually: 60–70 tons of potatoes, with other root crops, 25,000 cabbages but also lettuce, broccoli and green beans. Substantial quantities of apples, plums and redcurrants contributed to the asylum dietary but who ate the 800lb of berry fruit produced in 1899 or the peaches and nectarines was unclear.[95] Allowing for price increases in the early 1900s, farm activities still increased substantially. Livestock was valued at over £2,000 in 1910 and £2,500 four years later and 800 pigs and 400 sheep were sold annually. General sales exceeded £3,550, with further direct sales to the asylum of £1,500 but, in further demonstration of sensibility to market prices, these proportions were reversed by 1914, with general sales worth £1,900 and asylum sales exceeding

---

[92] AR, 1903, MS, p. 10.
[93] Based on AR, 1910–13, financial tables.
[94] e.g. in 1892 asylum sales were £957 and general sales £260 whereas in 1894 the respective figures were £470 and £1,000.
[95] Farm Records 1892–9, SAH 110.

£3,900. In so far as the asylum made farm purchases at less than market rates and collected an annual 'presumed rent', it received additional subsidies.[96]

Although NCA finances were sound, its governing body and its reputation were briefly scandalised. The immediate origins seemed innocuous: two attendants were investigated on suspicion of taking food in 1908 and related inquiries revealed irregularities in stores and provisions accounts. Police searches revealed that a number of married attendants took home their rations, which they felt entitled to do, but two employees of the meat contractor were caught leaving the asylum with meat. They were prosecuted and sentenced to prison but the asylum committee divided over its response to further allegations concerning the removal or non-delivery of asylum goods. A majority and Thomson himself were unaware that a local solicitor and his agent were investigating matters more thoroughly. They supported an internal inquiry, open to the lunacy commissioners and held on 10 March 1909. The storekeeper, butcher, kitchen gardener and gatekeeper were charged with pilfering or collusion with contracting suppliers, but only the butcher was dismissed.[97] Meanwhile, a minority secured support from Norfolk County Council for a direct investigation by the lunacy commission itself and at a three-day inquiry, held in private from 17–19 May, wider allegations were made. These centred upon the behaviour of the committee, which 'lacked unanimity, firmness and directness' and was 'too lenient' on the personnel previously investigated.[98] New regulations, including stock and accounts inspections by independent outsiders, the separation of functions between storekeeper and clerk, and the reorganisation of central stores, became operative in 1910.[99]

Still more alarming was the alleged mistreatment of patients and use of galvanic batteries by the medical staff. Thomson argued that such applications were always given as treatments but conceded that he did not give special sanction and that they 'may have been applied to a patient for violence to an Attendant'. Medical officers applied the battery 'to patients capable of exercising self-control to deter them from dirty, violent, destructive and erotic practices . . . as treatment, and not as punishment'. Dr Law supplied a list of 20 women patients so treated over the previous three years, 'with the reasons for the application'. Dr Gavin merely listed 25 male patients: immediately afterwards he took his annual leave and obtained a similar post in York. When the commissioners allowed patients to give evidence 'without being overheard . . . most said they were sure it had been

---

[96] Based on AR, 1910–14, Farm and garden account. In addition to conventional rent and rates the farm paid an annual 'presumed rent' of £160 on asylum-owned land.

[97] CVIS, Oct. 1906–Dec. 1914, SAH 14, 17 Oct. and 7 Nov. 1908.

[98] Medical Superintendent's Journal, Feb. 1903–Feb. 1915, SAH 134 (CiL Inquiry, 3 July 1909).

[99] AR, 1908, MS, p. 10; 1909, MS, p. 10.

given to them in the way of treatment, not of punishment, several adding voluntarily that they did not think the doctors would do such a thing as to punish them'. However, patient C.S. 'had it three times. I think it was for breaking things up. It hurt me . . . I used to think it was for strengthening my nerves but now I think it was for punishment . . . Nurse S has been very kind to me since'.[100] Concluding that some usage was 'perilously near to punishment and . . . might open the way to the gravest abuses', the commissioners insisted upon full recording of any electrical treatment in consultation with the medical superintendent, and rules relating to medical procedure were duly changed.[101]

Major investigations exert strong pressure for accurate inventories and the 1910 NCA accounts were detailed to the last of 1,640 lemons or 150,147lbs of meat consumed. This may have been an exceptional year in terms of income from outcounty patients and farm surpluses, though there are no obvious indications. Whether through economies of scale or consequent upon modernisation, the asylum authorities – chiefly Thomson himself – had pared average weekly patient costs to 10s 2d. This comprised four shillings on food, three shillings to cover staff costs, 1s 7d for fuel and amenities, with sixpence for clothing, four and a half pence for furnishings and bedding and one pence for medicines. Spending on leisure amenities, entertainment, tobacco was a fraction of the nine pence allowed for miscellaneous items, almost half of which comprised local rates paid by the NCA. Meanwhile, 'Norfolk' weekly charges were set at 11s 1d. This suggests a considerable surplus on maintenance accounts but Norfolk agencies and ratepayers provided only 73 per cent of the NCA total income. Building accounts depended almost entirely upon the county council and local government board loans, but were augmented from the NCA's own operations. In financial terms the asylum was in good condition, to Thomson's credit, and making considerable headway as 'a going concern'. This may also explain why the asylum authorities later insisted upon control over its administration and finances, though not the patients, when it became a war hospital.

With the nurses' home completed, the NCA had 1,070 beds available from 1910. During the next three years patient numbers averaged 1,040 and the male asylum already had eight more patients than its stated capacity of 460. Such overcrowding seems surprising and partly reflected outcounty patients: 25 Great Yarmouth patients were transferred away early in 1914. The question of child patients was ignored, but there were then 9 girls and 13 boys at the asylum, the two smallest boys in the women's asylum because of overcrowding. Like his predecessor, Thomson looked to 'the removal of the Defective Children . . . to some other institution, more suitable for their care and training', as recommended by the lunacy commissioners and encouraged

---

[100] MS Journal, 3 July 1909.
[101] MS Journal, 2 Sept. 1909.

for adults under the 1913 Mental Deficiency Acts and for children under the 1914 Elementary Education Act.[102]

These difficulties were overlooked when the asylum celebrated its centenary on 10 May 1914 and in July hosted the annual conference of the Medico Psychological Association, which honoured Thomson as its President. His address, reprinted in the *Journal of Mental Science*, provided a whiggish account of improvements in professional practice and at Thorpe over the century. The 'dismal madhouse' had become 'a hospital for mental disorders, with all that the word hospital implies, in bright surroundings, light, air, sanitation and skilled attendance and nursing'.[103] Professional colleagues noted that the NCA was now the oldest extant public asylum and saw Thomson's achievement as its 'successful conversion . . . into one comparing favourably with the most modern of mental hospitals'.[104]

A substantial kernel of truth informed these pleasantries. Improvements at the NCA stemmed from Thomson's planning and direct involvement. He had begun the reform of nursing and was a 'pioneer in introducing a system of training and examinations for the nurses of mental hospitals'.[105] Yet significant problems had been revealed in 1909 and staff conditions had been addressed in the light of trade union activity and national pressures. More striking was the assumption that building improvements were an indicator of patients' health and well-being. The recreation hall would be a valuable amenity but there were few others beyond the sports field. Films were the major novelty for patients, who may have wondered whether there was more to life than work, inside or outside the asylum. And if Thomson was not responsible for perceptions of a well-regulated asylum in terms of church attendance, non-use of mechanical restraint or financial order, he did not criticise such yardsticks.

Latterly Thomson has been portrayed as the diligent medical super-intendent, not given to trumpeting his successes but quick to instigate practical reforms; one among those involved in 'rousing the conscience' of county authorities for financial and legislative support.[106] The description is recognisable, though Thomson's relationship with Norfolk County Council often centred upon his own role and wishes, presented as synonymous with

---

[102] AR, 1914, Cttee, p. 3, MS, p. 7.

[103] D.G.Thomson, 'Presidential address on the progress of psychiatry during the past hundred years, together with the history of Norfolk County Asylum during the same period', *Journal of Mental Science*, 1914, 60, pp. 541–72. The conference was held at the Guildhall, Norwich, and also included a reception at Norwich City Asylum, Hellesdon.

[104] AR, 1914, Cttee, cited p. 4.

[105] A. Rotherham, Board of Control inspector on his visit to the hospital in 1922.

[106] T. Turner, 'Public profile of the Medico-Psychological Association c. 1851–1914' in G. Berrios and H. Freeman (eds), *150 Years of British Psychiatry 1841–1991*, Gaskell, London, 1991, pp. 3–16. Thomson attempted the first demonstration of X-ray equipment at the Norfolk and Norwich Hospital.

patients' interests. His medical work suggests few affinities with patients as individuals, however, and he was increasingly preoccupied with questions of hereditary taint and national degeneration. Indeed, this aspect of Thomson's professional life reveals, arguably, how culturally constructed knowledge of 'race degeneration' influenced and in turn gained credence from appropriate professional and scientific opinion.[107] This episode in Thomson's career was abruptly ended by the onset of war, which placed new demands upon his organisational abilities. Almost as Thomson and the NCA had achieved a national profile, the asylum was required for military use during the war emergency. Its transformation as the Norfolk War Hospital produced a new public identity and featured in the unreported but life-threatening wartime history of asylum patients.

---

[107] The parallel example, involving women and hysteria, is less obvious at the NCA, however.

6

Two histories: the Norfolk War Hospital, 1915–19

The Norfolk County Asylum's centenary *Annual Report* noted that, although the institution was the oldest provincial public asylum in constant use, much of the physical fabric was new or had been renovated, 'comparing favourably with the most modern of mental hospitals'.[1] Like many other medical superintendents Thomson presented the institution as a community aiming for greater self-reliance and, increasingly, as 'a hospital for the mind'.[2] If less directly involved with individual patients, he sought to improve their physical environment and comfort and had improved nurse training and nursing standards. Correspondents for the *Journal of Mental Science*, visiting to mark the centenary, 'could not desire a better illustration of the march of modern ideas as to the treatment of insanity than to walk through the wards of the Norfolk County Asylum'.[3]

Attempts to continue in this progressive vein were disrupted by the Great War, which resulted in the evacuation of almost all the existing patients and the physical conversion of the asylum into a military hospital under War Office control. Key personnel associated with the asylum remained, providing some continuity, but most were faced with major and demanding challenges late in their professional lives and had little time remaining for peacetime reconversion.

Such work, as will be seen, involved fundamental changes. Existing accounts, based upon Thomson's own record, recognise the scale of the effort involved and present this in patriotic fashion but they are incomplete. Wartime changes also involved the partial reconstruction or different perceptions of mental illness and a significant proportion of the evacuated NCA patients had traumatic experiences, which for some ended tragically. A subordination of asylum facilities and staff to the war effort, along with subtleties in administrative and financial arrangements seeking to preserve the position of the asylum, are also noteworthy. The limited public recording of such features restricts a comprehensive view but it is possible to demonstrate the varying experiences of patients and staff and stark contrasts

---

[1] Annual Reports (AR), 1906–21, SAH 32; 1914, Cttee, p. 4.
[2] D.G. Thomson, 'Presidential address', *Journal of Mental Science*, LX, 1914, pp. 541–72 and see his obituary, *Journal of Mental Science*, LXIX, 1923.
[3] 'Occasional notes', *Journal of Mental Science*, LXI, 1915, p. 114.

between public presentation and private realities. It is difficult to escape the conclusion that, for all the efforts and achievements surrounding the Norfolk War Hospital, consideration of the needs of asylum patients slipped disastrously in 'meeting an unprecedented national want'.[4]

The Norfolk War Hospital

As with much else in civilian life, the running of asylums was initially regarded as a matter of 'business as usual' after August 1914. By the following January the Army Council was already faced with mounting casualties and issued a request for some 75,000 additional hospital beds. Although the use of socially stigmatised facilities for military personnel aroused considerable misgivings, poor law institutions and asylums were the most likely providers of emergency beds on the scale envisaged. Asylums in particular offered space and recreational facilities for recovering troops and, as virtually self-contained institutions with staffs and amenities, they could serve at short notice or be modified and incorporated within revised arrangements relatively quickly.[5] The Board of Control, responsible for asylum supervision since 1913, planned to release 15,000 beds by pooling asylum facilities on a regional basis. One asylum in each of nine regions was made available for conversion as a war hospital along with its staff complement, excepting volunteers and enlisted territorials. All asylum medical officers were temporarily excused from the preparation of annual reports and detailed case records and were also allowed to reduce post-mortem investigations in order to offset anticipated increases in their workloads. As the Board's own medical commissioners were seconded to the War Office and to war hospital administration, its legal commissioners were left with responsibility for reduced levels of supervision in the remaining asylums.

Thomson was among the senior medical superintendents who met with the Board of Control to consider these arrangements on 1 and 8 February 1915, on the second occasion with Robert King, Chairman of the Committee of Visitors. A week later King chaired a meeting at the Shire Hall, Norwich, of medical superintendents from all eleven asylums of the East Anglia region (Group Five). This confirmed the NCA as the regional War Hospital and made plans for the remaining asylums each to receive roughly 10 per cent of its patients.[6] The choice reflected recognition that medical staff at the

---

[4] Sir Marriot Cooke and Hubert Bond, *History of the Asylum War Hospitals of England and Wales*, Cmd 899, HMSO, London, 1920, p. 2.

[5] Lieutenant Colonel Thomson, 'Norfolk War Hospital', Part 1, *Eastern Daily Press*, 4 June 1919. Lakenham School and Attleborough Poor Law Infirmary were similarly converted.

[6] AR, 1920, D. Thomson, 'Conversion, organisation and work of the institution as a war hospital', pp. 11–26.

Norfolk and Norwich Hospital, which had received military casualties into a mixture of hutments and marquee tents since October 1914, were readily available.[7] Moreover, the Norwich City Asylum at Hellesdon could accommodate some NCA patients at less inconvenience to their visitors and serve as an appropriate admissions centre for new Norfolk county patients for the duration of the war. Although an evacuation of mental patients on the scale envisaged would entail significant overcrowding at receiving institutions, the Board of Control had indicated its tolerance of rates of up to 20 per cent during the wartime emergency.[8] It was further agreed that 'a certain number of quiet, useful, insane patients' would be retained at Thorpe to work the asylum's West Farm.

There was little time to complete let alone fine-tune these arrangements. On 1 March telegrams from the War Office triggered the evacuation and conversion plans at the NCA with 'all haste'. Local poor law guardians were instructed to send new patients to Hellesdon and relatives of existing NCA patients were notified of likely transfers and destinations and allowed to make visits, though they were not encouraged or given financial help unless the patient was dangerously ill. Sixty patients were selected for discharge to the care of relatives or friends, partly to reduce the number of transferees and overcrowding at the receiving asylums. Whether on the grounds of familial concern, a desire to contribute in some way to the war effort, or the pragmatic acceptance of the cash allowance involved, the relatives of 53 patients were persuaded to accept them at home. Seventeen patients, in poor health or not meeting the usual criteria for probationary discharge, were temporarily accommodated at West Farm. While they awaited transfer to Hellesdon or other care in the Norwich area, they were looked after by the matron and her assistant, patient Emma H—, but a further 23 male patients were to live and work at West Farm for the duration. The remaining 960 patients were evacuated between 19 and 31 March, 'safely and without the least mishap or accident', according to Thomson's account.[9] Although each departing group supposedly represented a cross-section of NCA patients, he also claimed that 'patient's predilections' were recognised, for example in cases where a relative lived in the vicinity of a receiving asylum. Such claims contrasted with the hasty despatching of patients, without adequate records

---

[7] The first 97 light cases arrived from France on 17 October 1914. Some 7,880 war casualties in all were treated at the Norfolk and Norwich. A.J. Cleveland, *History of the Norfolk and Norwich Hospital 1900–46*, Jarrold & Sons, Norwich, 1948, pp. 131–7.

[8] Cooke and Bond, *War Hospitals*, pp. 4–6.

[9] Thomson, 'Conversion', p. 12. In addition to Hellesdon, the eastern area asylums receiving NCA patients were Severalls (171), Brentwood (154), Melton (107), Three Counties, Arlesey (95), Cambridge (95), Hill End, St Albans (80), Ipswich (65), Buckingham (65), West Ham (54) and Colchester (13). In addition, six of the private patients were transferred to the Bethel Hospital, Norwich, and the remaining five went to Severalls.

of their conditions or treatments, just as national procedures for monitoring their welfare were relaxed or dismantled by the Board of Control.

Conversion of the physical fabric of the hospital involved the immediate removal of obvious asylum features, such as door and window locks and padded cells, the widening of corridors and doorways to accommodate stretcher parties, and the installation of lifts in lieu of unsuitable stairways. Some 1,050 beds were available, which was less than initially envisaged. Smaller rooms in the old asylum could not be crowded with still more beds and the retention of an administrative centre dealing with mental patients meant that War Hospital offices had to be dispersed around the site, encroaching upon ward space. Hutted accommodation for additional stores, soldiers' packs and equipment was erected on the main site, next to the laundry. Only one-sixth of the enlarged nursing staff could be placed in the existing nurses' home and most of the remainder were housed in two parallel rows immediately north of the main road, one row of which was still on active service in 1990, and patient bed space on the wards was now at a premium. Temporary blocks housed operating theatres, sterilising, anaesthetising and X-ray facilities, one located behind wards D and E on the north side, the other with adjacent medical officers' huts on the lawns in front of the main building. These were to standard army design and provided after Thomson had visited the Woolwich, Cambridge and Edinburgh military hospitals and discussed requirements with military surgeons.

Accompanied by the matron and clerk and steward, Thomson also attended Woolwich for briefings on War Office administration and regulations. As space for patients was at a premium, he regretted that 'the existing asylum mess rooms have to be given to the large number of house, kitchen and laundry servants who have to be engaged, housed and fed, to supplant the lost Asylum patients' labour'.[10] This acknowledgement was overlooked as preparations went on but Thomson would have further cause to reflect on the contribution of asylum patients as wages and general costs rose rapidly later in the war.[11] Meanwhile, he resisted pressure to convert the recreation hall into mess-room facilities, correctly anticipating its potential value to recuperating patients, but his request for a designated electrotherapy room was to go unanswered for three years. After just eight weeks of frenetic activity and at a cost to the War Office of £16,000, the Norfolk War Hospital was ready to receive patients by the last week in May.

Now enlisted as Lieutenant-Colonel in the Royal Army Medical Corps, Thomson became Officer Commanding and Administrator at the hospital. He retained day-to-day control of the enlarged hospital staff but, although he maintained his links with the asylum Committee of Visitors and the Board of Control, he was ultimately responsible to the War Office and to the senior

[10] Thomson, 'Conversion', p. 15.
[11] ibid., p. 15.

officers of Eastern Army Command who carried out periodic inspections. Medical attention was primarily provided by a core staff of five young doctors, on temporary commissions as majors in the RAMC and paid £1 4s 6d per day, all found. Charles Noon and Douglas Home were surgeons in the main and annexe hospitals respectively; they and A. Humphrey, the registrar, had all been house surgeons at St Bart's. Dr Spence Law, formerly the asylum's assistant medical officer, became registrar at the main hospital and Arthur Cleveland arrived from the Norfolk and Norwich hospital to take charge of the X-ray and electrotherapy department. These five served throughout the war and Thomson was sufficiently impressed with their work that he rarely called upon Norfolk and Norwich hospital consultants, except for Sydney Long, physician to the officers' wards from early in 1917.

Most of the clinical and clerical work on the wards was done by civilian medical officers, usually local GPs paid £1 per day, although five of these had themselves been called up by January 1917. Their replacements included the 'Allied doctors' Jouckheere and Briffaux, both Belgian refugees, six Americans and an Australian, Dr Huxtable, and Dr Irene Eaton, resident pathologist in 1915–16. These doctors were responsible for treatment and care but also for returning soldiers to duty and the detection of malingering, issues which became increasingly controversial as the manpower shortage and disillusionment with the war intensified. They participated at Medical Boards which assessed fitness for military duties and later civilian work or eligibility for war pensions. A further three army officers were attached to the War Hospital, respectively as inspector of the local auxiliary hospitals, officer for the convalescent camp and as an additional medical officer at the annexe.

The reorganisation of nursing posed major problems, for the War Hospital required a greatly increased staff at a time when the shortage of trained general nurses was acute. Mary Hamer was retained as matron with new assistant matrons Muriel and Hotine for the former main and annexe buildings respectively. Each ward sister was responsible for discipline and supervision and for the reduction of waste. All nursing staff in responsible positions also faced the additional army bureaucracy of requisition forms, dealing with leave passes and the visits of the War Office Inspecting Matron. An advertising campaign was used to recruit qualified hospital nurses, particularly as ward sisters and staff nurses, supplemented by Women's Army Auxiliary Corps, asylum and Voluntary Aid Detachment nurses.[12] By the summer of 1917, 'matron reports increasing difficulty in obtaining trained

---

[12] Among the nurse–soldier patient romances, Margaret Royal met an Australian soldier, wounded in France. He returned home and she married locally. Fifty years later he contacted her via the *Eastern Evening News* and, in 1976, several years after her husband died, she went to Australia at the age of 80 to be reunited with her wartime sweetheart (personal communication, Mrs V. Roberts of Thorpe St Andrew whose father, H. Pull, was a hospital attendant in the early 1920s).

nurses and . . . has to further dilute skilled labour with partially-trained and untrained women'.[13] At this point the nursing complement reached a peak of 320, including 39 ward sisters, 77 staff nurses and 16 masseuses, but most were probationers. Six months later there were 300 nurses, but also 125 male orderlies and 150 women 'servant' helpers.

There were particular problems for the former asylum nurses, many of whom were trained and certified as mental nurses and experienced in nursing bodily ailments, but not qualified as general nurses and therefore retained on probationary grades at lower pay, often on wards where they had formerly been in charge. To suggest that such nurses 'patriotically sank their rank and experience and acted as "probationers" under the hospital trained nurses' was simplistic and optimistic.[14] Thirty of the asylum's male attendants had volunteered at the outset of the war or were later conscripted but the remainder were temporarily enlisted, along with ward orderlies, into the RAMC as part of No. 9 Company. A few were given non-commissioned rank, primarily to help maintain ward discipline, but the majority were seen as low status half-civilians, half-soldiers. Thomson, taking his military duties very seriously but revealing something of his former regime, regretted that many of these men were older or not fully fit and that 'the slackers and inefficient could not be dismissed as in civil life'.[15]

Soldier-sufferers

Despite the appalling loss of life and severe casualties, one of the most remarkable features of the war was the increasing role and scale of medical effort. While prodigious numbers of soldiers were sacrificed, even more were protected from infectious disease by rudimentary sanitary measures and vaccination, which controlled typhus and typhoid. Moreover, roughly four-fifths of those wounded and nine-tenths of the sick and injured were returned to military duty in some way.[16] Developments in blood transfusion, plastic surgery, radiology and orthopaedics were stimulated by wartime experience, though not all were immediately applied in war hospitals let alone in civilian life.[17] Some important treatments, of gas-asphyxia or trench foot for example,

[13] Norfolk County Council Minutes, Asylum Quarterly Committee Minutes (AQC, held at Drayton Old Lodge), 7 July 1917, p. 7 and 5 Jan. 1918, p. 8. The matron's efforts had been approved by the Inspecting Matron.

[14] Thomson, 'Conversion', p. 18.

[15] Ibid., p. 19.

[16] A. Hardy, *Health and Medicine in Britain since 1860*, Palgrave, Basingstoke, 2000, pp. 59–60.

[17] R. Cooter, 'War and modern medicine', in W.F. Bynum and R. Porter (eds), *Companion Encyclopaedia of the History of Medicine*, Routledge, London, 1993, Vol. 2, pp. 1536–73, 1550–1.

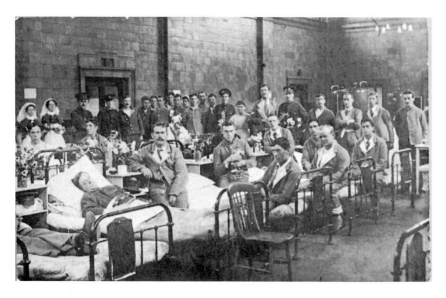

Figure 6.1 Soldiers' ward, Norfolk War Hospital (Roberts)

had limited civilian applications and, arguably, the systematisation of basic hygiene, medical records, the referral and transfer of the wounded and the rationalisation of medical expertise within teamwork were to prove of greater importance in the long term.[18] Medical facilities were initially overwhelmed by machine gun and shell casualties, which involved complex wounds made 'dirty' by heavily manured ground. Delayed treatment was associated with extensive levels of blood poisoning and the amputation of affected limbs became almost standard.

The modified system rested upon prompt first aid whenever possible at dressing stations before casualties were sent 'down the line' to a casualty clearing station. Here surgical teams undertook basic work, for example setting fractured bones and the debridement of wounds, removing shrapnel and bone fragments. Decisions to refer those requiring further treatment to a base hospital in France or a hospital ship for transportation to Britain were normally based upon the severity of the case and an assessment of the patient's ability to withstand a hazardous journey. Batches of casualty or sick cases, arriving at Dover or Southampton, were conveyed by ambulance trains to the Norfolk War Hospital and similar institutions. Local arrangements at the NWH sufficed for roughly seven months. Three convalescent cases were admitted on 26 May but the first convoys of injured men arrived on 9 June. Ambulance trains usually reached Norwich in the small hours of the morning

---

[18] R. Cooter, *Surgery and Society in Peace and War*, Macmillan, Basingstoke, 1993, pp. 105–36.

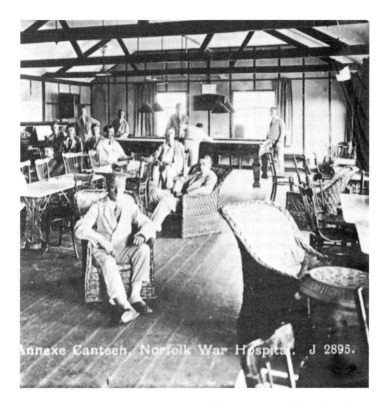

Figure 6.2 Annexe canteen, Norfolk War Hospital (Roberts)

and casualties were conveyed by the volunteer Norwich Transport Corps in Red Cross and Army ambulances to the NWH. There they were assessed by the hospital registrar and allocated to wards at the rate of roughly one per minute.[19] Some 400 patients arrived in June, with 350 still under treatment at the end of the month and 3,100 more admitted before the year's end. Inpatient numbers averaged between 600 and 800, considerably below the existing bed capacity, with 633 servicemen remaining on Christmas Day 1915.

Early in 1916 the NWH was designated a general hospital, to receive 'any and all cases', and Thomson was informed that its capacity must be substantially increased.[20] In practice the most desperate cases, such as shrapnel or gunshot wounds to head, chest or abdomen, were either 'not viable' or deemed unfit for evacuation to England. However, a high proportion of men

---

[19] Thomson, 'Norfolk War Hospital', Part 2, *Eastern Daily Press*, 5 June 1919.
[20] This was in anticipation of the Somme offensive that July.

with bullet wounds to their limbs, shattered bones and fractures and severe flesh wounds was received and the condition of many would have deteriorated substantially on the journey to Norfolk. Thomson's plans included the crowding of 400 additional beds into existing wards, day rooms and corridors and the erection of ten hutment wards, each containing 62 beds. Four of these were placed on the main site, wards 15 and 16 immediately east of the main building, wards 17 and 19 west of the church with staff mess and recreation rooms on its eastern side. Six other wards were set out in parallel pairs just to the north-east of the former male asylum, with additional bedrooms for medical officers and patients' recreation rooms.[21] With the addition of a few outdoor shelters, mainly for TB patients, the bed capacity was virtually doubled, to 2,000. All these beds were needed: the Somme offensive produced vast numbers of casualties as well as deaths and, as field facilities failed to cope, injured troops were evacuated directly to coastal ports and the UK. The NWH received 888 wounded in the first week of July and 2,000 by the end of the month. The average number of inpatients still exceeded 1,700 early in November, with nearly 1,200 remaining at Christmas, when there were 'almost continuous entertainments in the Great Hall', a facility now fully appreciated.

In 1917 the hospital's services clientele expanded further. Officers' wards, opened in the main building in the spring, eventually contained 100 patients. With the belated acknowledgement that military casualties included those suffering from forms of mental illness or breakdown, ward block 6 at the main building was set aside for their reception and 70 patients were under care by November 1917. Many of these were 'home troops' who had not completed military training or who were not thought fit for front line service; a few were former asylum inmates caught up by conscription. In practice, these patients were nursed by former NCA staff and placed under Dr Spence Law. By now the hospital was designated a 'Central' hospital, responsible for administrative arrangements and inspections of the county's auxiliary hospitals, for the reception of 'crash' cases from local aerodromes and for channelling infectious diseases cases to Norwich Isolation and other hospitals.[22] But the build-up of general patients went on, culminating in the admission of 1,410 casualties, following the Ypres offensive, in August 1917. Over 1,670 were still resident for the Christmas festivities that year, with some of the proceedings disrupted by the arrival in Norwich at 10.00 p.m. of casualties from the Cambrai front.

New pressure to expand accommodation, this time occasioned by the German spring offensive, led to the establishment of a hospital camp, using

---

[21] Plans of Norfolk War Hospital, held at Drayton Old Lodge.
[22] Some 20 auxiliary hospitals in Norfolk were maintained at roughly £35,000 in 1919. *British Red Cross and Order of St John, Joint War Committee and Finance Committee 1914–19*, 1921, pp. 611, 629.

over forty ten-bed marquee tents in a field to the north of the annexe buildings in 1918. This was intended for recovering convalescent and slight cases 'able to fend for themselves' and no regular nursing was provided. As the German attack literally overtook the allied forces and their medical personnel in some areas, the assessment of casualties could not proceed and overwhelmed base hospitals had to forward new patients en masse to Britain. Some 500 of these arrived at the NWH, raising the patient total above 1,500 in April and beyond 1,800 in June, including 300 in tents. Shortly afterwards the influenza pandemic struck. Initially, locally stationed troops were admitted, but the 'severe and alarming' complications, the rapid development of broncho-pneumonia often followed by death, soon necessitated more emergency measures. Wards were set aside for flu victims and by 1 September, 2,035 patients were under treatment. In October and November at least 160 severe cases were admitted, again mainly from local units, with 43 deaths in a five-week period. Half the nursing staff were affected and three died. Thus the end of the Great War was associated with the hospital's sternest test. As Thomson put it, 'had it not been for the admirable volunteer help we got from convalescent soldiers, I don't know how we could have "carried on" . . . I wish never to have such an experience of hospital life again'.[23] Of the 423 patients who died in the NWH, 132 succumbed to influenza strains.

Altogether 44,651 patients were treated at the NWH, almost 90 per cent of them admitted after evacuation to England, and 419 of them died there. Of the 8,657 major surgical procedures carried out from 1915 to 1919, nearly 3,000 involved the removal of bullets or shell shrapnel, including 1,232 severe flesh wounds, 956 cases of compound fracture and 808 for 'removal of foreign body'.[24] Cases of gangrene, gas gangrene or trench foot necessitated almost 500 amputations and a greater number of operations for 'removal of dead bones'. Surgical work also included over 400 herniotomies, 300 appendectomies and relatively minor procedures. These addressed conditions which might be expected in civilian life but they were undertaken so that servicemen could function at some level within the war machine, rather than on general health grounds. Recoveries were promoted through techniques of manipulation, massage and 'more electrical work . . . one of the lessons of the war'.[25] Electrotherapy became extensive, although a specialist unit was not established until the summer of 1918, and the production of plaster pylon artificial limbs designed by Major Noon became a workshop industry using patient labour in the best asylum tradition.

Medical cases included victims of poison gas, sometimes relieved by oxygen treatments or steam sprays in high temperature wards, and a range of

---

[23] Thomson, 'Conversion', p. 23.
[24] Thomson, 'Conversion', p. 24.
[25] Committee of Visitors, Emergency Sub-committee, 1914–1922, SAH 25, Thomson, 10 April 1919.

common infectious diseases, although there were no references to venereal diseases cases in local accounts.[26] Nor was publicity given to the treatment of over 500 men suffering from varying forms of disorder, often officially grouped as 'confusional insanity' and from early 1915 generally referred to as 'shellshock'.[27] By November 1918 at least 80,000 British troops were affected in this way from their subjugation to the extremes of war, too many to be treated as long-term patients at special military hospitals for 'war neuroses' at Napsbury, Netley and Warrington.[28] Their distressing symptoms confounded pre-war assumptions that mental illness could be explained largely in terms of hereditary factors or predisposition in women and effeminate men. With officers even more affected than men in the ranks, such assumptions were increasingly viewed as a 'slur upon the noblest of our race'.[29] Doctors prepared to look beyond suspicions of cowardice or malingering were faced with the apparent contradiction of attempting to promote recovery of their patients in order that they could be returned to the conditions associated with their breakdown.[30] Many 'service patients', who were differentiated by their military status and supporting payments from the Ministry of Pensions from the rate-funded pauper lunatics, were transferred to war hospitals and county asylums. Some benefited from relatively new techniques of psychoanalysis, which gained further credibility, but most at Norfolk War Hospital and similar institutions received versions of psychotherapy based upon exercise, rest, baths and also bromide. Later, they were sent on to their local borough or county borough asylum, but 21 service patients remained at Thorpe after the war and their number soon increased.

Post-operative and convalescent cases at the NWH were managed through a daily cycle dominated by the morning medical round and oddly spaced meals, a 6.30 a.m. breakfast, 9.00 a.m. 'lunch', dinner at midday and supper at 7.15 p.m. Those designated 'up' or 'out' were to be out of bed or outdoors respectively and they were encouraged to participate in entertainments, sports and light work. From November 1915 a Voluntary Amenities Committee provided newspapers and books, pianos and gramophones. It also ran two canteens, raising more funds for entertainments, notably a twice weekly film show and more occasional concerts. A hospital orchestra and choir were sustained, despite the turnover of members, and ward classes in arts

[26] Under the 1917 Venereal Diseases Act a clinic had opened at the Norfolk and Norwich Hospital in April 1917.

[27] The term was introduced by Charles S. Myers, then serving in the Royal Army Medical Corps in France, in C. Myers, 'A contribution to the study of shell shock', *The Lancet*, 1, 1915, pp. 316–20.

[28] M. Stone, 'Shellshock and the psychologists' in W. Bynum, R. Porter and M. Shepherd, *The Anatomy of Madness: Essays in the History of Psychiatry*, Tavistock, London, 1985, Vol. 2, pp 242–71, 249.

[29] ibid. p. 252.

[30] See J. Busfield, *Men, Women and Madness*, Macmillan, Basingstoke, 1996, pp. 212–18.

and crafts were organised. Walking parties, under the charge of a properly mobile NCO, supplemented wandering the grounds and canteen visits as routine activities. Most prized was the reception of a visitor or a pass out, the latter awarded only to 'every way satisfactory patients' and conditional upon the written invitation of a friend or relative. Some ingenuity here could result in a trip into Norwich, although pubs and cycling were prohibited and the high-profile 'sick' blue uniform with its white shirt, red tie and identity disc was a further restriction. An interval away from war fronts was probably reward enough for most soldier-patients and public goodwill generated towards wounded heroes probably provided a variety of treats and compensations. After assessment at medical boards those discharged from the NWH but not rejoining their units were likely to be sent on to auxiliary hospitals for further convalescence, sent home as invalid cases or referred to asylums as 'service patients'.[31]

No soldier-patient or later service patient records are available, but letters from those dispersed from local war auxiliary hospitals provide a fragmentary and subjective source. There were simple letters of thanks to matrons, commandants or attendants, often coupled with apologies for a belated response but citing addresses which included training camps, barracks, Dublin and, presumably from a French Canadian soldier, 'au front'. One letter, signed by John Mann and sixteen others from eleven different regiments at Brundall Auxiliary Hospital at Christmas 1915, illustrates the mixing of patients and offered the matron 'heartiest wishes for a speedy recovery'. Canadian Sgt H. Williamson was now at Woodcote Park Convalescent Camp, Epsom, with 'at least 4,000 patients'. His daily routine still began with a 6.30 a.m. breakfast but was then more arduous: 'training camp would, I think, be a more appropriate name as nearly everyone does physical drill and route marches almost every day.' Even among the small sample of letters it is apparent that other patients were not nearly so well and possibly were traumatised by their war experiences. In May 1916 Captain Wagstaffe wrote, 'since I have been home I have got such terrible headaches it is unbearable sometimes . . . I really have not been well enough for anything'. 'Baby', now in ward 11 at the Norfolk and Norwich Hospital, regretted that he had been injured 'so long' and suspected that he still had bone fragments in his leg: the nurses 'cannot see any bone but they can feel it, I am now waiting for the doctor to see it'. Private Elliot wrote several undated letters. Transferred to an infirmary ward at Britannia Barracks, Norwich, he found: 'it is very cold. It is more like a union workhouse than it is a hospital.' Apparently at home in Belfast, he later complained that 'one of the small

---

[31] See H. Bettinson, 'The Norfolk War Hospital', M.A. dissertation, UEA, Norwich, 1999, for detailed discussion. She examined the Norfolk War Hospital Magazine, SAH 340, 1916–18, but 'no criticism of army severity appeared in its columns, any more than did poetry of the calibre of Sasoon or Owen'. See p. 40.

bones in my foot is broken again it is sticking out of the side of my foot' but 'I am not going to report sick I am going to let my ankle stop as it is now'.[32]

A hidden history: the asylum patients

What of the former asylum patients? Published accounts of the Norfolk War Hospital paid little attention to their fate but the available evidence from local and central sources is disturbing. Among the matters discussed by the asylum committee on 10 April 1915, after the asylum had been cleared, was the report by the inspector for the Board of Control. At the time of his visit fifty-three asylum patients were confined to bed, mainly with influenza although fourteen were suffering from dysentery.[33] It is doubtful that these patients, particularly the latter group, could have recovered by the time the asylum was cleared or that other patients were not about to fall sick. Their evacuation threatened their own health, that of other NCA patients and those in the receiving asylums. Although some patients were moved across the city to Hellesdon, almost 900 left Norwich by train for other asylums. Many went to Essex, 154 to the county asylum at Brentwood and 171 to the recently opened Severalls asylum. Suffolk County Asylum took 107 patients, with a further 65 at Ipswich Borough Asylum, and the asylums at Fulbourn (Cambridgeshire) and Arlesey (Bedfordshire) took 95 each.[34] Thomson described how:

> to many the asylum had been their home . . . many even had never been in a railway train . . . the whole gamut of emotion was exhibited by the patients on leaving, ranging from acute distress and misery, through gay indifference, to maniacal fury and indignation. I did not realise the strong mutual attachment till it was severed.[35]

More of this distress originated in physical illness than Thomson's account allowed, however, and his pressing responsibilities for the war hospital left little time for further 'asylum matters', as his medical reports showed all too clearly.[36]

---

[32] These letters were sent to matrons at Brundall and Hunstanton war auxiliary hospitals and the Norfolk and Norwich hospital in 1915 and 1916. I am grateful to Margaret Hewitt, completing her M.Phil. thesis, 'Efficiency not dependency: the social rehabilitation of World War I veterans in East Anglia' (UEA, Norwich, 2003), for making them available.

[33] Committee of Visitors Minutes, Jan. 1915–Feb. 1923, SAH 15, 10 April 1915 (BoC inspection).

[34] The remainder were Hill End 80, Bucks County 65, West Ham 54 and Colchester 13.

[35] Thomson, 'War Hospital', p. 13.

[36] Medical Superintendent's Journal, March 1915–April 1922, SAH 135.

Nearly 8 per cent of the NCA patients in 1915 were sent to their relatives or moved to West Farm, where alterations costing £400 were made to provide their accommodation. Although a small proportion of patients might have had probationary discharge in normal years many were essentially cleared out of the asylum on 25 March 1915. Henry G—, for example, was wanted at home. He suffered from recurrent mania but repeated requests by his father, 'anxious to take him home', were refused because Gray was 'very delusional and does not seem to have improved'. There was still 'no change' in his condition but the war emergency meant that he 'was today discharged in care of his father'. Gertrude H— wanted to go home. Her insanity was linked to 'moral imbecility/congenital mental defect' and she needed 'constant super-vision on account of her objectionable habits'. In wartime this behaviour was evidently more tolerable and, following a slight improvement, her request to go home meant that she was discharged 'relieved'. It is not clear who was to care for Daisy E—. Her father was in the asylum himself as a patient and her mother was 'said to be queer'. She was evidently ill-suited for domestic service because her problems were seen as hereditary and compounded 'at menstrual periods when she cannot be kept from the men servants'. This had been the cause of her admission and in December 1914, seven years later, she was 'quite unfit to look after herself'. The following February she showed 'no mental change' but she too was discharged 'relieved' on 25 March.[37]

These patients had their physical health but some clearly did not. Frances C—, then aged 81, was also among those sent home. She had been admitted in 1912 suffering a fourth bout of recurrent melancholia, which dated from 1873, and had attempted to hang herself. She failed to improve and was described as 'very helpless now' just one month before she was discharged 'relieved'. Rebecca N—, aged 67, was a similar case; at the end of February 1915 she was 'very dull and feeble' and even on 20 March there was 'no mental or bodily change to report', yet she was discharged 'relieved' five days later. William B—, aged 84, had been admitted in 1914 suffering from epilepsy and senile dementia. His elderly wife could no longer cope and she reported that she found him 'beyond control, very violent'. In February 1915 he 'had 2 fits in the evening . . . and very restless' but on 25 March 'was today discharged in care of his wife'. Henry J— had enjoyed better physical health during his twenty years in the asylum helping in the wards and kitchen, though there had been spells when he required force feeding and his one period of probation had ended when he was brought back 'violent and unmanageable'. By 1912 Dr Flynn considered him to be 'the best worker in the house' but in December 1913 he had a stroke, which paralysed his left side. His recovery was limited

---

[37] Case Books, males discharged 1910–15, SAH 282, H.G. 1910–15; females discharged 1910–17, SAH 302; G.H. 1913–15; D.E. 1907–15.

and a year later there was 'no change'. Nevertheless, on 25 March he 'was discharged today in care of his son. Recovered'.[38]

Among those patients sent to West Farm, Thomas P—, aged 46, suffered from chronic mania but was also considered to have a congenital mental defect. During his six years in the asylum he had attended to the medical superintendent's garden which may explain why, uniquely among the farm patients, his case notes continued to be updated annually. He was 'simple minded . . . very talkative but industrious' but was discharged to the care of his 'comfortably off 'cousin in 1918. Arthur T—, formerly a carpenter, was another long-term patient. He had already been in Surrey County Asylum before he was transferred to Norfolk in 1903 and, after a 'very troublesome' beginning, seems to have settled well, working in the carpenter's shop. Later he was allowed weekly parole; his skills were valued and this possibly explains his presence at the farm, where he worked until 1919. He escaped on 23 May 1919, though he must have had ample opportunities to do so earlier and, having avoided recapture for fourteen days, 'he was accordingly discharged . . . Relieved'.[39]

Some patients were quite desperately ill when they were evacuated. Sophia R—, then aged 76, had been in the asylum for twenty-five years and in late February 1915 was put to bed with bronchitis. She was transferred to Ipswich Borough Asylum on 29 March, though her case notes stated 'Bronchitis, emphysema and weak heart . . . very feeble and demented', and she died there five days later. Arthur G—, brought to the NCA as a child of six, was now 44 years old, epileptic and suffering from ulcerated legs. Two days after he was moved to Brentwood Asylum he was 'in bed . . . in very feeble health . . . able to take liquid food'. However, the cause of his death, five days later, was 'phthisis; duration some months'. The upheaval of evacuation may explain why Ernest J—, 33 and epileptic, became violent and irrational following his journey to the Suffolk County Asylum. He died after a 'prolonged condition of marked epilepsy with great violence' lasting one month. What killed William M— shortly after he arrived at Brentwood is also unclear and there is some ambiguity surrounding the deaths of NCA patients at Severalls Asylum, Colchester. Within four days of her transfer Hannah S—, aged 28, went down with dysentery, from which she died on 6 April. The same cause of death was recorded for Jenny D— (80) on 17 April and Richenda P— (50) on 26 April. Some infections may well have been contracted at the NCA but others arose within the host asylums. Jessie W—, a 21-year-old epileptic, died from broncho-pneumonia one month after

---

[38] Case Books, females discharged 1910–17, SAH 302, F.C. 1912–15; R.N. 1909–15; W.B. 1914–15; males discharged SAH 282, H.J. 1895–1915.
[39] Case Books, males discharged, 1916–23, SAH 283, A.T. 1903–19; T.P. 1909–18.

her transfer to Severalls and Ellen W—, aged 45, appears to have contracted tuberculosis there before her death in July 1918.[40]

If the NCA had evacuated some very sick patients, the transfer process itself produced further traumas and at least three long-term patients, reportedly 'in good health', soon died afterwards. Suffolk County Asylum protested that 30 of the 107 Norfolk arrivals were in acute stages of infectious disease, colitis and dysentery and, significantly, its medical superintendent received a formal apology from the NCA.[41] With the initial evacuation completed, any new Norfolk admissions to the Hellesdon, Norwich asylum could only be accommodated if it transferred longer-term patients to other eastern region asylums. As these were also overcrowded, any additional space was most likely to arise as members of the initial groups of Norfolk evacuees died. Yet 424 more patients were transferred from Hellesdon after the March 1915 evacuation, suggesting extensive mortality in these asylums.

Table 6.1 summarises a reconstruction of NCA patient deaths in other asylums, based on information returned to Thorpe asylum for compilation in case notes. This may be incomplete but it suggests that delayed returns

Table 6.1 Norfolk County Asylum patient deaths in other asylums, 1915–18

	1915	1916	1917	1918	Total
Norfolk County Asylum	63	–	–	–	63
Hellesdon, Norwich	37	32	51	59	179
Brentwood, Essex	13	23	39	27	102
Severalls, Essex	19	19	24	30	92
Suffolk County, Melton	12	13	14	12	51
Three Counties, Arlesey	6	7	17	16	46
Fulbourn, Cambridge	8	8	12	9	37
Ipswich Borough	7	8	11	11	37
Goodmayes, West Ham	5	3	12	6	26
Hill End, St Albans	2	3	4	8	17
Buckinghamshire County, Aylesbury	2	1	5	8	16
Colchester Hospital	–	1	–	–	1
Annual total	174	118	189	186	667
(Death registers)	(174)	(103)	(162)	(141)	(580)

Notes: Norfolk County Asylum, Case Books, Males, 1915–18, SAH 279; Females, 1914–18, SAH 299; Register of Deaths 1907–21, SAH 223.

[40] Case Books, male deaths, 1915–17, SAH 279, A.G. 1878–1915; E.J. 1913–15; W.M. 1894–1915. Female deaths, 1914–17, SAH 299, S.R. 1890–1914; H.S. 1914–15; J.D. 1906–15; R.P. 1895–1915; J.W. 1910–15; E.W. 1907–18.
[41] Suffolk County Asylum (SCA), *Reports of the Medical Superintendent* (J.R. Whitwell), March 1915.

resulted in some underestimation in the annual Register of Deaths, shown for comparison, for 1916–18 at least. In all, 667 patients died by the end of 1918, 602 of them after they had been transferred from the NCA in March 1915. An average of 106 patients died annually in the immediate pre-war period 1910–14 and 101 for the period 1900–09. With fewer patients in total during the war years, some 400–450 deaths might reasonably have been expected, suggesting an 'excess' mortality of between 150 and 200 in the evacuated asylum population.

What light does this throw upon national explanations of asylum mortality during the Great War? Considerable debate surrounds the alleged impact of the war upon the health of the civilian population generally but the national asylum death rate increased from 12 per cent in 1915 to 17.6 per cent in 1917 and it exceeded 20 per cent in 1918.[42] In acknowledging this 'disquieting' trend, the Board of Control still maintained in 1917 that 'no definite conclusions could be arrived at' and it linked further increases in 1918 to the influenza pandemic.[43] Table 6.2 shows influenza to be significant at Brentwood asylum, but this accounted for less than one-tenth of NCA patient deaths. A study of Buckinghamshire County Asylum has noted

Table 6.2 Infectious diseases mortality in Norfolk County Asylum patients at receiving asylums in 1918

Asylum	All NCA deaths	TB	Influenza/ pneumonia	Dysentery	% deaths from diseases
Severalls, Essex	30	14	–	1	50
Hellesdon, Norwich	59	6	1	3	17
Melton Suffolk County	12	5	1	–	50
Brentwood, Essex	27	4	10	1	56
Fulbourn, Cambridgeshire	9	3	1	–	44
Buckinghamshire County	8	–	–	–	–
West Ham	16	3	1	–	25
Ipswich Borough	11	1	3	–	36
Three Counties, Bedfordshire	16	6	1	–	44
Hill End, St Albans	8	5	–	–	63
Total	196	47	18	5	33

Note: Sources as Table 6.1.

[42] See B. Abel-Smith, *The Hospital, 1800–1948: A Study in Social Administration in England and Wales*, Heinemann, London, 1964, p. 286; J.C. Drummond and A. Wilbraham, *The Englishman's Food: A History of Five Centuries of The Englishman's Diet*, Jonathan Cape, London, 1964; J.M. Winter, *The Great War and the British People*, Macmillan, London, 1986, pp. 105–6, offers a positive interpretation but see L. Bryder, 'The First World War: healthy or hungry?', *History Workshop*, 24, 1987, pp. 141–55.

[43] Reports of Board of Control (BoC), 1914–25, SAH 141, 1917, Part 1, p. 14.

increasing patient mortality 'consistent with food deprivation' and linked this with tuberculosis, although no NCA patients featured among the 68 deaths from tuberculosis there in 1918.[44] In the other receiving asylums TB caused one quarter of the NCA patient fatalities, however. The Board of Control acknowledged food shortages and semi-starvation as wartime facts of life in asylums but high levels of stress, associated with the disruption of evacuation and strange, overcrowded surroundings, may also have featured in TB mortality.[45] With daily convoys of wounded soldiers arriving, tuberculosis was sometimes regarded as 'a civilian and therefore an irrelevant problem' and mentally ill civilians who had been uprooted from their asylums were not a major concern.[46]

These transferred patients possibly fared worst of all. Suffolk County Asylum, affronted that its dietary was linked with the rising incidence of TB, maintained that the latter could be 'sufficiently accounted for' solely among its Norfolk evacuees, of whom '15 per cent were suffering tubercular disease' when they arrived. TB deaths there occurred solely among Norfolk patients and mortality among the Suffolk 'residents' was at its lowest for eleven years.[47] All NCA patients were kept separately from Suffolk patients, whom the asylum authorities felt duty-bound to protect. In 1919/20 just 40 of the 129 patients transferred to the SCA were returned to Norfolk. Another 19 had been discharged but 70, or 54 per cent of the total, had died.[48] Whatever the initial embarrassment or explanation for this mortality, expressions of gratitude to the SCA for the great care and attention which had been bestowed on the Norfolk patients seem wildly inappropriate.[49]

Some 33 per cent of the Norfolk evacuees who died in other asylums in 1918 did so from infectious diseases, but the variable experiences at these asylums suggest features beyond infection and malnutrition. Only at Suffolk County did mortality among women transferees exceed that of men, for example, and male NCA patient death rates were twice those for females at six institutions.[50] Serious staff shortages may have been a feature: 42 per cent of male asylum attendants nationally had volunteered for military service by

---

[44] J.L. Crammer, 'Extraordinary deaths of asylum inpatients during the 1914–18 war', *Medical History*, 36, 1992, pp. 430–41, 435. With an average daily intake of 1,580 calories in 1916 and supervision disrupted by staff shortages many patients were half-starved and prone to TB.

[45] BoC, 1918, Part 1, p. 24. Stress as a contributing feature in TB among the civilian population is noted in Hardy, *Health and Medicine*, p. 53.

[46] T.Dormandy, *The White Death: A History of Tuberculosis*, Hambledon Press, London, 1999, p. 225.

[47] SCA, Report, 1918, MS, p. 12.

[48] SCA, Report, 1920, MS, p. 12.

[49] Suffolk County Asylum Committee of Visitors, *Minute Book*, Jan. 1919–Sept. 1922.

[50] BoC, 1917, Part II, Appendix B, Table II. N.B. Crammer, 'Deaths', p. 430 maintains that male and female patients died in equal numbers at Buckinghamshire County Asylum.

1915 and more were later conscripted.[51] The Board of Control argued that such shortages, along with overcrowding, had 'less serious consequences than might have been anticipated'. Yet it had abandoned the usual statistical analysis of medical staff, explaining that 'large withdrawals' meant that such data was 'valueless for comparison with ordinary years'.[52] Even by 1915 asylum authorities were employing temporary staff, 'many of whom are entirely unsuited for the position which they hold'.[53] As the release of additional asylum facilities to the War Office increased ratios of asylum patients to medical and nursing staffs to unprecedented levels, inexperience, the lack of training and deteriorating working conditions were likely to take their toll.[54] Signs of poor health in patients went unrecognised or remedial action was not taken, recovery rates declined and mortality, especially male mortality, increased. Yet many patients, such as H.M., aged 67, going blind and no longer able to work, required constant attention, war emergency or not. His depression had already led to a suicide attempt before his admission to St Andrew's and transfer to the Norwich City Asylum in May 1915. He was 'a nicely behaved old chap except over his food and one cannot help pitying his distress for he says he has done very wrong by giving so much trouble . . . he believes his bowels are obstructed and that his food sticks inside him'. This delusion meant that 'every mouthful of food has to be placed in his mouth' and it is uncertain what level of staffing would have been required to avert his increasing feebleness and eventual death in August 1917.[55]

What happened to the transferred asylum patients constitutes one of the hidden histories of the Great War. The war effort shifted the goals of the Board of Control and of asylum medical and administrative authorities, resulting in more relaxed definitions of mental illness, lower levels of staffing and reduced standards of patient care. The profile of the mentally ill and concern for them was reduced and, within the asylums, those patients transferred from other institutions received even less priority, if the experience of Norfolk evacuee patients is any guide. On a more general note, the official number of insane persons fell by 23,673 during the Great War, the first reduction in more than a century. The number of asylums in use was also reduced, from 97 in 1914 to 88 in 1915 and to 81 in 1918.[56] There was a consistent average of roughly 1,100 patients per asylum and, although medical superintendents at receiving asylums did not relinquish control over

---

[51] K. Jones, *Asylums and After*, Athlone, London, 1993, p. 124.
[52] BoC, 1915, Part 1, pp. 21–2
[53] SCA, Report, 1915.
[54] BoC, 1918, Part 1, p. 3; SCA *Minute Book*, 19 Oct. 1918. SCA nursing staff worked an average 81-hour week.
[55] Case Books, male deaths, 1915–17, SAH 279, H.M.
[56] BoC, 1918, Part 1, Summary of Insane Patients, 1914–18, p. 3.

patient numbers, in practice they reduced local admissions to accommodate the transferred patients. Annual average admissions for male and female patients in Norfolk fell by 20 and 10 per cent respectively, comparing the period 1915–19 with 1910–14.[57] The Board of Control explained such reductions as 'influenced by the increase in employment and resulting improved conditions amongst the working population, leading to an actual diminution of nervous mental disorders'.[58] If true, this explanation had major implications for peacetime policy; otherwise, it confirmed the social, medical or legal redefinition of insanity on a national scale under wartime conditions.

Administration and reconversion

Administrative arrangements for the asylum and war hospital were handled by Tom Parry, the asylum Steward, and John Middleton, its Clerk of Works, under the direction of Thomson and the Committee of Visitors. The latter maintained contributions towards the upkeep of NCA buildings and staff pensions and set the charges made to Norfolk poor law unions for their patients. Significantly, these charges were not necessarily determined by current maintenance costs at the various receiving institutions. West Farm became a major supplier to the war hospital and the working patients there made a considerable contribution within these arrangements, as will be seen.

Information relating to the hospital finances in this period is difficult to unravel and is based on accounts, published retrospectively in 1921 and summarised in Table 6.3. Such public records reflect compromises repeatedly reached between a commitment to the war effort and to the NCA and local ratepayers. They also include the cumulative effects of wartime inflation, which were only partly offset by a decline in the number of NCA patients over the period 1915–19. A brief review covers only the main account headings and comments inevitably include a speculative element. As seen in Table 6.3, payments for patients and the farm account comprised the bulk of the NCA maintenance accounts. The relatively static income derived from poor law unions between 1915 and 1918 suggests that the Committee sought to limit charges in a period of rising costs. It had the benefit of a relatively large surplus in 1915, reflecting the reduction in patient numbers and the substantially lower charges agreed with the receiving asylums. With low admissions and higher mortality, patient numbers continued to fall and the 1915 surplus was sufficient to cover increased charges by host asylums until the end of the war. Only then were NCA charges to Norfolk raised significantly, to meet increased costs as the asylum reopened.

[57] AR, 1921, Table II; Norwich City Asylum 1915–19, SAH 199, Summary of Admissions.
[58] BoC, 1915, Part 1, p. 9.

Table 6.3 Norfolk County Asylum, maintenance accounts, 1915–20

	All payments			Payments for patients Income from Norfolk poor law unions	Net figure	Payment to other asylums		Farm accounts		
	Receipts	Expenditure	Surplus				Sales	Payments	Net
	£	£	£	£	£	£	£	£	£
1915–16	43,933	39,609	4,324	31,590	+8,469	23,121	10,807	12,717	–1,900
1916–17	60,998	60,540	458	31,185	–229	31,414	24,282	27,230	–2,498
1917–18	67,554	66,515	1,039	31,209	–2,245	33,454	31,150	31,200	–50
1918–19	63,981	59,008	4,973	31,249	–4,861	36,610	26,296	21,428	+4,868
1919–20	61,148	53,694	7,454	40,183	–3,502	43,685	11,104	7,840	+3,264
					(net £2,368 1915–20)				

Source: Annual Report, 1921, summary, pp. 35–6

The financial position was considerably enhanced by the contribution of the farm and its patient labour force, whose numbers were augmented by suitable Norfolk patients brought from Norwich City Asylum. At least one of the latter replaced escaped farm patients like A.J.T., mentioned above, and C.W.A., who 'wandered off home' in June 1916. Under new wartime standards these were simply designated 'discharged', presumably because staff resources were too stretched to allow further investigation or pursuit.[59] Allowing for wartime inflation, there was clearly an increase in farm live-stock, activity and production for the war hospital until some point in 1918 when this eased off, falling sharply in 1919–20 as patient numbers at the war hospital declined and before the asylum had fully reopened. By then, livestock and foodstuff sales had produced substantial surpluses on the farm account. All this suggests astute financial management in an inflationary situation. In manipulating patient charges and then farm surpluses, the Committee achieved positive balances on the asylum maintenance account, annually carrying forward a small element and transferring the remainder to the building fund account, consistent with pre-war practice. In this way a substantial part of maintenance account surpluses, totalling £18,248 by the end of 1919–20, benefited the building fund.

Between 1915 and 1921 the Committee received a total of £109,291 for the adaptation and repair of existing buildings and necessary additions for war hospital purposes. Inevitably, some of this money also maintained the physical fabric of the asylum and offset the depreciation and wear of wartime use. Meanwhile, the separate asylum building account was continued on a reduced basis, supplementing a balance of £396 after repairs at the end of March 1915. However, by 1918, the committee recognised that, 'since military occupation excessive wear and tear has taken place', some of which was felt to be 'undue'.[60] Further compensation would be sought but the building account must be strengthened. Transfers from maintenance accounts became substantial; £4,501 for 1919–20 and £2,877 the following year. With minor on-going expenditure on the asylum offset by rents and other income, a net balance of £13,194 remained at end of the 1919–20 financial year. The real value of this sum was partly eroded as the costs of scarce building materials rose but, with a depreciation settlement for buildings, plant and equipment still outstanding, members of the Committee may have been quietly satisfied with the immediate financial position.

With the end of hostilities the war hospital briefly took on the further role of 'dispersal hospital' from December 1918, acting as a clearing-house for injured troops returning to Britain and for those requiring longer-term care

---

[59] Medical Superintendent's Journal, 1915–22, SAH 135. Having 'wandered off home' C.W.A. was discharged on 6 June 1916. A.J.T. escaped and was 'discharged' on 6 June 1919.

[60] AQC, 5 Jan. 1918, p. 8.

than could be provided in auxiliary hospitals. As many of the latter were closing and the influenza outbreak continued, the number of patients passing through the NWH for treatment and assessment at medical boards of injury or disability and for entitlement to invalid pension remained high. Over 1,200 patients remained in March and still 700 early in April 1919, with something of a scrambled dispersal as the Board of Control pressed for the return of the hospital to its peacetime role. Understandably, Thomson regarded the administrative arrangements required for this additional and unfamiliar work as 'the last straw'.[61]

On 10 April the Committee of Visitors convened to consider the restoration of the NCA and the question of depreciation. The War Office had offered all host institutions compensation for reconversion work and for depreciation of mechanical and engineering plant, based upon 5 per cent of original capital costs for each year of use by war hospitals. Reinstatement costs of £7,500 were agreed but, armed with additional reports from its original engineering contractor, the committee sought enhanced compensation payments of £8,994, based upon four and a half years' depreciation. The Army Area Quartering Committee could not see why it was liable for expenses after it had quit the site and the committee was unwilling to bear such costs before its own patients had returned.[62] In addition, although Thomson was still under the terms of his commission, he had already identified the war hospital operating and dental theatre and X-ray facilities as 'extremely useful and desirable adjuncts to a mental hospital'.[63] With G.S. Smith, the NCA architect and surveyor, he drew up a list of purchases, which included hutments earmarked for use as stores, nurses' accommodation and isolation wards. In the end the committee compromised on four years' compensation for wear and tear of boilers, engineering equipment and drains amounting to £7,318 and paid £3,406 for the additional facilities, after which the war hospital account finally closed in November 1921.[64]

As the last years of the war were associated with industrial unrest, labour relations also assumed new significance. The generalised nursing shortage was particularly acute in mental hospitals and the Board of Control had acknowledged in 1918 the need for a 'definitive and friendly settlement' in order to retain qualified staff and to maintain standards.[65] Disputes in a number of asylums occurred around the National Asylum Workers' Union's

---

[61] Thomson, 'Conversion', p. 21; War Hospital Orders 1918–19, SAH 339, 15 Jan. 1919. Most of those requiring further treatment were sent to military hospitals at Colchester and Cambridge and convalescent cases went to Brighton (officers) and Eastbourne (other ranks).

[62] CVIS, 10 April, 7 Aug. and 2 Oct. 1919.

[63] MS Journal, 3 April 1919.

[64] CVIS, 24 June 1921; Special Business CVIS, Sept. 1919–April 1925, SAH 22, 19 Nov. 1921.

[65] BoC (date unknown), 1918.

demands for a 48-hour working week with minimum wages of £2 and 36 shillings respectively for qualified male and female nurses.[66] For the time being the war hospital was not directly affected, but a strike by domestic staff in April 1918 was resolved through the payment of temporary war bonuses of 12 per cent in June.[67]

Upon closure of the war hospital, many staff were dismissed with one month's wages, a further £5 and a 'civvy suit' or additional money in lieu of notice. With reconversion and an eye to the national situation, the former NCA attendants and nurses could not be dealt with in summary fashion and they were offered paid leave, with a 10 per cent war bonus on their salaries, pending a planned resumption of work on 1 September 1919. A meeting of senior personnel in July concluded that improved working conditions, notably the implementation of the 48-hour week, would require an expansion of staff numbers by 25–30 per cent and would add £4,000–£5,000 to pre-war salary costs. Additional nursing staff accommodation, met by the purchase of war hospital hutments, was a further requirement. Staff were re-employed on weekly wages of 42 shillings for men and 36 shillings for women, with bonuses approaching two-thirds of pay available for war service, seniority and the MPA certificate. However, men no longer received meals and women nurses and domestic staff were deducted up to 23s 6d weekly for their board, lodging and laundry.[68] Moreover, the committee was reluctant to accept wages negotiated nationally by the Mental Hospitals Association and the NAWU, even at the reduced settlement for rural areas. Thomson acknowledged the previous deficiencies facing nursing staff but stated publicly that 'the pendulum has swung too much the other way . . . juniors have too much leisure and too much pay . . . some more reasonable means will have to be arrived at in days to come'.[69]

Under its new title the Norfolk Mental Hospital reopened on 18 November 1919. Male patients began to be readmitted almost immediately and their hospital wards reverted to their pre-war usage except for the first-floor ward B, which was now reserved for service patients. Former 'main' buildings were not available until 3 January 1920, after which 445 women were admitted within the month. Not all were survivors from among the 564 women who had been evacuated from the NCA in 1915, for additional Norfolk patients had arrived via Hellesdon hospital in the intervening period and a few had been cured or discharged. More ominously, 461 male patients left in March 1915 and the official 1920 figure of 327 returning males included 21 new service patients in addition to the post-1915

[66] Also overtime payments, NAWU recognition for indoor staff, epithet 'nurse'. *History of the Mental Hospital and Institutional Workers Union 1910–31*, Manchester, 1931, p. 24.

[67] MS Journal, 8 April 1918. An indicator of deteriorating conditions was the strikers' demand for a daily meat meal, which could not be met.

[68] CVIS Special, 3 June 1920; CVIS, 9 Nov. 1920.

[69] AR, 1920, MS, p. 10.

admissions.[70] It was only to be expected that some patients would die during any four-year period, but 667 deaths had occurred. The asylum population had consisted of 1,025 initial and 424 subsequent transferees: a few patients were admitted and retained at Hellesdon until 1920, but many had been transferred twice, to Hellesdon and then to another asylum. This suggests a cohort group mortality approaching 45 per cent for the period 1915–20 with a great deal of 'excess mortality' and a disparity of male over female deaths.

National explanations offered by the Board of Control referred to tuberculosis, the severe winter of 1916–17 and influenza outbreaks, although lower standards of care and nutrition were also acknowledged. Thomson avoided the mortality question by arguing simply that the lower number of admissions to the reopened hospital reflected wartime experiences, which had increased 'the financial prosperity of all classes, particularly the working classes', and produced 'the lessened incidence of insanity in the population generally'.[71] Although referred to in disingenuous fashion, these experiences were significant, indicating the importance of economic well-being to mental health and the possible influence of a sense of purpose imparted to people's lives in wartime. They also suggested the role of social factors in defining insanity, not least in wartime, when fewer resources were available for the processes of committal and retention of the mentally ill and other priorities loomed still larger.

Reconversion marked not only the end of the war hospital but also the passing of the pre-war county asylum regime. Key staff personnel, many of whom had spent almost their entire professional or working lives at the asylum, continued to be prominently involved after 1915 and some were now literally exhausted. Thomson had forgone the option of retirement in 1917 but resigned after 36 years' service on 1 May 1922 and he died on 4 January 1923. His obituary notice combined references to his patriotism with the telling comment that 'apparently he stood the strain, but his tall spare frame grew gaunter, and it is very certain that his life was shortened by those years of stress when he gave of his best in his country's need'.[72] At the end of 1919 Dr Spence Law also retired from his position as Senior AMO after 28 years. He was replaced by Oliver George Connell, then a Captain in the RAMC at the Ashurst Military Hospital for War Neuroses, Oxford.[73] Matron Mary Hamer underwent major surgery late in the war and, 39 years after she began as an asylum nurse at Thorpe, she retired on the same day as Thomson. Assistant matron Louise Shulver also retired in 1922 with 28 years' service

---

[70] Of 406 male patients sent beyond the Norwich area only 215 returned. Thirty-five also returned from Hellesdon.

[71] AR, 1920, MS, p. 10.

[72] Obituary, *Journal of Medical Science*, LXIX, 1923, pp. 259–60.

[73] CVIS Special, 4 Dec. 1919. Connell, one of three candidates considered, was paid £450 p. a. with board, lodging etc. for himself and his wife, the appointment to commence on his demobilisation at the year end.

and Charles Fox, head male attendant, left after 34 years. The achievements and sacrifices of a long working life were denied to seven of the 32 attendants who were killed on war service and Thomas Flynn had been too badly wounded at Gallipoli to resume work as a medical officer.[74]

Any record of this period needs to acknowledge the extraordinary efforts required to establish the Norfolk War Hospital and auxiliary institutions and the sudden upheaval which this entailed for NCA, with the concomitant uncertainties and hazards for its own vulnerable patients. What happened to them has been one of the hidden histories of the Great War. Their privations were compounded by some abrogation of responsibilities by the Board of Control and NCA authorities, accepting that both bodies were fully engaged in making their best contribution, as they saw it, to the war effort. The dual administrative roles performed by former NCA staff encompassed some astute financial management, such that levels of debt were restrained and the pre-war upgrading of NCA buildings was either further enhanced or financially compensated. On reopening, the mental hospital included new facilities previously mentioned and additional improvements were under way, notably the 'quasi-temporary' isolation block for ten male and ten female patients, erected at the eastern edge of the hospital site. Additional accommodation for nursing staff was similarly provided, not least to address the problem of staff shortages. Rising staff costs posed a problem, but this was a national feature and greater rewards for mental hospital staff were long overdue. The hospital derived further benefit from the voluntary efforts of the wartime Amenities Committee, notably the provision of film projection equipment, so much a feature of interwar patients' lives.[75]

Less tangibly, it is possible that the war years raised the public profile and perception of the hospital, given its role and the increasing contact which had ensued.[76] If this was later eroded as the mental hospital was re-established any net enhancement was valuable and the change of name, first to Norfolk Mental Hospital in 1920 and then to St Andrew's Hospital in 1923, was a significant and positive contribution. It was a suitable epitaph also to Thomson, a feature he had come to emphasise as medical superintendent and one which epitomised the idea of improvement rather than the simple or direct restoration of the asylum. But cautionary notes must be sounded. With the passing of Thomson and many key personnel, much depended upon the ability or eagerness of Connell and a new regime to deliver improvements in the longer term. It is also difficult to resist the conclusion that, in 1920, the enhanced, renovated and restored hospital fabric had apparently fared better

[74] AR, 1920, MS, p. 8.
[75] Thomson, 'War Hospital', Part 2.
[76] Bettinson, 'Norfolk War Hospital', p. 27. This account makes favourable comparisons with similar institutions; see also Abel-Smith, *The Hospitals 1800–1948*, Heinemann, London, 1964, p. 271.

than many of the evacuated patients through the Great War. Alongside the public history of Norfolk War Hospital and its achievements, what can be gleaned of their experiences constitutes a disturbing story and a sad commentary upon the low social priorities attached to those identified as mentally ill.

7

St Andrew's Hospital: innovation and constraints, 1920–39

The inter-war years mark a period of contrasts in the treatment of mental illness, as in many other aspects of economic and social policy, between the best intentions of policy formulation and the delivery of services for large numbers of people. Although the 1890 Act remained on the statute book, it was considerably modified and partly supplanted by new legislation. Material provision for 'idiots' or 'the feeble minded', specified under the 1913 Mental Deficiency Act and the 1914 Elementary Education (Defective and Epileptic Children) Act, had barely begun.[1] The 1913 Act also triggered administrative and legal changes, notably the replacement of the lunacy commissioners at the Lord Chancellor's department by the inspectors of a Board of Control, first under the Local Government Board and then from 1919 under the new Ministry of Health. Conventionally the onset of war is seen as masking the significance of these developments, although the experiences outlined in the previous chapter should warn against presentations of the new Board as the champion of the mentally ill.

Post-war planning featured a new emphasis upon appropriate forms of treatment rather than upon the proprieties of committal procedures, however.[2] The Board sought to promote inpatient treatments, which bypassed the stigma of certification wherever possible, and also outpatient clinics, held in general as well as mental hospitals. Ministry concern with the poor reputation and the sheer scale of asylums, now typically accommodating over 1,000 inmates, produced attempts to reorient treatment in smaller mental hospitals. Ideally these were to have villa-style accommodation and smaller wards to facilitate an improved classification of patients, with specific admission/reception wards provided and the general promotion of face-to-face relationships and treatment. These objectives were elaborated in Board inspectors' reports following visits to Norfolk even before the 1924–6 Royal Commission on Certification, Detention and Care of Persons of Unsound Mind. The Commission also emphasised links between mental and physical illness in further justification of the need for an interactive approach to

---

[1] The 1914 legislation required the application of permissive terms of the 1899 Elementary Education Act. See M. Jackson, *The Borderland of Imbecility*, Manchester University Press, 2000.
[2] K. Jones, *Asylums and After*, Athlone, London, 1993, p. 114.

treatment, the adoption of the universal term 'hospital' and the abandon-ment of the stigmatised terminology of asylumdom.

Although the 1890 Act and its certification processes remained, the 1930 Mental Treatment Act set out alternative procedures and a future model. A patient willing to undergo treatment and making written application for it was seen as 'voluntary' and could then discharge himself or herself from a mental hospital at 72 hours' notice. Unwilling patients deemed likely to benefit from treatment could be given 'temporary' status under a special order, effective for up to six months and renewable for two further periods of three months if the Board of Control approved, thereby avoiding full committal.[3] There was no guarantee that voluntary patients would have control over their hospital treatments, however, or that if they chose to discharge themselves they might not later be certified and readmitted. Nevertheless the 1930 Act suggested a degree of empowerment for some patients and the possibilities of greater co-operation between patients and doctors in the quest for cure. Arguably, voluntary status, outpatient clinics and the possible use of general hospitals for treatments also suggested de-institutionalisation and even prototype forms of community care.[4]

Signs of a new approach in Norfolk, superficially at least, had included Thomson's own use of the term 'mental hospital' from 1910 and the official renaming of Norfolk Mental Hospital in 1920. Oliver George Connell, who became medical superintendent on 1 May 1922, had been Thomson's deputy since January 1920 and had a year's war service at Ashurst Military Hospital for War Neuroses, Oxford. He had previously been a medical officer at the Napsbury, Middlesex and Bicton, Shrewsbury asylums. In December 1923 Connell suggested the title St Andrew's Hospital, because 'to the public . . . the words "mental hospital" amount to "lunatic asylum"', and this was approved 'for local purposes only' in January 1924.[5] Connell, who gave evidence to the Royal Commission, immediately encouraged a parole system, which reduced the restrictions placed upon trusted patients, and tried to develop outpatient clinics. Board inspectors soon reported that, 'in discussing numerous matters with Dr Connell the progressive lines on which he wishes to develop the medical work here are very manifest'.[6] He later also promoted voluntary attendance and, with little success, the use of temporary patient status.

---

[3] Jones, ibid., pp. 120–40, surveys relevant legislative changes 1913–30.
[4] This supplements discussion in J.V. Pickstone (ed.), *Medical Innovations in Historical Perspective*, Macmillan, Basingstoke, 1992, pp. 186–9.
[5] Medical Superintendent's Reports, May 1922–March 1927, SAH 136, 13 Dec. 1922; Committee of Visitors (CVIS) Special business, Sept. 1919–April 1925, SAH 22, 3 Jan. 1924. The Suffolk County Asylum had already become St Audrey's Hospital, Melton, and the title 'St Andrew's Hospital, Thorpe, Norwich' appeared on the 1923 annual report, published in 1924.
[6] Board of Control Inspectors' Reports (BoC) 1926–59, SAH 142. Copies are cited with page numbers as they appeared in published versions in the hospital's annual reports.

Innovations are often restricted by financial and other constraints and in Norfolk, as elsewhere, public spending curbs followed the Great War and the 1931 financial crisis. Although Connell and the committee of visitors operated under these restrictions, stop-gap measures and an atmosphere of 'make do and mend' seem to have applied throughout the inter-war period. With a range of facilities from the former war hospital available on-site for purchase second-hand and the pressing needs of major capital projects, notably the renewal of boiler house equipment and new drainage and sewerage arrangements, this was to an extent understandable. As will be seen, Norfolk County Council also made a substantial financial commitment in establishing the Little Plumstead Colony for Mental Defectives between 1929 and 1933, although the long-term problem of overcrowding at St Andrew's was addressed cheaply. However, Board inspectors became frustrated at the slow pace of local improvements. By 1930 they were openly critical of the hospital's admissions facilities and its failure to reorganise men's wards to improve the classification of patients and provide a less barrack-like atmosphere. Similar dissatisfaction with overcrowding on the women's side, inadequate occupation therapy for male patients and poor facilities for visitors did not augur well for a wholly progressive outlook.

Some other features merit further investigation. Greater importance was attached to appropriate forms of professional qualification and the Diploma in Psychological Medicine, introduced in 1910, was increasingly required and rewarded in new medical officers. Any contribution to the retention of good appointments and reduced medical staff turnover was likely to work to the patients' advantage, if more regular face-to-face contact was the goal. Attendants and nurses were also expected to obtain nursing qualifications: in Norfolk the emphasis remained on the (Royal) Medico Psychological Association Final Certificate.[7] Successful outcomes were publicly equated with improving standards but these were undermined by the continuing high turnover of newly trained staff. Connell's own reports as medical super-intendent were cursory, predictable and suggestive of routinism: the contrast with an eye for detail and the encouraging or even campaigning tone adopted in corresponding reports by Board inspectors is noticeable. A novel feature was the arrival of women on influential bodies: Isabel G.H. Wilson visited the hospital twice as a Board inspector in the 1930s and from 1931 Mrs G. Cook and Miss M. Couzens-Hardy joined the committee of visitors in response to a stipulation of the 1930 Act. Although Connell was sensitive to the inspectors' criticisms, his efforts were dogged by financial restrictions and he adopted a lower profile than his predecessor. If these impressions are

---

[7] After the 1919 Registration of Nurses Act the General Nursing Council introduced its own Mental Nursing Certificate and the RMPA certificate was eventually phased out in 1952. R. White, *The Effects of the National Health Service on the Nursing Profession 1948–1961*, King's Fund, London, 1985, chapter 6.

misleading, patient case notes, the less constricted actions of voluntary patients, and the earliest oral testimony of people associated with the hospital offer additional pointers to any change in treatments and attitudes towards patients.[8]

Improvements and overcrowding

The return of fewer existing and new patients than might have been expected in 1919 meant that the reopened hospital initially had some spare capacity, its 1920–21 average of 855 resident patients appreciably less than the pre-1914 maximum of 1,050. By 1923 there were over 1,000 patients and their number expanded steadily, reaching an average of 1,205 in 1930. A solution to these overcrowded levels rested upon the belated establishment of what was described as a colony for mental defectives four miles away at Little Plumstead and the use of still more detached workhouse accommodation as hospital annexes. Even with patient transfers, the number resident at any one time at St Andrew's continued to exceed 1,100 (see Table 7.1) with roughly 1,400 under treatment in the course of each year.

In 1919 the use of former war hospital equipment represented an economical means of improvements when materials were in short supply and costs were high. X-ray, dental care and operating theatre equipment had already been purchased when ward 1 in the women's hospital was converted into a treatment centre with examining rooms and additional offices in 1920. Mr Charles Noon and Dr H.J. Starling were also engaged to attend monthly and in emergencies, respectively as consulting surgeon and physician.[9] The longer-term disadvantages of conversion or a patchwork approach could not be calculated, although Thomson's emphasis upon sexual segregation led to some duplication when better centralised facilities might have been provided. Foresight remained that most scarce of resources, however, and if the Board of Control was in possession of a blueprint for improvement, this was not revealed locally before the mid-1920s.

Yet Connell and the hospital committee were soon faced with other pressing demands, which swallowed up much of the hospital's accumulated funds and jeopardised further expansion. With thirteen deaths from TB and

---

[8] Mrs Doris Rose, who nursed on the women's wards from 1931, had fewer recollections of Connell than of Dr Livesay, at the women's hospital until 1935, or even Dr Morris, in the men's hospital until 1933. I am particularly grateful to Mrs Rose and her daughter Mrs Louise Fitt for a detailed transcript of Mrs Rose's recollections and other information on the asylum/hospital.

[9] MS Journal, 7 Sept. 1922. Connell's first request (4 May 1922) was for improvements to his house, after which the senior medical officer occupied the original master/superintendent's rooms, recently used for office space.

twelve active cases reported in 1922, some former hutments were moved across the male hospital approach road and converted as a 'quasi-temporary' isolation hospital for twelve male and twelve female tuberculosis patients in 1923.[10] Male ward F and the former women's isolation hospital were refurbished and verandahs added for use as admission hospitals. However, committee minutes and Board inspectors' reports suggest that the planned size and purpose of these buildings was subjected to repeated revision and delay.[11] The intended women's admission hospital was used merely as an additional dormitory until 1926, for example, and that on the male side was not ready until 1927. Other war hospital hutments were earmarked as additions to the 'tubercular hospital' in 1924 and as a male parole ward in 1925 before they were adapted as a fifty-bed women's ward in 1926.

How did this situation arise? First, the hospital committee became preoccupied with two capital projects. Following complaints by the nearby Blofield rural district council, it emerged that the expanded war hospital had overwhelmed the former asylum sewerage and drainage system and had been allowed to discharge raw sewage into the river Yare. Although the hospital sewage plant was overhauled, it was in poor condition and lay in close proximity to the intended women's admissions hospital. Connell warned that 'a visitor from the Board of Control . . . will raise some adverse comment about patients sleeping . . . so near the sewage beds. I would like the committee to bear this in mind should such trouble occur.'[12] As a major sewerage scheme linking Thorpe village with the Norwich area system was in progress, the committee decided to connect the hospital and estate cottages, at a cost of £7,500.[13] Along with a reservoir to ensure ample water supplies in the event of fire, these measures disrupted both hospital sites for three years before their completion in 1926. Acknowledging its 'inestimable value', Board inspectors nevertheless felt that 'this expensive work has . . . delayed improvements that would otherwise have been undertaken'.[14]

Meanwhile, the hospital committee divided over a second problem, the condition of boilers and generating equipment, before it decided upon a five-year replacement programme rather than reliance upon outside sources of electricity. In 1927 the first phase of work, with additional pumps and emergency generators, cost £11,500, fully one whole year's spending on capital account.[15] In addition, £8,000 was requested from Norfolk County

[10] Annual Reports, 1906–21, SAH 32; 1920, MS, p. 10 and CVIS, 1915–23, SAH 15, 16 Feb. 1922.

[11] CVIS, 16 Feb. 1922; BoC, 17 June 1924, p. 11, 27 April 1927, p. 12 and 17 March 1926, p. 12.

[12] MS Journal, 3 May 1923.

[13] CVIS, 1 June 1922 and CVIS Special, 2 Dec. 1926.

[14] BoC, 17 March 1926, p. 12.

[15] CVIS Special, 7 Feb. 1924, 31 March 1925 and 1 April 1926. The third replacement boiler was finally installed in 1932.

Council for the first post-war redecoration of the hospital. Spending on these items effectively precluded any major recommendation by Board inspectors. When Neville Chamberlain, Minister of Health, visited on 28 October 1926 he found the hospital suitably spruced up and duly expressed his 'entire satisfaction with the organisation and general care of patients'.[16] This was not wholly unexpected, but it echoed the general tone still being taken by Board inspectors. Perhaps in recognition of the investment at the hospital, their suggestions were modest and Connell was able to respond. Thus a 'small but quite nice laboratory' was established in the women's hospital in 1926, followed by the renewal of X-ray and introduction of ultraviolet light equipment and improvements in dental and operating theatres.[17] A former glasshouse was also converted as an outdoor ward for fifteen women patients in 1927.

These piecemeal improvements and shuffling of ward accommodation occurred in the context of an unrelenting rise in patient numbers and corresponding efforts by Board inspectors to tackle overcrowding and to prepare for new treatment procedures. Admissions increased further from 1920 under contractual arrangements with poor law and borough authorities in Great Yarmouth for the reception of 100 patients. Thirty women patients were also transferred from Napsbury Hospital, Middlesex in 1923 and, though St Andrew's was full on the women's side the following year, their return 'at no distant date' was delayed until 1926. Board inspectors also 'saw several patients who appeared to us to be suitable for detention in a properly equipped Poor Law Institution'.[18] They suggested for the first time the possibility of outpatient clinics, using the hospital's medical officers and honorary consulting staff at the Norfolk and Norwich Hospital. Even after the Napsbury patients departed Board inspectors criticised the 'distinct overcrowding' in female dormitories. They also 'had some conversation with Dr Connell as to what may be considered day accommodation' and felt that 'there may have to be some re-adjustment of the figures given to us'.[19] Outbreaks of paratyphoid, linked to the drainage alterations, raised their anxiety in 1928 and fears grew that smallpox, prevalent in the area, would appear at the hospital despite a substantial re-vaccination effort. A number of typhoid 'carriers' were identified as the laboratory came into its own but they remained with other patients because 'the excess of patients over the authorised space has increased somewhat alarmingly'.[20] By now the men's

---

[16] AR, 1926, MS, p. 9.
[17] BoC, 7 March 1927, p. 14 and 14 March 1928, p. 14.
[18] BoC, 17 June 1924, p. 11.
[19] BoC, 7 March 1927, p. 13.
[20] BoC, 14 March 1928, p. 13; 26 Nov. 1929, p. 11. Excesses of over 60 women patients on authorised day and night space and over 30 men on day space did not prevent the renewal of contracts for 100 Great Yarmouth patients.

hospital was also overcrowded, frustrating Connell's plan to subdivide the large wards and improve the classification of patients. As he had pressed for new buildings 'within the next two or three years at the most' in 1926, the committee was understating matters early in 1929, when it acknowledged that 'some scheme for the provision of further accommodation will have to be considered in the near future'.[21]

As yet there was no clear plan. Faced with overcrowding, the committee remained reluctant to cancel the lucrative accommodation of Great Yarmouth patients. While it sought low cost alternatives, Connell urged poor law medical officers 'to refrain from sending to this hospital chronic or harmless patients'. He reminded the Thetford guardians that their pneumonia or typhoid patients might become delirious but were not insane and that some senile patients might 'reasonably be retained at the workhouse'.[22] Poor law unions were also circularised with regard to suitable accommodation and Connell, accompanied by a Board inspector, actually visited Thetford workhouse in September 1926. However, the building was eighty-five years old, its wards were 'not attractive', it had 'old type prison windows' and was considered unsuitable. Lingwood workhouse was also considered as a hospital annexe in 1928 but Connell was again ordering forty extra bedsteads for St Andrew's the following year. With 1,230 patients resident in June 1930 it was decided that 'patients suffering from congenital mental defect . . . should not be detained in this hospital and that such cases should be brought before the committee at subsequent meetings with a view . . . to their discharge'. This matter was already the concern of the Norfolk County Council Mental Deficiency Acts Committee (see below) but the full council was asked 'if steps can be taken at an early date to provide accommodation for at least 100 senile cases'.[23]

Under the 1929 Local Government Act local authority public health and public assistance committees took over poor law arrangements and Norfolk County Council was among the bodies empowered to appropriate former workhouse accommodation. Swainsthorpe Public Assistance Institution, five miles south of Norwich, was set aside 'to accommodate senile cases in Poor Law institutions and the mental hospital in order to relieve overcrowding there'.[24] Its existing inmates were transferred to Wicklewood PAI and 37 senile women patients were sent from St Andrew's by the end of 1931. Patient M.D. was among the group transferred together on 11 January 1934. Then aged 71, she was first admitted after her fiancé emigrated and had been a working patient since 1889. E.F., admitted in 1901, had been transferred to

---

[21] MS Journal, 6 May 1926; AR, 1928, Cttee, p. 5.
[22] CVIS Special, May 1925–Aug. 1930, SAH 23, 7 Jan. 1926 and MS Journal, 3 Dec. 1925, 11 Jan. and 4 Feb. 1926.
[23] CVIS Special, 5 June 1930.
[24] CVIS Special, Sept. 1930–Dec. 1931, SAH 24, 4 Sept. 1930.

Brentwood in the Great War and did not wish to return; she was now 75 and had been 'unemployable' since 1920. C.P., admitted after her baby died in 1914, had been discharged because of the war but, according to her sister, 'had always been queer' and was in Thetford workhouse prior to her read-mission to St Andrew's. Three other patients simply had no one to care for them. E.B. was 84 years old and bedridden; F.B., aged 80, was a former midwife who had no children of her own; and M.H., aged 61, was a retired school teacher who had always lived alone but was now melancholic.[25]

In the men's hospital Board inspectors found evidence that overcrowding and large wards had produced a situation in which 'restless' patients annoyed quiet ones, who sometimes 'retaliated' before the attendants could inter-vene.[26] A major reshuffle followed in the next two years, with 320 male and female patients discharged 'relieved' from St Andrew's, two-thirds of them to Swainsthorpe. Fifty of the Yarmouth women patients moved in 1932 to Hellesdon Hospital, where they were joined by the remaining 10 women and 40 men in 1934. Afterwards the annual average of patients discharged 'relieved' exceeded 60, roughly three times the 1920s' level, and included additional transfers to Thetford PAI. On average, twelve more patients were discharged 'not improved' each year in the 1930s. Such measures helped to keep patient numbers fairly constant, with roughly 450 men and 680 women in residence for the remainder of the 1930s, although admissions and the total number of treatments and numbers 'relieved' had increased with the growth of voluntary attendance. Yet overcrowding on the women's side still featured, there was no reorganisation of male wards and the PAI accommodation provided for the transferred patients was unlikely to represent an advance on that at St Andrew's.

The issue of admission hospital facilities demonstrated a more dramatic shift in the attitude of Board inspectors. In 1926 they considered makeshift arrangements 'a very satisfactory indication of the progressive policy of those responsible for the management of this large hospital' but, two years later, stated that 'a properly equipped admission hospital with its ancillary villas' was needed at 'the first favourable opportunity'.[27] By 1930 'their provision is more urgent now that the Mental Treatment act is passed' as new accommodation, 'quite apart from those whose mental disorder is long standing and where behaviour is in any way of disagreeable character', was essential.[28] For example, use of the male admission ward verandah for TB cases was now unacceptable. While 'sympathetic' on this question, the

---

[25] Examples drawn from Case Books SAH 603.
[26] BoC, 20 Oct. 1932, p. 11. This followed a 'noisy' patient's complaints concerning his rough treatment in the 111-bed male C ward.
[27] BoC, 17 March 1926, p. 12 and 14 March 1928, p. 12.
[28] BoC, 17 Sept. 1930, p. 11. Inspectors also criticised use of the male admission ward verandah to accommodate TB cases.

hospital committee could not 'at present recommend the building . . . owing to the financial stress in the county' and soon afterwards it received a circular from the Ministry of Health calling for economies in the face of the 1931 national financial crisis.[29]

Board inspectors reiterated their opposition to proposals involving the conversion of existing buildings and stated that 'the matter will be kept in the forefront of the list of necessary works to be done'.[30] With Norfolk County Council financially committed to the Little Plumstead project and keen to economise elsewhere, there was deadlock. The committee at St Andrew's could not even consider conversion work and in 1934 Connell's rather desperate suggestion, that the production of breeze blocks in occupational therapy could be utilised in building an admissions unit, suggested labour camp economics. No other proposals were made and committee minutes indicate that the next capital project under consideration was for nurses' accommodation.[31] Still the Board inspectors persisted that 'the provision of more modern facilities for treatment . . . [is] undoubtedly desirable' and that 'accommodation for newly-admitted patients is not now up to present day standards'.[32] Their complaints suggested that, when compared with similar institutions, the hospital fabric was less satisfactory in 1939 than in 1914. Although important, it was not the sole determinant of standards of care. These are next examined using broad indications of hospital policy, published results and treatment records, the influences upon nursing staff and standards and more fragmentary evidence of hospital life.

Responses to national legislation

The better care of vulnerable individuals was always desirable, but much of the pre-war political and medical establishment was increasingly influenced by the concept of deficiency in the national population and its association with economic, social and even racial degeneration. David Thomson's concern with 'hereditary defect' in some asylum patients or their 'tainted progeny', noted in Chapter 5, would not have seemed odd, still less offensive, to many of his contemporary professionals. Legal confusions – the 1886 Idiots Act differentiated idiots from lunatics and the 1890 Act did not – compounded broader disagreements over the appropriate sites of care, particularly for the young. Thomson and his predecessor Hills wanted to remove 'idiots' or

---

[29] CVIS Special, 6 Aug. and 5 Nov. 1931.

[30] BoC, 29 April 1931, p. 11; 20 Oct. 1932, p. 13.

[31] CVIS, 4 Aug. 1934; 6 Oct. 1938. Responses to a Ministry of Health circular on capital projects indicate no funding for an admissions unit until 1941–2 at the earliest, even had there been no war.

[32] BoC, 21 May 1937, p. 12; 20 April 1939, p. 12.

'mental defectives' from asylums and workhouses but, like the authors of the 1913 Mental Deficiency Act, their motives were hardly humanitarian. Under the 1914 Elementary Education Act, local authority Education Committees were required to provide a suitable secure environment with appropriate help or training for 7- to 16-year-olds, with half the cost to be met by central government. In institutions or colonies sexual segregation was to be enforced and definitions of protection were sufficiently wide as to include, for example, the detention of pregnant but unmarried girls.

There were 22 children in Norfolk County Asylum when the 1913 Act came into operation and the new Board of Control urged their removal.[33] The Norfolk Education Committee also dealt with a small number of children under the 1899 Elementary Education (Defective and Epileptic Children) Act: most were at home, subject to domiciary visits and supervision, but six had been sent to the Royal Eastern Counties Institution at Colchester. A new Mental Deficiency Committee, comprised mainly of the asylum committee with Thomson as medical adviser, was charged with providing a plan for Norfolk, using the services of medical officers of health, poor law doctors and relieving officers.[34] More children sent to Colchester were joined by thirteen evacuated from the asylum in 1915 and, with parental consent, all remained there when the Norfolk Mental Hospital reopened. Nevertheless, with transfers, new admissions and overcrowding Connell complained in 1926 that 'a certain number of children, low grade mental defectives, who should not be sent here at all . . . take up adult beds'.[35] With marginally more concern a Board inspector noted, in a 111-bed male ward, 'several quite young patients, who I am glad to hear will, as soon as possible, be moved to a home for mental defectives'.[36]

The search for suitable accommodation ended when Norfolk County Council purchased Little Plumstead Hall and its estate, then the home of Major D.G. Astley, chairman of the St Andrew's hospital committee, for £14,600 in 1922. This was adapted to provide initial accommodation for 70 patients at a cost of £5,100 and, while suitable facilities were planned and constructed, 105 acres of land were temporarily leased to the St Andrew's hospital farm. The hospital also contributed personnel and facilities in this inaugural phase, notably Maud Gibbs, formerly assistant matron at St Andrew's, who became matron-superintendent after eight weeks' additional training at the Royal Eastern Counties Institution, Colchester. Dr Morris acted as visiting medical officer under Connell's supervision and was then

---

[33] BoC, 11 June 1914.
[34] Norfolk County Council Mental Deficiency Act Cttee (MDC minutes at Drayton Old Lodge), 10 April 1915.
[35] MS Journal, 11 Jan. 1926.
[36] BoC, 17 Sept. 1926, p. 11.

appointed as medical superintendent in 1933.[37] In May 1930 the first children were admitted and 48 girls were resident in December, but accommodation for boys remained incomplete.[38] Little Plumstead was intended as a mental defective colony for all Norfolk, including Norwich and Great Yarmouth, and local estimates envisaged up to 1,300 patients if adults were also included.[39]

Accommodation for 300 and facilities for 500 patients to allow further expansion was agreed upon, with segregated villa blocks for 60 adult males and females, boys' and girls' villa blocks of 50 beds each supplemented by two 20-bed homes. Other provision included accommodation for 40 nursing staff, a school hall and workshops along with boiler-house, kitchen, stores and laundry. With capital costs estimated at £105,000 in January 1931, economies were soon made. Using the 1929 Local Government Act and 1930 Public Assistance Act, Norfolk County Council earmarked the Heckingham PAI as a suitable annexe for 'low grade defectives'. This was fifteen miles from Little Plumstead, which would accommodate children and 'higher grades' suitable for training.[40] Construction work was delayed by a revised schedule, searches for lower cost materials and difficulties with sewerage arrangements but by March 1934 over 180 young patients were resident at Little Plumstead, with room for 150 more and a further 169 at Heckingham.[41]

With this rationalisation of the county's facilities St Andrew's could, in theory, focus upon the mentally ill. Although implementation of the 1930 Act was patchy and delayed, even earlier initiatives seem to have anticipated conceptions of community care. Some existing patients had already benefited from the modification of older systems of trial and parole. In the early 1920s Board inspectors noted 'a comparatively large number' of patients out on

---

[37] CVIS, 2 Jan. 1930. A. Roddick, assistant secretary at St Andrew's, became clerk and steward at Little Plumstead in April, though provisions, etc. were initially ordered via St Andrew's.

[38] NCC MDC (MDC) minutes, Oct. 1930–March 1934, C/C/10/370, 1 Jan. 1931. One child had died from TB and one was transferred. Residents included 20 girls aged under 16 years, 8 epileptic patients and 2 'cot and chair or idiot' patients. At least 4 girls arrived from St Andrew's, others returned from Colchester.

[39] MDC, 1 Oct., 6 Nov. and 4 Dec. 1930. The NCC (excluding Norwich and Gt Yarmouth) had 120 children or juveniles at Colchester or in PAI accommodation and 200 under supervision in their own homes. Over 300 adults were in public assistance or special institutions or on outdoor relief.

[40] Objecting that Heckingham would not be a single-sex institution, the Board of Control granted only temporary approval. It was told bluntly that 'Norfolk was a poor county . . . it would be more practicable to deal with a single institution rather than ask for too much'. MDC, 6 Nov. 1930; 4 June 1931. Former Heckingham inmates were transferred to Lingwood PAI and Pulham St Mary PAI.

[41] Capital spending was £81,250 and net maintenance costs roughly £20,000. Norwich and Gt Yarmouth paid standing charges for a quota of patients, plus maintenance. MDC, 6 June 1933, 4 Jan. and 1 March 1934.

trial. Not all were practically recovered for the procedure was also 'used with a view to testing whether a patient is fit to reside at home, or with friends, though still far from mentally well'.[42] N.S., for example, had recurrent mania and underwent two periods of treatment in the hospital. Her husband was concerned that 'she may be taken by the police for some crime', as she was prone to purchase goods and bus rides without the means to pay. She was still 'excited and garrulous' four months after readmission but asked to go home and, after a week's trial, was discharged and 'waiting for her husband to take her'.[43]

Roughly 100 patients were granted periods of leave in any one year, though only a minority had a cash allowance, a defect in an otherwise progressive policy. Boards of Guardians were quick to focus upon the differential between hospital charges made on them and the actual expenditure incurred by the hospital in such cases. Loddon and Clavering guardians were reassured that leave and a two-guinea allowance to patient H.S. 'was made after enquiry and that the practice . . . is one which may result in real economy', but they were less concerned with the long term. The Erpingham guardians were more direct: when B.T. was sent on trial without an allowance, they threatened her return unless she was supported financially by the hospital or relatives.[44] Roughly 220 patients were also on parole, one-third of them allowed to leave the hospital, conditional upon their nightly return. The remainder, limited to the hospital estate, were usually working patients and three wards, male H, female 9 and the laundry ward, operated on an open-door basis. Window locks were also gradually removed, though small blocks were retained to ensure adequate ventilation on the wards. Such measures, the Board inspectors felt, did 'a very great deal to promote general contentment . . . remove the idea of imprisonment and to increase . . . individual responsibility'.[45]

A second initiative lay in hospital committee support for the Mental After-Care Association. Founded in 1879 to help former asylum patients, this had little presence in Norfolk until 1924 when a group of prominent local ladies, including wives of committee members, presented plans for secure cottage homes for older patients and suitable positions for recovered patients. Connell enthused over their request for philanthropic and local authority help, not least because 'it would greatly be to our advantage, in view of the Royal Commission . . . if we are asked what steps we take with such cases'. 'Financial assistance from all the Norfolk Boards of Guardians' and private donations were obtained along with 'considerable help . . . in finding homes for a number of senile cases who were suitable for discharge to cottage

---

[42] AR, 1921, BoC, p. 10; BoC 25 Nov. 1922, p. 12.
[43] Case Books, SAH 603 (N.S.).
[44] CVIS Special, 4 Jan. 1925; 5 Aug. 1926.
[45] BoC 17 June 1924, p. 10.

homes'.[46] Connell's subsequent reports suggested that the Association's more ambitious plans were dependent upon hospital appeals to a reluctant Norfolk County Council for financial aid under the terms of the 1930 Act.

Shortly before he retired, David Thomson had concluded that nearly one-third of his patients were 'obviously incurable', that one-third were 'paranoic/delusional/hallucinatory cases of long-standing' and that the remainder were experiencing acute or prolonged stress. He felt that post-war reform efforts should address pre-hospital stages of treatment, using outpatient clinics without certification, to avoid stigma and secure prompt attention 'for the obviously curable cases of short duration'.[47] This anticipated the Board inspectors' suggestion and in July Connell was authorised 'to take such steps as is deemed necessary towards establishing a mental clinic at the N&N hospital'. Having requested information he was already aware of successful precedents at Radcliffe Hospital, Oxford and Queen's Hospital, Birmingham and hoped 'to see and treat patients with a view to preventing certification'.[48]

Connell encountered some lack of co-operation and had anticipated problems over the use of the voluntary hospital's facilities. He was positive that short-term costs arising from 'these positive ideas' would be more than offset in the longer term, though he was also motivated by the belief that 'the Royal Commission will comment adversely if no attempt is made to establish such a clinic'.[49] By the time a delegation comprising Connell, the medical superintendent at Hellesdon hospital (the former city asylum) and representatives from their hospital committees formally approached the Norfolk and Norwich hospital the 1930 Act was imminent. They successfully proposed outpatient clinics at the N&N, where city and county patients would be seen by the relevant medical superintendents. 'Defectives and chronic cases of insanity formed the majority of those attending' but Connell felt that the experiment was 'justified by the fact that a proportion of borderline cases have derived considerable benefit'.[50] The number attending increased slowly to 47 in 1939 with additional clinics held at St Andrew's and King's Lynn from 1937.

Meanwhile, voluntary patient numbers rose from 24 in 1930 to exceed 80, over one-third of the new admissions, in the late 1930s. Few could be considered less serious or complex than the patients who were certified. Among the first was J.E., a young woman of 20 whose depression over a love affair was not helped by her father's beatings, which may have triggered her decision to be admitted. Feeling better, she discharged herself a fortnight later, her 72-hour notice stating, 'I have a situation to go to, it was quite my

---

[46] MS Journal, 3 July 1924; AR, 1926, Cttee, p. 5, MS, p. 10.

[47] AR, 1921 MS, p. 5.

[48] MS Journal, 3 July 1924; CVIS Special, 3 July 1924.

[49] MS Journal, 3 July 1924.

[50] AR, 1931, MS, p. 8. Twenty-nine outpatients were seen in the first year of the scheme.

fault that I came here'. Connell was less convinced and wrote to her GP: 'I suggest that if you find her certifiable at any time it would be as well to certify and send her back.' After five years as companion/maid she returned as a voluntary patient in 1938 and Connell diagnosed her schizophrenic. She was then placed under the novel and risky cardiazol shock therapy. Her voluntary status did not prevent this essentially experimental treatment but, in conjunction with her contacts with the outside world, limited it. When her former employer offered her work and her father requested her discharge, Connell reluctantly agreed.[51]

Another patient, M.F.,was admitted in a depressed state following a hysterectomy at the age of 38. Rather quickly her doctor decided that she was 'self-centred, hypochondriacal and dissatisfied . . . has many unreasonable complaints' and she, equally rapidly, felt better and left the hospital 'recovered' within the fortnight. V.C.'s illness was associated with the shock of finding her five-month old baby dead. After three months she became a voluntary patient, then resumed eating and slept better in hospital, although she had 'delusions of unworthiness'. She prayed a great deal and claimed to hear God's voice, though this was the only answer she found in hospital before she discharged herself, 'relieved' after two weeks.[52]

More voluntary patients contributed to the growing numbers 'relieved' in the 1930s. Admissions fell slightly in 1939 but almost all were directly from patients' homes and 39 per cent were voluntary. It was premature to ascribe great significance to these figures but, if they reflected the value of early contact and the success of outpatient clinics, they were encouraging. In contrast, plans to admit temporary patients failed completely. Relieving officers showed little inclination to deal with orders for the 'rate-aided class', local general practitioners seemed unaware of or unenthusiastic about such plans and patients or their relatives saw little difference between 'temporary' and 'committal' status in cases where attendance was involuntary. Connell relayed critical observations by Board inspectors and the contents of a Board of Control circular on the subject to all relieving officers and GPs in Norfolk to no avail, as the only temporary patient admitted to St Andrew's in the 1930s was transferred directly from Hellesdon hospital.[53]

---

[51] Case Books, SAH 650 (J.E.), covering the period 1933–8. Connell's letter was dated 30 May 1933. Cardiazol, a noxious chemical, was administered to induce epileptic fits on the dubious observation that epileptics were not schizophrenic. J.E. returned again to St Andrew's in 1944, see Chapter 8.

[52] Case Books, SAH 603 (V.C.).

[53] CVIS, 7 Feb. 1935 (BoC circular no. 805).

Patients and treatments

Hospital reports in this period offered little comment on the social background of patients. There were virtually no private patients, although the fifty or so long-term 'service' patients, maintained by the Ministry of Pensions and paid a small weekly allowance of 2s 6d, were regarded as such. Before the 1929 and 1930 Acts St Andrew's remained closely associated with the poor law and patient transfers frequently involved the workhouse. Afterwards there were still many 'rate-aided persons of unsound mind' like A.H., aged 53, on poor relief for twenty years and admitted from Downham PAI in 1931 in a manic condition. She was sedated initially, then became a working patient and four months later asked to leave, but was 'quite unfitted to live alone and no relative has offered to take her . . . says she would like to go to Downham workhouse'. After repeated requests she was transferred there on trial but soon returned, 'quite impossible – noisy and interfering'. Fifteen months later she was again discharged, this time 'relieved' to Swainsthorpe PAI. Most patients had poor labouring and domestic service backgrounds or were currently, if not formerly, dependent or destitute. E.B., aged 73, only became 'restless and confused' after her husband died but was in poor physical health. She was also moved to Swainsthorpe but, becoming more ill and anxious, was returned to St Andrew's and died from heart disease a year later. W.A. had been in the Royal Navy during the war and was evidently if not officially traumatised. He spent the 1920s in workhouse wards and the Yarmouth Infirmary until an assault upon a fellow patient led to his arrival at St Andrew's in 1933. Six months later he was again in transit, the hospital secretary's letter to his mother stating merely: 'I beg to inform you that the County Borough of Gt Yarmouth has arranged with Norwich City Council for the future treatment of their patients at the Norwich City Mental Hospital, Hellesdon.'[54]

With the limited diversification of occupations in inter-war Norfolk, links between rural labour, poverty and mental illness remained. The reason for S.A.'s discharge from the army in 1916 was unknown, but he was a farm labourer until he became unemployed in 1932. This triggered his depression and he was seriously ill when persuaded to enter hospital two years later. 'Coaxed to eat', he soon refused food and an attempt at tube-feeding led to his collapse. He remained feeble, was notified tuberculous and died a week later in 'depressive stupor with hypostatic congestion'. W.T. had been a farm labourer and completed his military service but then became 'peculiar . . . and a nuisance to the neighbours'. He was admitted after assaulting a relative in 1921 and quickly became 'a useful member of the farm gang'. He had a hernia but was always 'in his usual health' until he was quite unexpectedly found dead in bed one morning in December 1944. A third farmworker, W.H.,

---

[54] Case Books, SAH 603 (A.H.); 600 (E.B.); 607 (W.A.).

'could give no account of himself' when found wandering by Norwich police in 1929. As a Norfolk patient he was moved from Hellesdon to St Andrew's and worked well in the farm gang, Dr Morris noting that he always described himself as 'Chief constable of the hospital'. He was allowed parole, re-graded as a voluntary patient and eventually discharged himself in 1945, his notice stating that 'he had a job to go to'.[55]

If family breakdowns often led to admissions, family ties and close rural communities were a significant feature in recoveries. E.E., a 26-year-old farmworker, became manic after his mother was paralysed in June 1929. He had a very difficult year in hospital, at first requiring spoon-feeding, with spells on paraldehyde and bouts of bronchitis and pneumonia. Throughout, he was regularly visited by his father, sister, brother, other relatives and the local vicar. He gradually became 'brighter and free from delusions . . . works quite well now about the ward' and was discharged 'recovered' in December 1930. Patient E.A. was left with three children when her husband was killed in France in 1916. The family was increasingly impoverished; she constantly told her daughter 'all the money is gone and we will all starve' and she weighed 5 stone 12 lbs on her admission in August 1934. Over the next five months, she was regularly visited by all three children, she gained almost a stone in weight and 'worked very well' in the sewing room. On her recovery, her daughter wrote simply to the matron: 'I shall be coming for mum on Saturday . . . I thought I would let you know so mother don't have to be downhearted . . . I hardly know what to write because I am so happy please let mum see this.'[56]

With a large number of long-term patients and reasonable efforts to contain mortality the age profile of the total hospital population was naturally advanced. Patient F.A., for example, was suicidal on admission but then recovered her bodily health and considered herself 'boss of the workroom'. There was some basis for her claim for when she died in 1930, aged 90, she had been in the hospital and its wartime substitute for forty-eight years.[57] The year 1930 represents a suitable mid-point for the period and the last before the transfer of older patients to Swainsthorpe or of younger ones to Little Plumstead became established. One-fifth of all patients were then aged 65 years or more and almost one half were aged between 45 and 64 years. Less than one-third were under 45 years old, only one-ninth of the total were aged 25–34 years and just one in thirty patients was less than 24 years old.[58] When admissions are compared over three sub-periods, 1922–5 marking Connell's first years, the early 1930s and later 1930s, the initial breadth of the patients' age profile is noticeable, though there was some ageing of admissions groups

[55] Case Books, SAH 590 (S.A.), 606 (W.T.); 591 (W.H.).
[56] Case Books, SAH 650 (E.E.), 607 (E.A.).
[57] Case Books, SAH 607.
[58] AR, 1930, Table IV, p. 17.

later on. Until 1935 there were roughly as many patients aged 25–34 years as in any other ten-year cohort group above the age of 25 years, each group comprising 17–19 per cent of total admissions. Afterwards, 40 per cent of admissions were aged 55 years or more, compared with 34 per cent in the early 1920s.[59]

Connell also provided a summary grouping of the causes of insanity, which covered about two-thirds of new admissions. In the early 1920s 'insane heredity' affected over 30 per cent of admissions, while 13 per cent suffered from 'acute or prolonged stress' or senile decay and just 2 per cent had alcoholic intemperance or had syphilis. Hereditary features remained prominent in the early 1930s and were cited in 25 per cent of admissions by the late 1930s. 'Senility' accounted for 11 per cent of admissions in the 1930s but the gender dimensions of 'acute or prolonged stress' were revealed even in summary information. Nearly 10 per cent of all admissions were affected but a similar proportion had 'climacteric' disorders and another 5 per cent were evidently affected by 'puberty'. These latter categories were confined to women patients, who comprised 60 per cent of annual admissions and residents (see Table 7.1). Life-cycle features and social status were routinely cited in explanation of their insanity: for every twenty-five women admitted, four had conditions related to the menopause, two to puberty and one to childbirth. Four more were considered 'senile' and three were noted as 'widowed'. These defining characteristics were retained during the 1930s, with a slight increase recorded in the proportion of widowed women patients.

Hospital admission was a questionable procedure for women who lacked emotional or economic support in periods of crisis. Their illnesses and needs were defined by a male-dominated profession, largely in the absence of suitable alternative personnel or facilities. For example, patient E.S., who lived with her parents, had an illegitimate child brought up by them but always regretted sending away her lover. She was admitted some twenty-two years later as a 'climacteric/melancholia' patient and attempted suicide on her second day in hospital. With pleurisy and suspected tuberculosis, she was placed in the open-air ward where her subsequent weight gain was interpreted as a sign of recovery until her visiting sister mentioned the family history of oedema. She was given a diuretic but developed pneumonia and died eight days later. B.S. was more fortunate; her 'change of life' made her depressed but a combination of extra diet, sleeping draughts and nights in the open-air ward produced sufficient improvement for her to be discharged 'relieved' to her husband. A third patient, A.M., was admitted into St Andrew's when her husband died but she recovered and went to work as a housekeeper for the next eleven years. After she 'had suddenly taken against

---

[59] Calculated from annual reports 1922–5, 1930–4 and 1936–9, Table IV. Younger patients may have featured in voluntary attendance, with some at outpatient clinics or Little Plumstead in the later 1930s.

. . . her employer without reason' she was readmitted as a 'climacteric/ recurrent mania' case. Because she was debilitated, doctors assumed that her allegation, that her employer quarrelled because she had refused to sleep with him, 'hardly seems credible and is probably a delusion'. With thyroid treatment she gained weight and worked in the laundry for eighteen months before she was discharged recovered after a successful trial.[60]

Four contrasting examples illustrate very different problems affecting women patients. G.N., aged 27, was certified after an apparent suicide attempt in June 1933. She was married with two children but was now pregnant by another man and, as she explained to Dr Livesay, was trying 'to get out of it'. With no medication required, she felt better and worked until her baby was delivered at the end of October. In November she was 'up and well' and was discharged 'recovered' two months later. I.M.'s second child was born just two days before she was admitted with 'recent mania' and a temperature of 103 degrees. She was put on a catheter and given an enema for her distended abdomen and hyoscyamine to promote sleep. Her death the following day was partly ascribed to 'Part II mania', but this was probably an attendant feature upon the puerperal toxaemia also cited. Mrs Y—. was a victim of another sort: she had recovered but was transferred to Downham workhouse, accompanied by a letter stating that she was not insane and requesting the guardians to employ 'the kindest methods . . . to influence her husband and restore Mrs Y— to her home'.[61] Lastly, M.S. aged 70, was married but had no children and had led a comfortable life until her husband died. She became increasingly depressed and after six weeks was admitted to hospital. A trial with relatives was quickly arranged but her condition deteriorated further and she was re-certified. Now 'very feeble', she was spoon-fed and given medinol to help her sleep. Her death, within thirteen days of first admission, was ascribed to a rather broad interpretation of senile dementia.[62]

By the early 1920s all wards had a clinical or doctor's room where patients could be individually interviewed or examined and their records maintained. Diagnoses and treatments were facilitated by general improvements in medicine and related technology, notably X-ray diagnosis of fracture after falls or accidents and in general monitoring for tuberculosis. Blood, faecal, urine and spinal fluid testing became routine in the earlier identification of disease, though a full-time laboratory assistant was not appointed until 1933. Induced malaria treatment for general paralysis was offered, though the hospital had few cases and little came of an offer to make this available to patients from other hospitals, as suggested by Board inspectors.[63] Connell had secured financial support for his subscriptions to the Royal Society of

---

[60] Case Books, SAH 600 (E.S,); 603 (B.S., A.M.).
[61] CVIS, 5 March 1925.
[62] Case Books, SAH 603 (G.N., I.M.); 600 (M.S.).
[63] BoC, 14 March 1928, p. 12.

Medicine on the grounds that the availability of new research findings would improve laboratory work and treatments.[64] However, he also implemented measures such as an extra padded room for elderly women who, 'because of their restless condition are liable to fracture a limb or bruise themselves, which in a case of death would mean unnecessary inquests'.[65] Rest days in bed 'about once a week' for these patients were cited as a feature in their better health in 1934 and, as with other patients, the monitoring of any weight loss was usually followed by transfer to the ward verandahs or the women's 'greenhouse' ward.

Dentistry at the hospital became extensive, if rudimentary: all new patients were routinely examined and treated, but a large number of extractions and emergency treatments were undertaken using general anaesthesia at weekly clinics. Major surgical operations were also carried out by Mr Noon. Patient M.L., aged 42 and in poor health, had liver extract to counter her anaemia and had most of her teeth extracted. In March 1933 Dr Livesay noted a discharging swelling on her breast and Noon advised its amputation. With the permission of her nearest relatives obtained, a mastectomy was performed at the hospital and, two days later, Livesay noted, 'Tube removed. Wound looking well'. The medium-term success of the procedure was indicated by her transfer 'relieved' to Swainsthorpe ten months later. However, little could be done for E.B. who, at 58, had confusional insanity, heart disease, breathing difficulties and oedema of both legs. Over an eight-month period he also collapsed and had a stroke, but was revived by medication which included digitalin, brandy, atropine, coramine, strychnine and oxygen administration. If the imminence of his death was predictable, hospital staff had attempted a range of treatments to forestall it.[66]

Table 7.1 suggests some improvement on pre-1914 experiences, with a greater percentage of admissions later discharged 'recovered' and lower overall rates of mortality. Sustained improvement during the inter-war period is less noticeable, however. The decennial average number of residents for the 1920s masks a real increase, from 822 to 1,205, between 1920 and 1930. Recovery rates on admissions were sustained, although annual fluctuations were amplified by voluntary attendance after the 1930 Act. For example, in the sub-period 1930–34 annual male recovery rates varied between 18 and 40 per cent and female rates between 30 and 46 per cent. The increasing number of those discharged 'relieved' reflected the ability of voluntary patients to discharge themselves and the transfer of older patients to public assistance accommodation. Similarly, more patients were discharged 'not improved'. Given these trends, an increase in readmissions, from one quarter of all

[64] CVIS, 4 April 1934. Possibly associated with new treatments (e.g. induced pyrexia) and drugs (tryparsamide in late 1930s).
[65] MS Journal, 7 Feb. 1924.
[66] Case Books, SAH 603 (M.L.); 590 (E.B.).

Table 7.1 Average patient admissions, recoveries and mortality by decade, 1920–39

	Average no. resident			Admissions			% admitted recovered			Mortality %		
	Total	M	F	Total	M	F	Total	M	F	Total	M	F
1910–4	1035	453	582	225	103	122	31.5	28.1	34.4	11.2	11.4	11.0
1920–9	1009	412	597	233	96	137	39.0	32.9	43.4	7.4	8.6	6.6
1930–9	1141	458	683	244	103	141	40.0	35.0	43.6	6.2	7.8	5.1

Note: Admissions figure for 1920s excludes patients returning to the re-opened hospital in 1919–20.

admissions in the early 1920s to almost one-third in the 1930s, was not unexpected. However, mortality rates were significantly reduced, if at a decelerating rate and with a marked gender imbalance. Despite the particular difficulties faced by overcrowded women patients, their death rate fell below 6 per cent from 1922 to 1930, with low points of 3.4 per cent in 1935 and 3.8 per cent in 1939. This compared very well with a national mental hospital average of around 7 per cent, but male rates were higher and fell more slowly. Their low point of 5.5 per cent in 1938 was more satisfactory, but was immediately followed by a sharp rise reminiscent of pre-1914 levels in 1939.

Detailed study of changing causes of death over time is marred by alterations in the classification. Thus, broad reduction in 'senile decay' and greater emphasis upon diseases of the nervous system might indicate the changing role of St Andrew's or more determined efforts to present information felt appropriate to the public records of a mental hospital. Nor was it always clear whether pneumonia was the principal cause of death or a fatal associate of another deep-seated illness. Barely one quarter of deaths led to post-mortem investigations in the early 1920s and the proportion in the 1930s rarely exceeded one-third. Five or six broad forms of illness were routinely cited in four out of five deaths. Before 1925 24 per cent of deaths were attributed to 'senile decay', over 13 per cent to cerebral haemorrhage, 12 per cent each to TB and respiratory illnesses, mainly pneumonia, and 7 per cent to disease of the heart or circulatory system.

In the 1930s cerebral haemorrhage, cited in 25 per cent of deaths, was matched by heart and circulatory diseases. Pneumonia or bronchitis consistently caused 20 per cent of deaths, and cancers became more frequent, accounting for 10 per cent. Tuberculosis now killed less than 5 per cent and deaths associated with general paralysis and epilepsy, respectively 8 and 3 per cent of all fatalities before 1925, became infrequent. Whether prophylactic measures or earlier medical attention reduced the incidence of syphilis is uncertain, but the infrequent malarial treatment carried high risks.[67] The use

[67] Calculated from annual reports 1922–5, 1930–4 and 1936–9, Table III, Causes of death.

of phenobarbital greatly assisted in the management of epileptic conditions: when L.G.'s medication was suspended, because he was in such poor health and anaemic, he again experienced 'fits frequent and severe, at least five per day since Luminal has been stopped'. His death after ten more days was a reminder of earlier patterns of illness.[68]

Staff: conditions, qualifications and standards

There were few changes to the principal medical staff between the wars, though junior appointments arrived and left. Dr A.W. Livesay became senior medical officer on Connell's promotion in 1922 and occupied the position until his retirement in ill-health in 1935. George Goolden, the junior medical officer from 1919, was possibly overlooked and left in 1923, to be followed by R.E. Jenkins. Compared to Connell, whose salary was raised from £900 to £1,000 with emoluments worth £200 in 1923, Livesay and Jenkins were not overpaid even when £25 was added to their respective salaries of £400 and £350. When Jenkins resigned his post in February 1925 a locum was paid for three months while Connell sought a suitable applicant with the Diploma in Psychological Medicine. Finding none, he suggested that any successful junior should begin with a lower starting salary of £300, with £50 to be added on successful completion of the DPM. Dr J.V. Morris, appointed from three candidates interviewed, passed the preliminary part of the DPM in 1928 though his salary had already been raised to £400.[69] If familiarity aided treatment and medical management, having the same three medical officers for eight years probably benefited patients. When Morris became medical superintendent at Little Plumstead in 1933 his replacement, W.J. McCulley, already had the DPM and was quickly promoted as senior medical officer on Livesay's retirement. Drs T.A. Radcliffe and P.A. Heath then held the junior post before A.J. Crossley arrived in 1939.

On the retirement of Miss Hamer in May 1922 Miss R. Wheatley became matron until her death in 1936, after forty-two years at the hospital. Florence Thorpe and Maud Gibbs were appointed as her assistants, respectively in June and August 1922, the latter returning from a period as matron superintendent at Little Plumstead (1933–6) to become matron at St Andrew's. Percy Keeble, who had ten years' experience as a charge attendant and three as a temporary sergeant in the RAMC at the war hospital, became head male attendant in 1922; he and matron Gibbs remained in their posts until 1947.[70] The

---

[68] Case Books, SAH 590 (L.G.).
[69] MS Journal, 5 March and 7 May 1925; AR, 1928, MS, p. 10.
[70] After Mr Fitt retired in 1922 the hospital had women dispensers; Gladys Hughes 1922–3, Elizabeth Fitzgerald 1923–6, Miss Wagstaffe 1926–7, Miss Wilson 1927–8 and Dorothy Robertson 1928–30.

improved training of attendants and nurses, flagged to indicate rising standards, was somewhat undermined by staff turnover, itself suggesting continued problems notably during periods of retrenchment.

Because of its wartime status the hospital largely avoided an industrial dispute which was settled with the introduction of a sixty-hour working week including meal breaks, the payment of war bonuses, and wages based on prevailing rates in urban or rural areas. As a constituent of the Mental Hospitals Association the hospital committee implemented this settlement but was 'of the opinion that the present rates were equitable and that no action would be taken' regarding further increases. Wage costs represented 60 per cent of hospital spending. Most attendants were then earning between 46 and 56 shillings weekly and nurses from 36s 10d to 44s 9d, but the maximum figure for qualified senior staff was 62 shillings for women and 79 shillings for men.[71] An increase in board and lodging charges to nurses to 23s 6d per week in August led to the temporary resignation from the committee of George Edwards, its sole trade unionist and Labour councillor.

Against a backcloth of national wage reductions the following year, most rural mental hospitals cut attendants' wages by three shillings and nurses' pay by one-fifth, with holiday entitlement also curbed and the working week increased to an average of sixty-six hours.[72] A four shillings reduction at St Andrew's affected nurses particularly badly, as their board charges were not reduced by a similar amount, despite the general fall in living costs, for over a year. Corresponding pay cuts ordered for daily workers, engineers, porters and stores personnel were usually accompanied by the comments; 'if not accepted, his services to be dispensed with' or 'engagement of another man at reduced wages'.[73] The eight women daily helpers were dismissed 'as their work can be done by patient labour', saving £400, with works and engineering department staff numbers reduced by June 1922.

With patient numbers considerably less than pre-war averages and high maintenance costs the hospital undertook major cutbacks in nursing staff by 1922, confirmed in Table 7.2. Those such as nurse H—, dismissed on the spot for theft of patients' and nurses' clothing, and nurse D—, given notice as 'unsuitable for the service' after assaulting a patient, would have gone in any event. More marginal cases, for example attendants L— (neglectful of duty), A— (asleep on duty) and nurse C— (alleged misconduct), were expected to leave 'owing to reduction of staff' rather than on disciplinary grounds and their pensions contributions were reimbursed.[74] This deteriorating working

---

[71] CVIS Special, 6 May, 3 June and 9 Nov. 1920. Nationally, there had been strikes in Lancashire, a union recognition dispute in Cornwall and the extension of the union in Scotland.

[72] *History of the Mental Hospital and Institutional Workers Union 1910–31*, Manchester, 1931, pp. 54–5.

[73] CVIS, 16 Feb. 1922.

[74] MS Journal, 1 June 1922; CVIS Special, 7 Dec. 1922, 4 Jan. and 1 Feb. 1923.

Table 7.2 Nursing staff: numbers, qualifications and ratios to patients, 1922–39

	Day staff		Night staff		Qualified staff (preliminary)				Day staff: patients	
	M	F	M	F	M	(M)	F	(F)	M	F
1920	86	117	11	15					(1:3.8)	(1:4.4)
1921	78	98	7	13					(1:4.7)	(1:5.3)
1922	67	65	9	13	21	(20)	9	(8)	1:5.5	1:8.1
1926	65	78	10	13	34	(19)	14	(5)	1:6.7	1:8.2
1930	66	97	10	16	38	(13)	22	(20)	1:7.5	1:7.4
1934	65	87	10	17	47	(14)	37	(9)	1:6.6	1:7.8
1939	71	86	13	21	50	(16)	24	(19)	1:6.5	1:8.1

Notes: Staff to patient ratios for 1920–21 in parentheses are not directly comparable with later figures as the hospital then had greater spare capacity and a shorter working week. Information calculated from Annual Reports.

environment also produced extensive resignations as the hospital filled and by 1923 problems with nurse recruitment led Connell to investigate comparative rates of pay in other hospitals, locally and nationally. Concluding that 'we are on the lowest scale' he proposed an economy-conscious solution, which substituted a light supper for the nurses' evening meal, thereby allowing a four shillings reduction in boarding charges.[75] 1926 was not the best year for the union to campaign for a 48-hour working week and in 1930 the hospital committee resolved to take 'no action' in response to local requests for a 53-hour week. Four more years elapsed before two sympathetic committee members forced a vote on the issue and the Mental Hospitals Association itself recommended a maximum 54-hour week, exclusive of meals in February 1935, which meant the recruitment of additional staff at St Andrew's.[76]

The immediate post-war ratio of staff to patients could not be sustained with staff cuts and increases in the patient population. Table 7.2 suggests that nurses on overcrowded wards were under pressure throughout the 1920s, even as more were recruited, and that the situation for male attendants also deteriorated, albeit more slowly. Inevitably, there were dangerous moments. At the peak of an influenza outbreak in February 1922 67 of the 152 nurses and attendants were themselves in bed, along with 168 patients. During another outbreak in March 1924 the hospital was again short-staffed and the

[75] MS Journal, 5 July 1923. St Andrew's provided nurses with five meals, compared with three or four at most hospitals.
[76] CVIS Special, 7 June 1934; 1 April 1935. G. Hewitt and J. Weatherbed were union sympathisers; their resolution failed by 6 votes to 2 in 1934. George Edwards, the earlier union advocate, had died in 1933.

attendant running J.R.'s bath was called away. J.R. scalded his foot and ankle and his leg soon became infected. Connell was fearful that, 'in the event of the patient dying an inquest will be held', adding 'although he might die from some other cause'.[77] Additional staff were engaged as the women's wards became overcrowded but, although patients were transferred away after 1930, renewed economy measures meant that nurse to patient ratios again deteriorated. By 1939 extra night staff had been recruited in response to shorter working hours but the day staff were only 'just up to the figure regarded as necessary'.[78] Staffing levels on the men's side were better but the introduction of training in air raid precautions in 1937 was ominous and, almost immediately in 1939, numbers were 'seriously depleted owing to the calling up of those liable for service'.[79]

Typically Board inspectors remarked that: 'a very large proportion of members of the staff have long service to their credit . . . they appear generally to be well-trained and kindly in their behaviour to patients.'[80] These were not platitudes: adverse comments were made regarding other aspects of hospital life but never against the nursing staff. Features from the lack of bedsores among patients to the deployment of female nurses in the men's infirmary were cited as evidence of good nursing practice. Discipline also remained tight: attendant Ernest P—, 'found in possession of two bars of soap belonging to the hospital on his leaving duty', was dismissed and a similar fate awaited nurse A—, who overstayed her leave of absence. Less surprisingly, the hospital committee confirmed the dismissal of 'Harry C— . . . such negligence enabling a patient to escape', while attendant W—, dismissed for striking a patient and reapplying for work six months later, met with the unanimous response 'that his request could not be entertained'.[81]

When it chose to do so, the hospital committee tried to retain and reward suitable staff, offering a two shillings weekly proficiency payment to all who obtained their preliminary certificate and a similar addition for final certificate holders, while long-service bonuses were extended to domestic and laundry staff.[82] The proportion of male attendants who held the RMPA Final Certificate roughly doubled to two-thirds over the period, with most of the remainder taking the preliminary certificate (see Table 7.2). Nurses tended to be less qualified, the number taking the preliminary certificate was erratic and staff turnover was higher. In 1937, for example, Connell noted the nurse shortage and the need for fourteen more probationers. These problems were compounded by inadequate accommodation: 137 nursing staff slept at the

---

[77] ibid., 22 March 1924. Shortly afterwards R— died from acute nephritis.
[78] BoC, 20 April 1939, p. 14.
[79] AR, 1939, MS, p. 6.
[80] AR, 1921, BoC, p. 11.
[81] CVIS Special, respectively 6 March 1924, 2 May 1928, 5 Feb. 1925 and 3 Nov. 1927.
[82] ibid., 6 March 1930; 5 July 1928.

hospital but only 44 were at the nurses' home, with 21 in rooms on the wards, 9 in the laundry block, 7 in a detached block and 56 in hutments.[83] Unlike the majority of patients, nursing staff could vote with their feet and the hospital committee had to accept that, even with electric lights and hot water, wooden huts were still huts and now more than twenty years old. A proposed extension to the existing nurses' home, adding 70 more rooms at a cost of £17,500, was abandoned in favour of more radical plans for a completely new building for 150 nurses and costing £65,000, the former home to be used for patients' accommodation.[84]

Before she married, Mrs Doris Rose nursed at St Andrews from 1931 to 1936, working mainly on wards 5 and 6, and her recollections offer a valuable insight into ward life.[85] Seven day nurses dressed and washed approximately 60 patients each morning for an 8.00 a.m. breakfast. Some patients had to be spoon-fed bread and milk by nurses because they were invalid, others because they were unco-operative. Particularly difficult patients were temporarily sheeted in a chair and held by two nurses while the medical officer force-fed them one pint of milk mixed with a proprietary 'complete food' and delivered via a funnel and stomach tube. This procedure was traumatic and potentially dangerous, with the risk that the struggling patient's airways might become blocked.[86] Later, 'each patient had to spend one hour each day outside, whatever the weather; in the case of bad patients a nurse would take charge . . . walking them around the exercise area'. Twice weekly the patients were bathed and had their hair washed. Violent patients might be given paraldehyde in a medicine glass during the day or put into a side room with one-to-one nursing, as they could not legally be placed in padded rooms between 7.00 a.m. and 7.00 p.m., a regulation 'which was taken very seriously'.[87] Similarly with patients who behaved 'out of hand (and there were many)', although those who tore off their clothes might simply be put into coarse linen suits, tied at the back. At night violent patients were put into padded cells, some of which contained a bed made from rope and coarse linen. These had double doors, the inner door fitted with a grille so that the patient could be checked hourly and, where necessary, attended by nurses working in pairs. Hyoscyamine was given by injection as a night drug

---

[83] MS Journal, 2 Sept. 1937.

[84] CVIS, 2 Sept. 1937, 4 Aug. 1938.

[85] Mrs Doris Rose, transcript, see note 8.

[86] A.C., aged 54, collapsed and died of a heart attack 24 hours after tube-feeding on 3 Feb. 1934. R.R., aged 50, had several alternations of tube-feeding and hyoscyamine before dying from pneumonia on 7 Mar 1934.

[87] 20 ml paraldehyde was given. 'It smelled horribly; when you administered it to the patients the smell got into your clothes and made you feel sick.' Wards 5 and 6-side rooms had drainage channels around the walls, though patients were given papier mâché pots. Doris Rose's first night duty involved scrubbing the 23rd Psalm, written in excrement, off the tiled white wall in one such room.

to such patients, with repeated administrations after about two hours, if required.

Attendant H. Pull trained at the hospital in the early 1920s. His daughter Vivienne recalls that 'to obtain a job at the hospital you either had to play a musical instrument or be a sportsman. My dad played cricket, so he was in'. His uniform consisted of 'navy blue tunic buttoned up to the neck, trousers and a peaked cap', later replaced by a navy suit and waistcoat, though the peaked cap remained.[88] Male attendants washed and dressed patients and made up coal fires on older wards which did not have steam heating. Student attendants and nurses spent more time on sick and infirmary wards where active nursing rather than supervision was essential. Food was collected from kitchens for those patients eating on the ward: 'after each meal all the cutlery had to be counted and nobody was allowed to leave the table until this had been done.' When patients were put to bed, their day clothing was removed and distributed again the following morning. Vivienne remembers; 'many's the time my Dad came home with a bloody nose or urine-soaked clothing.'

Hospital life

It is difficult to form, let alone convey, an accurate impression of hospital life generally, or to consider how this was affected, for example, in periods when additional economies were sought. There is no shortage of information concerning administrative and financial aspects, the frankness of which was often revealing, even if it was not given a high profile. A modest degree of 'reading between the lines' suggests an atmosphere of austerity once major capital commitments had been made. Comments were also made about patients and their amenities, but their own narratives are unavailable. Recollections of former staff or their families are optimistic and occasionally halcyon in tone but, in conjunction with official documentation, they suggest modest improvements in amenities and a part-liberalisation of hospital life, if only for some residents.

First, there were the practicalities of administration and finance. After 1920 membership of the committee of visitors expanded from fifteen to twenty-one and included the chairman and vice-chairman of Norfolk County Council, although Major D.G. Astley, who replaced A.G. Copeman in 1921 was the committee chairman for the remainder of the inter-war period. George Edwards, the farmworkers' union leader and Labour MP, sometimes played an oppositional role during his twenty-three years of

---

[88] Vivienne Roberts (née Pull), interview 20 May 1999. Mr Pull became deputy chief male nurse, working at the hospital for nearly 40 years before his death, aged 68. He persuaded her husband to become a nurse there in 1948.(see below), I thank Mr and Mrs Roberts for their help.

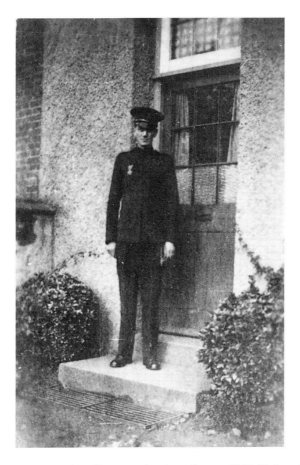

Figure 7.1 Jack Pull in attendant's uniform c. 1925 (Roberts)

membership before he died in 1933 and Councillor George Hewitt did so afterwards. Mrs G. Cook and Miss M. Cozens-Hardy, the first women members from 1931, brought no radical agenda with them, though both were involved in the Norfolk Mental Aftercare Association. Two members undertook routine inspections and visits at the hospital, monthly or more frequently, and further meetings to consider 'special business' were held every two months. Board of Control annual inspections normally lasted for two days and the Ministry of Pensions checked the service patients and their facilities. Between five and ten poor law guardians, later the members of public assistance committees, also visited each year, as did the Mental After-Care Association.

Table 7.3 sets out the main elements of hospital income and expenditure in selected years, beginning with 1921 as re-conversion work distorted comparable figures for 1920. Weekly maintenance costs per patient soared to 40s 3d in 1920 and spare capacity in the hospital did not make for maximum

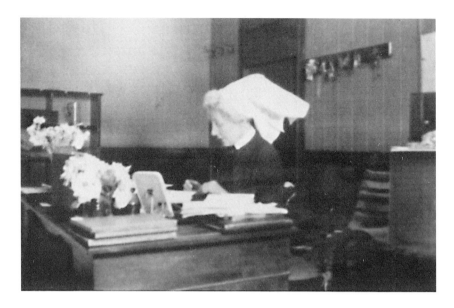

Figure 7.2 Maud Gibbs, matron 1936–47 (Drinkwater)

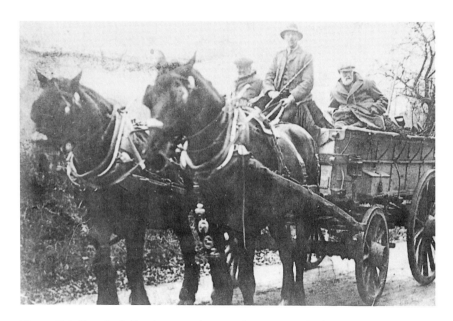

Figure 7.3 Farm bailiff and patient farm-workers c. 1925 (Roberts)

Table 7.3 Income and principal items of expenditure on maintenance accounts, 1920–39

	1921	1925	1930	1935	1939
Net income	£97,775	£64,812	£65,968	£66,899	£74,187
of which Norfolk	81.5	77.5	80.7	91.0	91.4
'outcounty', etc.,	18.2	18.1	16.9		
service patients (%)				5.0	4.5
Net expenditure	£77,962	£65,269	£63,933	£66,618	£73,908
of which (%)					
Medical salaries	5.2	5.4	6.1	4.1	4.1
Staff wages	34.6	32.6	33.4	37.5	36.1
Pensions	1.1	3.1	3.7	5.7	6.3
Provisions (of which	19.1	24.5	24.5	20.6	21.7
farm provides %)	(34)	(33)	(40)	(37)	(40)
Necessaries	19.2	13.3	10.2	10.6	11.7
Patients' clothing	1.3	4.4	4.0	3.2	3.0
Furnishing/bedding	1.5	4.0	3.9	3.6	2.2
Dispensary, etc.	0.8	0.8	0.7	1.1	1.2
Rates, taxes, sundries	5.1	8.4	10.6	9.3	8.4
Transfer to building account	£2,105	£2,268	£2,507	£923	£694
Balance b.f.	–£9,286	£37,263	£38,101	} +£334	} +£891
Balance c.f.	£8,593	£33,785	£36,847		

efficiency, but patient admissions were not so flexible and a sharp fall in costs could not be predicted. Substantial farm profits did allow a reduction in charges to 38s 8d but, with almost 60 per cent of spending consumed by wages and the necessaries of food, light and fuel, little remained for clothing or furnishings, let alone other patient comforts. A further reduction in charges, to 28 shillings by the close of 1921, reflected a general fall in the cost of living but also proactive measures by the hospital committee to reduce staff and other costs. The downward trend continued, stabilising at 19s 3d in the late 1920s and early 1930s, which considerably assisted the hospital during the national financial emergency of 1931–2. Even then, with the Ministry of Health urging economy measures and Norfolk County Council instituting pro-rata wage reductions, the prosaic Major Astley acknowledged 'a difficult and trying year'.[89] Charges remained below 22 shillings for most of the 1930s, before climbing to 24 shillings in 1939 and rising further with the onset of war.

[89] MDC, 7 Jan. 1932, p. 10; AR 1931, Cttee, p. 6. Norfolk County Council reduced wages and allowances and suspended new appointments under the 1931–4 National Economy Campaign.

The high level of charges for 1920/1 produced a substantial surplus as costs fell rapidly in the course of 1921, after which net figures for income and expenditure were relatively stable. This represented a managed outcome, for income from outcounty and service patients was a significant component in total income and produced a substantial annual surplus for the building account. Consequently, hospital authorities were keen to maintain service patients and their yearly contracts with Napsbury and Great Yarmouth, even as overcrowding increased. A request for accommodation from the London County Council had to be refused and Connell calculated, then fretted over, the lost annual surplus of £230 after the Napsbury patients were returned.[90] As the Yarmouth patients were removed to Hellesdon, leaving mainly the service patients, 'outcounty' income and allocations to the hospital building fund declined in the 1930s.

Special meetings of the hospital committee considered financial items as diverse as the bulk purchase of tinned meat, the stockpiling of more than 1,200 tons of coal in anticipation of the General Strike or legal actions to secure outstanding sums of money. For example, it invoked Section 287 of the 1890 Act in a dispute with London County Council 'to enforce payment of outstanding and future charges in the case of Henry Storey, a patient at present chargeable to that authority'.[91] A system of tendering for hospital accounts was routinely monitored; T.E. Parry, the hospital steward, regularly reported that goods supplied were of poorer quality than earlier samples examined and, just as regularly, the committee ordered their return or demanded additional discounts.[92] Among the major headings of expenditure itemised in Table 7.3, the control exerted over wage costs is noticeable, but the committee's efforts were frustrated by rising pensions contributions along with other overheads, such as local rates and taxes. A relatively small amount was spent on medical salaries, mainly as the hospital did not appoint the fourth medical officer favoured by Board inspectors, and on drugs and medicines. The combination of falling prices and enhanced fuel economy helped to restrain the cost of 'necessaries' and spending on clothing and furnishings, having increased after the immediate post-war restrictions, was carefully controlled.

Relatively low levels of spending on foodstuffs and provisions reflected the contribution of the hospital farm. After a period of extensive production for the War Hospital, the farm had one further year of large profits, exceeding £5,000, as most produce was sold at high prices. With the resumption of the mental hospital a new pattern emerged. Octagon farm and 49 acres of pastureland and marsh were purchased for £2,435 early in 1920 to develop a

---

[90] MDC, 2 Aug. and 7 June 1923; MS Journal, 6 May 1926.
[91] CVIS Special, 4 March 1920 (meat), 4 Feb. 1926 (General Strike), 1 Jan. and 7 May 1931 (LCC).
[92] CVIS Special, 3 March 1921 (change milk supplier), 7 April 1921 (3 coal contractors).

dairy herd to secure milk supplies.[93] With additional land rented from Norfolk County Council following its purchase of estates at Little Plumstead and Postwick, roughly 220 acres were available for a time in the early 1930s. Patient labour was already used to considerable effect: farm outsales exceeded £2,500 and direct hospital sales averaged £5,250 annually in the 1920s, the latter representing roughly one-third of hospital provisions in price terms. Farm livestock was usually valued at £3,000 and each year the farm paid an average rent of £200 and provided haulage for the hospital valued at £650. Annual farm profits between the wars averaged £675 and these were transferred to the building account. In the depressed conditions of the early 1930s farm production switched from less profitable outsales, averaging £1,750 annually, to hospital sales, which exceeded £5,600 and represented 40 per cent of all provisions. Farm-work could indeed be defended on therapeutic grounds, but its utilitarian value to the hospital was obvious.[94]

Hospital building accounts also suggest tight financial management. Following War Hospital settlements, the financial allocation from Norfolk County Council averaged £10,700 per year, a low point of £7,000 in 1933 reflecting the council's economy campaign. Almost 80 per cent of building funds were spent on repairs and 75 per cent of this amount went in salaries and wages for the engineering and workshop staff. In this sense, most of the building account was actually devoted to routine maintenance at the hospital. Annual spending on new building or alterations averaged £2,600 and also dipped noticeably in the early 1930s. Although the sewerage scheme and the phased renewal of boiler-house equipment were major capital projects, the building accounts were in deficit in only three years, again indicative of firm management and adherence to financial objectives. Combined surpluses generated from outcounty or service patients and from hospital farms provided an additional £2,500 each year. This figure was almost the equivalent of moneys allocated for new building, or one quarter of NCC contributions; it represented the hospital's own contribution and an amount not required from county ratepayers. No doubt the latter felt hard-pressed, but they had already been relieved as the hospital's post-war surplus was consumed by capital spending and they were not asked for contributions to much-needed items such as an admissions hospital or a new nurses' home.

These features had repercussions but other evidence, beginning with the equally important practicalities of food, clothing and work therapy, is more illustrative of life within the hospital. Faced with rapidly increasing prices in 1919 the hospital committee abandoned the set dietary regime so that the steward could 'take advantage of market fluctuations'. His purchases included

---

[93] CVIS, 3 Sept. 1919.
[94] Based on AR, Farm and Garden Accounts, 1920–39. Over £1,000 was written off or deducted from livestock values on comparison of totals 'carried forward' and 'brought forward' in 1931 and 1932.

a large consignment of '48 cases of tinned meat', possibly armed forces' surplus stocks, and the committee noted: 'frozen Argentine beef and frozen NZ lamb issued to the patients and staff with satisfactory results.'[95] The following year the dietary consisted of an austere tea, bread and margarine breakfast with cooked or tinned meat and vegetables or meat pies and dumplings prominent in the main meal. Soup, rice and fruit puddings featured heavily in a 'second diet' reintroduced for some women patients, which had barely one-third of the standard male meat allowance. Afternoon tea, again of bread and margarine, was supplemented by suppers of baked potato or bread and cheese, with cocoa. Board inspectors cited the patients' maintained weight as testimony to this 'excellent' diet, apparently unaware of contemporary dietary investigations which looked beyond the bulk intake of food.[96]

Fortunately, this situation did not last. Although Connell abolished the working patients' beer allowance in 1922, substituting lemonade or cocoa and saving an estimated £650, he responded to new Board circulars which emphasised a varied diet. Breakfast now consisted of bread and tea with another item: bacon, egg, fish or sausage, potted meat, or porridge. This was followed by a dinner of meat or pie and vegetables accompanied twice weekly by fresh fruit or fruit pudding, although women had smaller portions, particularly of the more necessary fresh meat and vegetables. Food for the remainder of the day was sparse: potted meat or jam was added to the tea, which once a week was merely 'cake', with a half-pint of cocoa for supper. Although working patients had additional bread and cheese and extras in the 'sick diet' included eggs, beef tea, milk puddings, port wine and brandy, Connell remained economy-conscious. When asked to provide two extra puddings per week, he looked for 'modification of the general dietary' to achieve this without extra cost and his introduction of fish represented a nutritional bonus.[97] A major innovation in 1937 was the adoption of a three-week cycle in the hospital menu, the introduction of choice of main meal for patients and the replacement of stewed fruit by fresh fruit at least once in the week. Board inspectors then considered the dietary 'particularly well-varied and generous', though Connell's matter-of-fact justification of the experiment was that 'a large demand for one dish by interested patients is counterbalanced by indifference of other patients to the choice'.[98] Even before this arrangement the diet provided represented a considerable improvement on that of the lesser-paid or unemployed between the wars.

---

[95] CVIS Special, 4 Dec. 1919; 4 March and 7 Oct. 1920.

[96] AR, 1920, Table 4, pp. 32–3; BoC, 1921, p. 10.

[97] MS Journal, 5 Aug. 1926.

[98] BoC, 25 May 1938, p. 11 and AR, 1939, MS, p. 13 One may speculate on how aficionados of *nouvelle cuisine* would have coped with a 'male' hospital dinner portion of 25 ounces of meat pie, potatoes and vegetables, 'extra bread served if required'. Its 'female' equivalent weighed a mere 18.5 ounces.

A literal interpretation of 'make do and mend' underlay the fractional spending upon patients' clothing in 1921 (see Table 7.3). Subsequent spending increased but the standard of clothing was variably interpreted, according to their own lights, by Board inspectors. For example, in 1927, 'dress and appearance were very satisfactory and we were glad to notice that several of the women were wearing their own clothing'. However, inspector Isabel Wilson felt that 'the women's headgear . . . leaves room for improvement; perhaps the ladies of the Committee could choose a better head covering than the male cloth cap now in use'. With no improvement a year later the inspectors considered that cloth caps for women gave 'a grotesque appearance to those wearing them'.[99] Clothing was probably adequate but drab, women's dresses based on navy pin stripe material, and general improvements were limited to alternative footwear and more changes of underwear. In the 1930s occupational therapy classes placed greater emphasis upon personal appearance, the individual labelling of clothing and underwear commenced and patients were encouraged to wash particular items for themselves. Men were provided with flannel trousers and pullovers, while 'clothing of varied pattern and modern design, approximate to that worn by women outside the hospital is now available [and] . . . much appreciated by the younger women'.[100]

'Work as a means of treatment quite apart from its utilitarian value is now generally recognised', although Connell kept the latter objective firmly in view.[101] Spending her childhood next to West Farm and then at Octagon cottage in the mid-1920s, Vivienne Roberts recalled the farmland and garden grounds at the hospital: 'The patients loved working on the farm for which they were given bacca [tobacco] money. The hedges at the hospital always looked very neat, these were also cut by the patients with shears, under supervision.' Extensive greenhouses were used to propagate flowers for wards, gardens and for more sombre occasions. 'When a patient died, the nurses laid them out and put them in the coffins, the gardeners dug the graves and the head gardener Mr Houghton would arrive with a glass hearse . . . the gardeners also had to supply a wreath of flowers.' Her recollections are also of some freedom for parole patients and a surprising degree of familiarity: 'My dad had one of the patients called Charlie help him in his garden; we often heard him talking to himself but he was quite harmless. As children we got to know quite a few and often talked to them.'[102]

However, Board inspectors wanted more male patients employed in workshops, 'with a view to helping or even learning some simple occupation there' and recommended the appointment of a hospital 'occupation

[99] BoC, 7 March 1927, p. 13; 20 Oct. 1932, p. 11; 21 Sept. 1933, p. 12.
[100] ibid., 25 May 1938, p. 12. Floral pattern dresses had been introduced.
[101] ibid., 29 April 1931, p. 12.
[102] V. Roberts' interview, 20 May 1999.

officer'.[103] An arts and crafts centre was established in 1932, an occupational therapist and two nurse assistants taking classes for 'hitherto unemployable' women patients in knitting and rug-making. Two years later over 280 patients were involved in craft sessions with music and physical exercise classes to good effect. That 'patients enjoy the change of surroundings in coming from the wards to the occupation room' was reflected in 'their response in improved behaviour and particularly in the care of their clothes and cleanliness'.[104] It may also have featured in the re-establishment of the patients' choir, which sang regularly at religious services and concerts in 1936. Nine-tenths of women patients took part in hospital work or in classes but progress was less noticeable on the men's side, where two-thirds of patients were so employed. Traditional tasks predominated here and, if basket weaving was seen as therapeutic, breeze block production was distinctly utilitarian. Connell was given the veiled reminder that it was 'of the uttermost importance that the male nursing staff should become interested', a criticism which led to the promotion of exercise classes and new work making playing fields, tennis courts and a bowling green by 1937.[105]

Some 300 patients attended religious services: Vivienne Roberts remembers men assembling 'at F ward court . . . they were ushered out through a small gate and counted as they went. On arriving at the Church . . . they were counted in . . . and the men sat on one side and the women on the other'.[106] Leisure time also remained highly organised, but there were modest developments. The interest from bequests such as the Johnson (1871) and Attwod Porter (Great War) funds was used for recreational purposes and Christmas celebrations now included a present for every patient and a dance which lasted until midnight. For patients and attendants' children

> one of the highlights of the year was the Sports Day . . . on the beautiful cricket field where all sorts of races were held. Side shows would be going on round the edge of the field including coconut shy, greasy pole, bowling for the pig etc. etc. They really enjoyed it.

More regularly, 'on fine evenings male and female patients are permitted to mix on the cricket field, where the band is in attendance and dancing, mixed cricket matches and other games are played'.[107] Other sporting spectacles were laid on by a highly successful attendants' football team, champions of the Norwich Business Houses League for the 1930–31 season, which had four

---

[103] BoC, 17 March 1926, p. 14. A number of hospitals had already made such appointments.
[104] ibid., 23 Feb. 1935, p. 13.
[105] ibid., 21 May 1937, p. 13.
[106] V. Roberts' interview, 20 May 1999.
[107] AR, 1923, MS, p. 10.

members who played at county level in the 1930s and another who played county cricket.

Those who were not voluntary patients had few rights or entitlements. However, the early combination of leave and parole offered greater scope for a significant minority and, from the outset, Connell encouraged patients to associate with those in other wards, allowing 'minor entertainments and tea parties'. Relatives, friends, ex-servicemen's organisations and others were invited to visit patients, although new admissions were not allowed visitors in the first month, as this was thought to be unsettling. Daily visiting hours of 10.00 a.m. until midday and 2.00 p.m. until 4.00 p.m. appeared convenient but on Sundays, perhaps the solitary free day for most people in Norfolk, the hospital was normally closed to visitors. They were allowed to bring cake, fruit and tobacco but were reminded that 'conversation should be of a cheering and hope-inspiring nature, especially when it relates to family matters . . . [those] scolding or blaming, or injudicious allusions . . . are liable to be stopped from visiting'.[108] The hospital's failure to introduce tea rooms for patients and their visitors, planned from 1930 but not achieved until 1939, was curious, not least because opportunities to supplement hospital income were normally grasped promptly and firmly. Another shortcoming was more predictable. Patients were allowed to write two letters per week and visiting relatives could take away additional family correspondence, but they were urged not to post any other letters. Connell was wary of patients' communications beyond friendship or family boundaries, arguing that 'the contents of letters mainly dwell upon their delusions'. Evidently this justified a system under which any additional letters were opened, made available for inspection by the hospital committee but, unless some item was to be investigated, then burned.[109]

Some essentials of inter-war life were assimilated at the hospital, notably weekly filmshows. Early projection equipment was another legacy from the War Hospital and features were supplemented from 1925 by 'the Pathe Topical Film', secured from the Haymarket picture house once the hospital had agreed to cover any damage. By 1931, however, 'we shall not be able to obtain silent films . . . and the question of installing a 'Talkie' apparatus will have to be considered'. Contrary to Board of Control opinion, which initially 'deplored' such expense, equipment was purchased for £396 in 1932 and the new films were 'greatly appreciated' by patients and by the committee, which thanked 'Messers Metro-Goldwyn-Mayer . . . for their generosity in providing Talkie Cinema Films free of charge . . . during the past winter'.[110] Radio sets were also installed in every ward by 1935 and increasing numbers of patients

---

[108] Rules for Visitors, St Andrew's Hospital, SAH 503, 1923.
[109] MS Journal, 3 May 1923.
[110] AR, 1931, MS, p. 9; MS, 1932, p. 9: CVIS 5 April 1934.

permitted in day rooms until 9.30 or 10.00 p.m.[111] Women were allowed to smoke which, in conjunction with choice of clothing, may have enhanced several interpretations of movie culture by the late 1930s. Their reading material was augmented by purchased and donated stocks of novels and, from 1933, by a central library run by voluntary patients. Conditions on the men's side were much less cosy; in one ward just 6 of the 74 patients used the library, the rest relying on newspapers and 'aged tracts which are never changed'. Smoking was well established here and, with male TB rates three times the national average for mental hospitals, 'there were more spitoons in evidence than were necessary'.[112]

If St Andrew's Hospital was a test-bed for new approaches to mental illness between the wars, the results were mixed and inconclusive. Connell was reputedly a progressive figure, with experience of the treatment of 'war neuroses'; his opinions were sought nationally and he was an advocate of precisely the voluntary and outpatient treatments which were flagged by the 1930 Act. He attempted to raise the number of qualified nurses and attendants staff and saw the DPM as a qualification to be encouraged in junior medical staff. Rather more slowly than had been anticipated, outpatient clinics were established and voluntary procedures featured in more than one-third of admissions by the late 1930s. Roughly one-fifth of the certified patients had parole, though there was no definite increase in this proportion over time. Occupational therapy was introduced with positive results, again with some lag in the men's hospital. A range of improvements in hospital life, including a modicum of free time, can be identified, but whether these were enjoyed by more than groups of trusted or working patients remains questionable. In so far as any of these measures undermined the concept of the hospital as 'total institution', the continued emphasis on work and the need for an economic contribution reinforced it.[113]

The latter feature was all the more important considering that external economic restrictions clearly affected the physical fabric and planned development of the hospital, with consequences for standards of treatment, care and the quality of life. Even where substantial spending occurred, efforts to upgrade the sanitary and power-generating infrastructure of the hospital were a poor justification for the failure to provide a new admissions hospital. The pursuit of qualitative improvements in the nursing or medical staff was also undermined by financial imperatives, notably with periodic cutbacks, the

---

[111] BoC, 23 Feb. 1935.

[112] e.g. Messrs Murdie were paid 'for the supply of 200 second-hand novels', CVIS Special, 4 Jan. 1925. The men's library opened in 1934. BoC, 7 Jan. 1936, p. 14; 25 May 1938, p. 13.

[113] E. Goffman, *Asylums*, Penguin, Harmondsworth, 1961. The term covered institutions where the rest, leisure and work of the inmate population were tightly organised by a single authority within a single place or site.

failure sufficiently to address staff turnover or to make additional medical appointments. Although it was most quantifiable, finance was not the only area of shortcoming. Case records for the service patients were not retained but most were regarded as long-term cases and a staple source of income; their number barely diminished but there is little evidence of new admissions. How Connell's war experience helped such patients, or any others, is unclear. His imprint – literally his handwriting – in patients' case records is minimal. He ran outpatient clinics and was involved in correspondence with other doctors concerning voluntary patients, but signs of regular face-to-face contact of the kind advocated in the inter-war period are very few. As a more remote interpreter of policy, Connell responded to Board inspectors' promptings and to the hospital committee, but he attempted few major initiatives.

It is difficult to generalise from the variety of patients' experiences as indicated in case records. Published summary information suggested improved recovery rates and a more considerable proportion of arrivals and departures when compared with the Edwardian era. There was a downward trend in mortality rates and by the late 1930s one half of those who died in St Andrew's were aged 65 years or more. Mortality patterns were consistent with some ageing of the hospital population, but they suggest some problems. Female death rates were 'remarkably low' compared with national equivalents, but male rates were considerably higher. Tuberculosis was not rife in the hospital but isolation facilities for women were more effective, if continuing male mortality from TB is any guide. With renewed outbreaks of influenza, diarrhoea and paratyphoid in 1938, Board inspectors noted that, for the second successive year, over 110 patients or one-tenth of the hospital population, were confined in bed.[114] Many were senile or infirm patients, although 239 of these, equivalent to one-fifth of the hospital's resident population, had already been transferred to Swainsthorpe or Thetford. Remarks that the admissions unit was 'not now up to present day standards', or that 'rather a lot' of patients were placed 'in single rooms for mental reasons', did not reflect positively on inter-war achievements. Nor did they suggest that the hospital was in a strong position before the trials of the Second World War.[115]

---

[114] BoC, 21 May 1937, p. 13; 25 May 1938, p. 12.
[115] ibid., 20 April 1939, p. 13.

8

Wartime and post-war crises, 1939–48

The association of 'total war', in which the civilian population is heavily and directly involved, with longer-term welfare arrangements is a familiar subject for historians. Links between the domestic war effort, the emergency organisation of national health services and the establishment of a welfare state in Britain are strong, if complex.[1] As the part of mental hospitals and their patients in this context is less obvious and local or grass-roots experiences are comparatively unexplored, St Andrew's offers the opportunity for a case study. There are fewer source materials, however, and wartime records were often compiled less accurately or comprehensively. Under the pressure of events, or from the need to pursue a particular agenda, the standard of 'on the spot' assessments may also have slipped. Recognising these deficiencies, this chapter aims to show how St Andrew's Hospital took on additional roles in adverse circumstances and the effect of upheavals and scarcity upon new, temporary and established residents. It suggests that overcrowding and staff shortages were so aggravated in wartime that they assumed crisis proportions in the early years of the National Health Service. Coping with these extraordinary difficulties whilst maintaining the semblance of routine was a demanding task for key hospital personnel. Yet they also began to appreciate that pressures for post-war reform, whilst not dealing fully and directly with mental health care, were nevertheless sweeping them towards an uncertain future.

In many respects the experience of mental hospitals and their patients in the Second World War resembled that of the asylums and their inmates in the First World War. Some hospitals were again evacuated and the essentials of accommodation, food, care and attention, and recreational space for patients were pared down, perhaps below officially acceptable minima, in the face of shortages and overcrowding. The national total of mental hospital patients fell from 133,000 in 1939 to 127,000 early in 1945 but these figures, which excluded armed forces' patients, reflected displacement by wartime Emergency Medical Service rather than any sudden improvement in treatments. Deprivation was one part of the war experience in which mental hospital patients fully participated, as reviewed in one hour of a parliamentary debate held in November 1945. Weekly maintenance costs per head averaged 30 shillings in mental hospitals and 90 shillings in general hospitals:

---

[1] R. Lowe, *The Welfare State in Britain since 1945*, Macmillan, Basingstoke, 1993, offers a good introductory survey.

the official allocation of space per patient was 50 square feet in mental hospitals, compared with 120 in general hospitals and 144 in fever hospitals. Perhaps not surprisingly, the incidence of TB in mental hospitals was fifteen times above the national average by 1942. Under pressures of overcrowding the classification of patients allegedly degenerated into one based in practice upon their degree of physical infirmity and propensity to noisy, disturbed or 'bad' behaviour or habits.[2]

Official references to the 'predisposition' of institutional populations to TB were hardly consistent with an acceptance of increased overcrowding. Assurances that such levels were curbed by 'scientific rationing' or because 'the Board of Control and local authorities have been specially vigilant' carried all the conviction of a junior minister under pressure.[3] However, the prompt rationing of food probably helped to restrain mortality rates in mental hospitals, despite considerable illness and disease, compared with the situation in the First World War. Vigilance on the part of Board inspectors and other supervisory bodies in wartime was less obvious, though little of it would be required to stand comparison with the levels displayed from 1915 to 1919 (see Chapter 6). With the intensification of 'total war', aerial attacks were more menacing and, while catastrophic mortality and physical destruction were widely predicted, there were also fears that much of the civilian population might experience mental breakdown. Large numbers of 'bad cases' might then swamp casualty and mental hospitals, which themselves were potential targets. In the event such casualties and fatalities, though not the physical destruction, were lighter than expected. This was fortunate, for the ability of mental hospitals to have coped then must be doubted. As it was, according to an otherwise broadly optimistic account of their longer-term history:

> those mental hospitals which continued in operation faced acute shortages of clothing, food and heating, with an unprecedented degree of overcrowding and under-staffing. This meant the return of the locked door, of inactivity . . . tuberculosis was still a killer and isolation was a necessity.[4]

Despite considerable preparations, the role envisaged for St Andrew's Hospital was barely determined before war began. Although the great majority of patients remained at the hospital site, roughly one-third of the accommodation was given over to the wartime Emergency Medical Service and used for the treatment of evacuee, military and civilian casualties until 1947. For much of this time the 'Emergency Section' in the north side

---

[2] Hansard's Parliamentary Debates, 6 Nov. 1945, Mental Hospitals. Mr J. Lewis (Bolton) and Dr S. Taylor (Barnet), 1188–1201.
[3] ibid., Parliamentary Secretary to the Ministry of Health, Mr Key, 1201–4.
[4] K. Jones, *Asylums and After*, Athlone, London, 1993, p. 142.

buildings required 362 hospital beds, which inevitably meant the disruption of patterns of hospital life and a great deal of overcrowding. These problems were compounded by other aspects of wartime experience, the introduction of the black-out and air-raid precautions (ARP), severe food shortages and the loss of nursing staff because of conscription and the competing demand for labour in the war effort.

War preparations and arrangements: coping under pressure?

At different points in 1939 and 1940 East Anglia was seen as a reception area for evacuees and a possible invasion site. The organisation of health care was a matter of some concern in the inter-war period and fears that peacetime health services might collapse under aerial attack in wartime were more widespread. Contingency plans from 1935 for the area surrounding Norwich were revised several times before the Norfolk and Norwich Hospital was identified as the main clearing centre for casualty cases. Although that hospital also retained 125 'civilian' beds, most patients were evacuated when war broke out; children to the city's Jenny Lind Hospital and nearly 300 adults to nearby hospitals. However, the shortage of hospital facilities in the surrounding area meant that mental hospitals and ex-poor law institutions were needed; St Andrew's and Hellesdon Hospitals and Wayland PAI, Attleborough and Bowthorpe Road PAI, Norwich were the respective local examples. State funding covered patient care under the Emergency Medical Service, subject to availability but offered as of right. There were air raids on Norwich in September 1940 but the more serious Baedekker raids of 28–30 April 1942 resulted in 377 casualties admitted to hospital. In these raids and again on 26–27 June 1942 the Norfolk and Norwich Hospital was itself bombed and the operating theatre block and nurses' accommodation badly damaged. Altogether 340 people were killed in air raids on Norwich and 401 of the 1,092 recorded civilian injured were hospitalised.[5]

At St Andrew's the hospital committee was initially concerned with air-raid precautions. It responded to circulars from Norfolk County Council and the Board of Control by sending the matron, head attendant and engineer to local classes for instruction in anti-gas precautions and by organising a series of lectures and demonstrations, given by the Area Medical Instructor to 124 medical and nursing staff.[6] Outline proposals for the evacuation of mental hospitals, issued by the Board of Control in conjunction with the War

---

[5] S. Cherry and B. Ross, 'The Norfolk and Norwich Hospital and the establishment of the NHS 1939–55' in D. Ralphs (ed.), *The Norfolk and Norwich Hospital, 1946–2001* (forthcoming).
[6] CVIS Minutes, Dec. 1931–March 1945 and April 1945–July 1948 (at Drayton Old Lodge), 6 Aug. 1936; 4 Feb. 1937.

Office early in June 1938, indicated that St Andrew's would again feature as a war hospital. By August arrangements were made to enlist hospital staff into the RAMC Supplementary Reserve and the committee had contacted the Territorial Association regarding the adaptation of hospital buildings. When the War Office stated its requirement of a 600-bed facility to provide a third Eastern General Hospital, the committee offered the whole north side site.[7]

However, the desirability of a rigid demarcation between civilian and military casualties, particularly when both might arise from the same air raids, was under national consideration and the differentiation of casualty from 'routine' patients was felt likely to be more appropriate. When Dr Alick Knight, the Hospital Officer for Eastern Region, visited St Andrew's in April 1939 his request was for up to 342 beds for the reception of casualty cases. Even then, the possibility of clearing the Little Plumstead institution as an emergency hospital and moving most of its patients to St Andrew's was raised in July before the 342-bed casualty hospital proposal was reaffirmed in September. With two modifications, the requirement that all casualty beds be located on ground floor wards to minimise difficulties for stretcher cases, and the provision of 20 additional beds, plans were finalised in November 1939.[8]

With ARP training under way, the familiar hospital steam hooter was first silenced except for air-raid warnings and in 1941 replaced by an electric siren. An inspection by the county architect recommended sandbagging of ground floor windows and corridors but concluded that first floor wards could not be protected, beyond the taping of windows to reduce the risk of flying glass. Hopes were pinned on light-proof blinds, though these were not fitted everywhere, and upon existing fire-fighting arrangements, relying on water hoses to quell incendiary weapons. Supplies of gas masks were sufficient, but concerns that these could not or would not be used by many patients remained. Cellars were cleared for use as shelters, although a system of trenches and nine new underground shelters was completed early in 1941.[9] Bombs did fall around the hospital site and the air attacks on Norwich in 1942 produced anxious moments in terms of near-misses with incendiaries and the likelihood of a surge in casualty admissions. In the event, the greatest threats to patients arose from their overcrowding and nursing staff shortages and both persisted long after the war.

---

[7] ibid., 2 June, 4 Aug. and 6 Oct. 1938.

[8] ibid., 3 Aug., 7 Sept. and 2 Nov. 1939. The Little Plumstead option, proposed by two regional officers of the Ministry of Health Hospital Department on 12 July, was formally adopted 'after a prolonged discussion' in August. Board of Control objections to this were apparently decisive.

[9] ibid., 6 July and 3 Aug. 1939. The Ministry of Health was asked for £990 for the nine shelters and additional fire-fighting equipment on 3 Oct. 1940. Work was complete when Board inspectors reiterated their concern over gas masks on 18 Feb. 1941.

Arguably the first casualty of the hospital's war was sustained in October 1939, when the Committee suspended plans for a new nurses' home, scheduled for completion in 1941 at a cost of £65,000. There was no other option, but delay brought additional and unforeseen costs.[10] Arrangements for the reception of real casualties did not work smoothly. In November 1939 Connell was instructed to open the Emergency section for up to 100 army sick cases, mainly local conscripts with relatively minor illnesses, and 60 were soon in residence. They were placed in accommodation normally used by laundry and other staff, as their number did not warrant the removal of mental hospital patients from designated wards. St Andrew's laundry ward nurses and staff were left to make their own provisions and new nurses for the Emergency section were billeted locally. As yet there was no resident medical officer for the army cases or for any civilian patients, although staff from the Norfolk and Norwich Hospital made visits. This was unsatisfactory and direct treatment by the St Andrew's medical staff raised all manner of professional and practical issues. Only after two months and a direct threat by the Committee to close the section was the situation remedied.[11]

Other difficulties arose from the number of external authorities involved. In November 1939 the Board of Control permitted hospital authorities to retain control and use of designated wards in the Emergency section, provided these could be transferred within 24 hours' notice. This allowed some flexibility, but the Ministry of War insisted that service and civilian patients be separately accommodated, which implied additional emergency section wards and space. Connell was forced to shuffle limited resources, grouping emergency beds in the north side and additionally using male ward E as nursing accommodation to resolve the problems experienced with the billeting. Displaced male patients were moved into the former female wards 11 and 12, which increased overcrowding throughout the south side. Ministry requests to the Committee to consider plans and the necessary arrangements for a fifteen-block, 600-bed temporary hospital on land adjacent to the hospital consumed considerable time and effort until they were abandoned in November.[12] These arrangements then sufficed for the Emergency section and were only under severe pressure in June 1942 when, following air attacks on Norwich and the bombing of the Norfolk and Norwich Hospital, fifty beds were earmarked for temporary use by that hospital.[13]

---

[10] ibid., 8 Oct. 1938; 5 Oct. 1939. A less definite commitment to building an admissions unit, costing £36,000, by 1943 was also suspended.

[11] ibid., 2 Nov. and 5 Dec. 1939; 1 Feb. 1940. Dr D.T. Brown was the first of many appointments here.

[12] ibid., 2 May, 6 June and 7 Nov. 1940.

[13] A.J. Cleveland, *History of the Norfolk and Norwich Hospital 1900–46*, Norwich, 1948, p. 174; CVIS, 6 Aug. 1942. In August the N&N was allocated the Emergency section of

The hospital was much less successful in finding suitable accommodation for some of its own residents. Vague pre-war assurances that Little Plumstead and its annexe, the former Heckingham PAI, might receive some St Andrew's patients failed to materialise. It was some relief that the feared upsurge in mental hospital admissions did not occur, whether or not this was because of the 'phoney war' period, as the pressure of numbers within the reduced number of wards was now inevitable. It was perhaps more than coincidence that there were just 75 voluntary admissions in 1941, arguably the darkest year of the war, but numbers then rose steadily, from 96 in 1942 to 137 in 1944. By 1945 two-thirds of all the admissions were voluntary patients, compared with just over one-third in 1940. Nearly one quarter of those admitted were patients who had previously been in the hospital and roughly one-fifth were aged 65 years or more.

No detailed classification of the illnesses of the new wartime patients is available, but that for 1945 gives some indications. In one-fifth of the admissions no principal causal factor was ascertained, but hereditary features were cited in one quarter of the cases, including some examples of neuroses and 'eccentricity'. One-fifth were women admitted with conditions associated with 'critical periods' in their lives and another one-fifth were admitted with forms of mental stress. Both categories were larger than in the late 1930s, perhaps reflecting the additional privations of wartime, while a lower incidence of senile cases may reflect the overcrowded state of the hospital and recourse to alternative public assistance accommodation. Most of the remaining new patients had associated bodily illness or injuries, notably heart disease (7 per cent), lesions of the brain (2 per cent) and epilepsy (2 per cent).[14] Just nine new service patients were admitted, in 1943 or 1944. A number of Polish soldiers were also admitted: their status is unclear but their presence was a factor in Dr Pietocha's addition to the medical staff.

Table 8.1 summarises the treatment record of the mental hospital wards over the war years. A greater emphasis upon voluntary treatment probably underlay the increase in the number of patients discharged, approaching 200 annually from 1943. Not all were recovered or relieved, but the proportion so classified appears to have exceeded 1930s averages: in 1940 68 per cent of admissions were stated to have recovered, the highest proportion ever recorded at the hospital. These particular figures reflected measures to pre-empt overcrowding, as they derived from reduced admissions rather than a sharp increase in numbers actually recovered. Subsequent admissions were only marginally less than in the 1930s, however. The incidence of recoveries after 1940 was variable but lower, between 20 and 47 per cent for men,

Hellesdon hospital, mainly for maternity and surgical cases, returning the 50 beds at Thorpe for other EMS use.

[14] Annual Reports, 1934–48, SAH 34; AR, 1945, MS, p. 9.

Table 8.1 St Andrew's mental hospital patients in wartime and peacetime

	Average no. resident			Admissions			% admitted recovered			Mortality %		
	Total	M	F	Total	M	F	Total	M	F	Total	M	F
1930–39	1,141	458	683	244	103	141	40.0	35.0	43.6	6.2	7.8	5.1
1939–45	1,076	421	655	234	86	148	48.5	39.5	54.1	6.0	7.9	4.8
1945–49	1,117	447	670	384	159	225	38.0	29.1	43.6	5.5	6.4	4.9

averaging 34.4 per cent, and from 41 to 58 per cent for women, averaging 51.2 per cent. Nevertheless the average recovery rate of 48 per cent on admissions from 1939 to 1945 compared with 40 per cent for the 1930s.

Each year also brought some life-threatening outbreak of disease, yet mortality rates were broadly contained. The immunisation of all patients offered some protection from paratyphoid, but influenza and pneumonia proved destructive. Ten deaths from TB contributed to the increased overall mortality rate of 7.6 per cent, almost half of which was linked with lung infections, in 1940. A similar number of deaths from TB and more new cases in 1941 were linked with overcrowding and, possibly, shortages in diets. With seventeen deaths from TB in 1942 the lack of verandah space for infected patients was a pressing deficiency and Board inspectors suggested the transfer of TB cases, though there was nowhere to send them. As with overcrowding generally, although this question was 'carefully considered . . . it has not been found possible to relieve it'.[15] Similar numbers of new TB cases remained 'a disquieting feature' until 1946, when Dr McCulley was finally able to report that 'the improvement in ventilation brought about by the removal of the black-out, together with reasonably good diet, are largely responsible for the reduced incidence of tuberculosis'.[16] Enteritis, dysentery and gastric flu were successively reported in years after 1941 but the 7 per cent overall mortality for 1941 and 1942 was not unusually high and mortality rates then fell.

An average male mortality rate of 10 per cent between 1939 and 1942 suggests real difficulties, but these were then contained. Board inspectors felt that overall mortality of 5 per cent in 1943 was 'remarkably low': this, the 4.3 per cent in 1944 and the 5.3 per cent in 1945 compared well with the 6.9 per cent average for mental hospitals in England and Wales. Whether these later mortality figures reflected an easing of wartime difficulties, for example with food supplies, or the improving medical management of illness, is unclear. It is significant that wartime disease did not routinely lead to death, particularly in the light of experiences in the rather different conditions of the Great War evacuation. Mortality rates are an ultimate indicator which does not convey

[15] Board of Control Reports, 1926–59, SAH 142, 1 April 1944.
[16] AR, 1946, MS, p. 8.

well all the problems associated with overcrowding or nursing shortages. Recovery rates – usually subject to a considerable readmission rate – may be more reassuring, but they are likewise not a sensitive pointer to conditions on the hospital wards, particularly for the majority of residents who were not expected to recover.

Yet alternative guides are in scarce supply. After 1939 the hospital did not publish a full annual report, although abstracts were compiled for the Committee, Norfolk County Council and the Board of Control. Board inspections, undertaken annually at some point between February and June, provide a series of snapshots of the state of the hospital. These were likely to be less critical during the war emergency, as seen in Chapter 6, particularly considering the additional role expected of St Andrew's. For example, the defective admission hospital facilities, persistently criticised in the 1930s, were not mentioned in wartime inspections. Thus the overcrowding and staff shortages highlighted by Board inspections may have been severe indeed, particularly as both attracted adverse comments from other observers. Remarks by committee members undertaking their own monthly visits are not wholly objective but, as they were intended for their fellows rather than a wider public, were often candid.

The onset of long-term problems

The hospital had not referred to overcrowding in its own report for 1940–41 but this was already a major concern.[17] An average of 1,137 patients had been resident in 1939, with 1,151 remaining on 31 December, excluding military patients in the Emergency section. On 20 April Board inspectors noted excesses of 56 women by day and 52 at night over their specifications for patient accommodation. The men's side was not overcrowded, but was completely full. Although 76 patients were out on trial over the year and some could be discharged, their overcrowding increased. From 1940 until 1945 totals of mental hospital residents fluctuated within a narrow range, between 1,050 and 1,079. On the average figure of 1,068 residents (416 men, 652 women), there was an excess of 129 women and 99 men on Board specifications for daytime accommodation, which was only marginally lower at night.[18] This situation arose principally because five of the larger wards, with 362 beds, were now in the Emergency section. Problems were compounded as ground floor day rooms were converted into dormitories to facilitate any night-time emergency evacuation; fewer first floor bedrooms

[17] CVIS, 3 April 1941.
[18] The excess on night accommodation was 117 for women and 88 for men. Figures based on BoC inspections 20 April 1939, 14 June 1940, 18 Feb. 1941, 19 Feb. 1942, 13 May 1943, 1 April 1944 and 5 June 1945.

and dormitories were used as day rooms and such conversions were less successfully achieved. Worse still, the shortage of space under revised arrangements meant that two women's wards were subjected daily to the upheaval of conversion from dormitory to day room and back.

With less space came greater risk of disease. Although admissions fell in 1940, at least one quarter of the new patients were aged over 65 years and many were sick or infirm. Board inspectors had already noted a tendency to cram beds, particularly in some male dormitories where patients were essentially confined to bed for nursing.[19] The prominence of tuberculosis within fatalities has already been noted and, in crowded conditions, the hospital's pre-war problem with paratyphoid carriers became more threatening. All patients were immunised but a 'large' number of intestinal disorder cases were reported among women patients in 1941 and among men in 1942. A tentative diagnosis of 'influenzal interitis' was made and Connell's further precautionary measures included the removal of wooden toilet seats throughout the hospital.[20] The following summer dysentery was prevalent and Board inspectors suggested improvements in the sterilisation of milk and dairy equipment at the hospital farm. Two visiting councillors also noted: 'inspected the kitchen at the annexe . . . the walls and ceiling should be attended to as early as possible . . . the kitchen is in a shocking state.'[21] Board inspectors were also perturbed by 'the unusually large number of disturbed women patients' in 1941, and concluded a year later that aggravated difficulties with the classification of patients and additional problems in infirmary wards led directly to the 'disturbed condition of the more difficult wards'.[22] They cited women's wards 3, 5 and 6, which then contained 257 out of the 633 female residents.

Generally, the sense of crowding was worsened by black-out arrangements and the strengthening and taping of windows, which made wards gloomy even in broad daylight. As early as May 1943 the Committee ordered the removal of some of the protective boarding and linen strips on windows 'in view of their dilapidated condition and unsightly appearance'.[23] It made no attempt to comment on the view from within. Visitors' reports for the war years were generally comprised of remarks such as 'everything in order', that patients were 'contented' or that wards were 'rather crowded but under existing conditions this is presumably unavoidable'. But many a dismal daytime originated in poor weather, overcrowding and staff shortages,

[19] BoC, 14 June 1940.
[20] BoC, 19 Feb. 1942.
[21] BoC, 13 May 1943; and Visitors Report Book (Visitors), 1903–55, SAH 140; 24 June 1943. The redecoration of the kitchen, both dining room ceilings and ward 16, was still being urged as a priority on 12 April 1945.
[22] BoC, 18 Feb. 1941; 19 Feb. 1942.
[23] CVIS, 6 May 1943.

epitomised in the perfunctory note: 'All patients indoors. Many in bed with colds. Several of the nurses away with influenza. Staff short on both sides.'[24] In a few wards where suitable blinds had not been fitted windows were simply painted over. This extraordinary measure increased dependence upon artificial light by day and forced the choice between ventilation and observation of the black-out in hours of darkness.

Connell was unhappy with his own arrangements and one of the visiting justices noted after a monthly inspection that 'most of the grumbling came from the Medical Superintendent – black out or talk of it sends him more or less mad'.[25] Infirmary and isolation wards were worst affected, offering no respite for more than 100 patients who were practically bedridden. In May 1943 Board inspectors finally noted that 'ventilation at night is poor' and that 'the sick wards and some of the dormitories appear to be severely overcrowded, with the beds almost touching'.[26] Some larger wards contained four rows of beds, arranged along the walls with a central double row packed so close that the only measure of immediate relief would be to alternate patients, 'head' and 'feet'. The situation was no better in smaller wards: in the women's admission ward, which measured 54 feet by 10 feet, there were thirteen beds.[27]

As early as 1941 one visitor commented: 'the female staff is roughly 25% short and it seems unfortunate that so much labour has to be expended on senile cases which might be accommodated in a PAI.'[28] Three years later Connell reported on overcrowding and the strains imposed by a large proportion of senile patients upon a diminished and overworked nursing staff.[29] The Committee duly requested the county Public Assistance Committee to provide accommodation for more of the senile cases but little was available, owing to other EMS requirements and parallel staff shortages. For example, the Swainsthorpe annexe attempted to clear sixteen beds for St Andrew's patients but the resident medical officer there could find no more than six patients well enough to be moved out. As there was some spare capacity within the Emergency section at St Andrew's the Committee requested the ministry to release beds and allow flexibility in nursing arrangements, so that Emergency section nurses could be used on the infirmary wards.[30] One hundred beds were made available but these could not

[24] Visitors, 25 Jan. 1940; 23 July 1942.

[25] ibid., 21 April 1943.

[26] BoC, 13 May 1943.

[27] Assuming 6' × 3' mattresses, this consumed 234 square feet, over 43% of available space, before door space, any facility or movement by patients or staff could be considered.

[28] Visitors, 25 Sept. 1941.

[29] CVIS, 5 Oct. 1944.

[30] The Committee supported a parliamentary lobby, led by Northumberland Mental Hospital, for the release of any servicewomen willing to take up mental hospital nursing. ibid., 5 Oct. 1944.

be used because of the increasingly serious shortage of nurses. Thus, the end of the war coincided with a deteriorating situation. Dysentery was again reported and, in addition to the 100 or so bed cases, more than 60 of the women patients in wards 3, 5 and 6 were confined to bed with gastric flu during the Board of Control inspection in June 1945. Evidently, 'in some wards we visited bed after bed was separated from the next by the space of one hand', while 'the wards in which most of the gastric influenza cases were today are so overcrowded that proper nursing for infection is impossible'.[31]

Arguably, there had been difficulties for some time in maintaining 'proper' nursing. The immediate pre-war complement of 107 women nurses was considered barely adequate and several of the 84 male nurses joined the armed forces or were called up before nursing was deemed a protected service. Former staff were brought out of retirement on the understanding that their pensions would be safeguarded, but it was soon recognised that staff losses would necessitate additional recruitment. After the Mental Hospitals Association requested that nurses' pay be increased to compensate for the rise in the cost of living, nurses living out were given a rise of three shillings and boarders 1s 6d per week. Weekly war bonuses of two shillings and 1s 6d were also paid to male and female nurses respectively, although half of this amount was deducted in increased boarding charges. In a further concession, V. Boyce, 'temporary pensioner attendant', became the first to receive an extra six shillings weekly 'on account of his holding the nursing certificate'.[32]

The Committee refused to adopt nationally agreed pay scales in 1941 despite the efforts of the Secretary of the Mental Hospitals and Institutional Workers' Union, which organised roughly one-third of the nursing staff, and the intervention of Col. Mendlicott, MP for East Norfolk.[33] Instead it offered an interim 5 shillings bonus only to women nurses and domestic staff, who were in short supply. Temporary male nurses' wages were raised to 70 shillings and new domestic staff were graded on rates from 10 to 25 per cent below those for women nurses but the award to permanent staff was roughly 2s 6d per week below national rates. Women nurses now earned from 57s 6d per week and charge nurses from 73s 6d, all with an additional weekly war bonus of 6s 6d.[34] The hospital did accept the sections of the national Rushcliffe inquiry into the pay and working conditions of nursing staff applicable to

---

[31] BoC, 5 June 1945

[32] CVIS, 4 July 1940; 3 April 1941.

[33] MHIWU Norfolk Branch Minutes 1941–58, 5 Nov. 1941 and 12 Jan. 1942. I thank Mr Trevor Pull, whose father was the union's branch chairman, for access to this source. Mr H.W. Pull's correspondence includes letters from two sympathetic committee members, Messrs Hewitt and Wetherbed.

[34] Hospital Wages Book. Female staff, April 1940-March 1945, SAH 93. Average increases of 35% were swallowed up by inflation and increased boarding costs. CVIS, 6 Nov. and 4 Dec. 1941; 5 Feb. 1942. The Committee divided 5:3 over national pay scales and raised weekly boarding charges to 21 shillings. MHIWU Minutes, 22 March 1943.

mental nurses and was later able to claim ministry grants towards the cost of implementation with effect from March 1943.[35]

Although national agreements on nurses' pay would now operate, other staff had already benefited. Laundry workers, displaced from their accommodation by the Emergency section nurses, were among the first to appreciate the appointment of Ernest Bevin as Minister of Labour and National Service in the coalition government. From 1940 their pay scales improved 'due to a recent award under the Laundry Trade Board' and the hospital also implemented the national Joint Conciliation Committee scales for female house and kitchen staff.[36] However, many nurses did not share the Committee's view that their wages were adequate and, in a more favourable local labour market, not all persevered with the trying conditions of wartime St Andrew's. Whether for patriotic or pragmatic reasons, male nurses continued to join the forces, even though they could be exempted, and the loss of women nurses became a longer-term problem, unresolved on the eve of the NHS.[37] Married women were allowed to return to nursing subject to a three months' gap, meant to deter those who might be pregnant, and they could not act as charge nurses.[38]

Table 8.2 indicates the shortage of nursing staff, particularly women nurses, by 1947. Throughout the war roughly 45 of the male nurses were fully qualified but less than 20 women were RMPA final certificate holders by 1945 and there was little time or recruitment for training. Nursing shortages, overcrowding and the lack of time and facilities for patients were part of a vicious circle and working conditions were not helped by cramped or antiquated accommodation. A visiting committee member observed in 1943:

Table 8.2 Nursing staff at St Andrew's, 1939–47

		Total	M	F	
June	1939	193	84	109	(includes 13 M, 21 F night staff)
June	1940	183			(use of retired/temporary staff)
May	1943	147	66	81	
April	1944	142	64	78	(further part-time staff)
June	1945	147	74	73	(includes 11 M, 3 F night staff)
Feb.	1946	123	70	53	(use of Red Cross volunteers)
April	1947	132	76	56	(plus 32 part-time and 6 Red Cross nurses)

Source: BoC Reports, SAH 142.

[35] CVIS, 7 Sept. 1944 and 1 Feb. 1945.
[36] CVIS, 1 Aug. 1940.
[37] CVIS, 4 April 1940.
[38] Mollie Middleton, interview, 2 March 2001. She was a student and nurse at St Andrew's 1940–44.

if some of the patients who were apparently doing nothing could have some employment . . . I think it would be all to the good, though I realise the difficulties with the shortage of staff. The accommodation provided for the nurses must have some bearing on the supply.[39]

There was little chance of reducing hours worked, let alone meeting the 96-hour fortnight suggested by the Rushcliffe committee. Some flexibility was provided by the use of part-time nurses and Red Cross volunteers, though the latter also confirmed the sense of a nursing crisis at the hospital. In April 1945 two visiting justices observed: 'we were struck by the shortage of nurses, particularly on the female side – this puts a big strain on the staff available'.[40] Advertisements for probationer nurses had failed to produce a single application and Board inspectors noted that just 22 nurses were attempting to care for 642 women patients during their visit. They stated frankly: 'we do not think it will be possible to carry on indefinitely with so few nurses.'[41] Difficulties were neatly illustrated by the V.E. day celebrations: staff entitled to two days' public holiday were still waiting 'at the convenience of the hospital' in September 1945.[42]

Mental hospital patients in wartime

The onset of war signalled the end of full parole for the 75 patients then free to come and go from the hospital site; they joined the 116 on part parole within hospital grounds. Some featured in the flurry of patients discharged early in 1940 and the part parole status granted to 160 patients offered some relief from overcrowded wards, as did the newly opened visiting and tea rooms.[43] Because the recreation hall was equipped with light-proof blinds, films and whist drives could continue; winter Holy Communion services also took place there as the chapel was not blacked out.[44] However, wider restrictions included a 7.30 p.m. curfew, which imposed on those formerly allowed up until 9.30 p.m. and may also explain why film shows were temporarily abandoned in the winter of 1940–41. Although the hospital reported difficulties with the supply of films, Board inspectors were

---

[39] Visitors, 25 March 1943.

[40] ibid., 12 April 1945.

[41] BoC, 5 June 1945, p. 13.

[42] CVIS, 6 Sept. 1939.

[43] AR, 1947, Cttee, p. 7. These were provided from the Johnson and Attwood funds and separately administered, their accumulated wartime profits eventually providing dual projector sound film equipment, portable gramophones and records for the patients, textbooks and reference works for the nurses' library and a £1,000 contribution towards additional staff tennis courts and bowling green.

[44] Report of Chaplain, Sept. 1939–June 1946, SAH 155; 29 Nov. 1939.

unconvinced and persuasively argued that 'the weekly Talkie is quite the most important relaxation which the average hospital patient enjoys'.[45]

Outdoors, Board inspectors noted with approval that 'a number of patients are provided with small gardens of their own and these are extremely well cultivated', but wanted these arrangements extended, not least to women patients.[46] In a less positive contribution to the 'Dig for Victory' effort, cricket and other day pastimes were sustained beyond 1940 by an ingenuous arrangement using 20 sheep from the farm, which allowed the cricket field to be retained as 'pasture' rather than ploughed up.[47] Although the farm and gardens were a vital source of employment in every sense, occupational therapy and recreation were greatly curtailed and more patient activities were geared to covering for staff shortages. Early in 1943, for example, almost one-third of the 670 male and female patients said to be occupied were essentially 'assisting in the wards'.[48]

Few in Britain early in 1939 had a long-term perspective concerning an impending war and the hospital committee, whilst recognising the need to stockpile provisions, appears to have begun with the purchase of 100 cases of condensed milk and deferred on other items.[49] Shortages of eggs, milk and supplements for invalid diets were already noticeable in 1940, although the supply of provisions generally was considered adequate and one unexpected effect of food rationing was that patients still had meat in their breakfasts twice per week. Supplies via the Ministry of Food Eastern Division were bolstered by farm-produced vegetables and cheese; soup featured regularly as supper and much use was made of suet puddings and dumplings to eke out meat rations. Cocoa supplemented the meagre tea allowance and any surplus sugar was made into boiled sweets for patients.

Nevertheless, in the two years before January 1942 the average hospital patient lost half a stone in weight, according to a 25 per cent sample monitored by Board inspectors.[50] The stockpiling of haricot beans and blue peas in August 1943 because of a 'shortage of winter vegetables' suggests recent experience or anticipation of hard times. Provided that patients had access to a variety of foodstuffs, weight loss was not necessarily entirely detrimental, but samples and averages may have masked a number of patients seriously at risk from tuberculosis, for example, in these years. Four daily meals were maintained, including a two-course midday lunch, although heavy reliance upon bread and soup afterwards is suggested by the 5.00 p.m.

---

[45] BoC, 18 Feb. 1941.

[46] BoC 19 June 1940; 13 May 1943.

[47] Eric Browne, electrician at St Andrew's 1946–88, interview, 19 Feb. 2001.

[48] BoC, 13 May 1943.

[49] CVIS, 2 Feb. 1939. This was not a quirky decision; tinned milk was almost unobtainable by 1941.

[50] BoC, 19 Feb. 1942.

tea followed by 7.00 p.m. supper. With food rations and the farm to support them, hospital patients did much better than in the Great War and in relation to much of the general population. As a young nurse Mollie Blanchflower was not that concerned about shortages of particular foodstuffs and felt that, relatively, 'we lived ever so well in the war'.[51] By 1945 McCulley considered most patients to be in reasonable health, given wartime conditions, although he did not elaborate on 'the general improvement in the weight of the patients'.[52]

Individual cases reveal the variable influences of warfare upon the complex of features surrounding patient admissions and discharges. There was no mass exodus of patients from September 1939 and the apparently premature discharge of some may have reflected their increased and reciprocated wishes to be with relatives. During her fifteen years at St Andrew's patient N.B. had been violent and suicidal: she was described as 'simple and childish and rather unstable but more settled at present' when she was discharged 'relieved' to the care of her sister. Since 1937 medical officers had raised with P.B. the possibility of her going home but her previous reluctance ended promptly in September 1939. Patient A.B. was also 'not anxious' to go home 'even for four days' in August 1939 but seems to have changed her mind after a brief trial, whilst M.P. who was 'rather depressed' in July was soon sufficiently 'relieved' to go home.[53]

Among wartime admissions, C.W., aged 33, was in great fear of conscription and had delusions that he was being poisoned and had 'bullets up his nose'. He was an early candidate for electro-convulsive therapy in 1943 but died from tuberculosis, possibly contracted during his two years' stay in the hospital. Twenty-two-year-old A.A. was a gardener and a voluntary patient in poor health who felt that he had been tricked into admission and 'that people all thought he was evading military service'. He deteriorated and became suicidal but then improved to the point where 'he feels quite well and would like to see how he gets on outside', after which he was discharged 'relieved'. G.P., just 19, had already been discharged from the army for nerves and depression and was identified as a male case of 'hysteria'. After six months in the hospital he asked to go home and Connell made arrangements for him to visit the local labour exchange and secure work prior to his discharge 'relieved'. G.W. had served with the RAF but was 'nervous and worried and constantly vomited'. Prior to his discharge from a military hospital he had been given ECT and he came as a voluntary patient to St Andrew's. He was very disturbed because 'he went with a woman in north Africa, since then his penis has felt cold and he thinks the blood has run away

---

[51] Mollie Middleton, interview, 2 March 2001.
[52] AR, 1945, MS, p. 9.
[53] Case Books, SAH 609. These patients were discharged 6–8 September 1939.

from it to his inside'. After two weeks he wished to return home and was collected, 'not improved', by his brother.[54]

B.W. was an older patient, aged 58, whose depressed state probably arose from being turned out of his home, which lay within a battle area required by the military. He had twelve ECT sessions, but he also took to the familiarity of farm work and was successively given part parole, allowed 'out for the day with his wife' and then for a four-day trial. Having expressed the wish to go home, he was discharged recovered. The farm presented a range of opportunities, not all of them positive. A.W., a farm labourer, returned to St Andrew's as a voluntary patient after earlier suicidal episodes. After a month he was 'on the whole fairly cheerful and says he is anxious to do farm-work', which appears to have contributed to his continuing improvement and discharge 'relieved' six weeks later. L.W.L. had also worked in the farm gang since his readmission in 1937, following his alleged abuse of his daughter and a suicide attempt. He was later allowed part parole, withdrawn after he attended public houses, and appears to have drowned himself whilst out doing farm-work.[55]

Another patient, H.A., was seen as an uncontrollable 27-year-old mental defective when he was admitted in 1938. He had tried brush-making and farm-work and was settled in his behaviour but was just 'very slow'. Under wartime conditions both features may have contributed to his discharge, after a successful trial, in 1942. A slight improvement in G.C.'s behaviour also seems to have been grasped by hospital authorities. He was affected by recurrent melancholia and had two spells in St Andrew's before returning in 1935 as a voluntary patient. He was very seclusive and complained that a range of activities, from listening to the radio to working, brought on stomach pains. In the wartime hospital he received little sympathy, Dr Crossley's notes stating: 'lies about indifferently and will not occupy himself: hypochondriacal.' When after four more years he spoke of returning home, he was rapidly discharged, leaving with his wife and daughter, and apparently all other parties, 'relieved'.[56]

Connell also sought the decisive resolution of complex situations in wartime. J.E., who had twice previously been a voluntary patient and dis-charged herself, consulted her general practitioner in regard to readmission in 1944. His request for advice led Connell to respond:

> I am quite willing to take her as a voluntary case but . . . she should remain here until we advise her . . . to return home, otherwise it simply means an expense and trouble . . . If you feel that her condition is bad . . . then I would advise you to certify without delay and send her in.[57]

---

[54] Case Books, SAH 591 (C.W.); SAH 592 (A.A., G.P., G.W.).
[55] Case Books, SAH 592, (B.W., A.W.), SAH 591 (L.W.L.).
[56] Case Books, SAH 607 (H.A.), SAH 592 (G.C.).
[57] Case Books, SAH 654 (J.E.) (see also Chapter 7, note 51).

Connell also tried to retain patients such as S.C., then aged 53 years, who had been at St Andrew's since 1920. He encouraged her sister to write, but obstructed a distant cousin who sought her release. At a Board of Control appeal, Connell stated that S.C. was unpredictable and that 'it would take more than two people to control her'. When the cousin persevered, trial visits were held 'to see if she can put up with S. for the rest of the time' and S.C. was eventually discharged 'relieved' to her care in October 1942.[58]

Among the patients who died during the war was R.W., an epileptic who spent forty-six of his 62 years at St Andrew's doing ward work when he was able, punctuated only by evacuation to the Hertfordshire County Asylum during the Great War. S.W., a sufferer from Friedrich's Ataxia also spent his life in poor law institutions and the hospital, where he 'required every attention' before his death from bronchopneumonia. At his burial service, T.B. was simply described as 'an ex-serviceman who had been in this hospital since 1918'.[59] Often the admission of patients was delayed until the last moment in wartime and some were dying when they were admitted. L.H., aged 71, died of heart disease. He was said to be senile but Dr Crossley noted: 'he does not want to take poison but wants me to give him something to finish him off.' The condition of F.H., aged 50, had deteriorated so much that he was certified, but Crossley's suspicion that he had an intracranial tumour was shared by the consulting surgeon and confirmed on his death a few days later. J.T., a retired farmer, was regarded as senile but had a brain haemorrhage and died within days; as did J.C., a former watchmaker aged 73, from congestion of the lungs. Elderly residents were particularly vulnerable in wartime conditions. They included H.B., a former railwayworker aged 80 and suffering from heart disease, and H.T., previously a poor law officer but now aged 81 and suffering from a persistent cough. E.E., an 84-year-old farm labourer, had neglected himself and was admitted with an ulcerated leg which turned gangrenous. H.W. was younger, aged 61, but certified because of his persistent delusions and bizarre behaviour when he 'feels insects crawling over him'. He also suffered from a severe cough, difficulty in breathing, oedema, and cardiac pains before 'he took a sudden turn for worse' and died.[60]

C.C. was among a group whose melancholia was probably associated with the heart disease later noted as their cause of death. He had been discharged from the army in 1918 suffering from neurasthenia and received a war pension, which allowed him to work part time. However, he developed chronic bronchitis and his renewed depression culminated in a suicide attempt and hospital admission, repeated when he was allowed out on trial after six months. He died from myocardial degeneration after three more years in hospital. F.H. had also been depressed and suicidal on completion of

---

[58] Case Books, SAH 603 (S.C.).
[59] Case Books, SAH 591 (R.W., S.W.); Chaplain, 20 Feb. 1940 (T.B.).
[60] Case Books, SAH 591, the deaths of all these patients occurred Feb.–Nov. 1944.

military service in 1918 but recovered until the death of his brother triggered a new attack. His year in the hospital was marked by increasing restlessness, sedation, repeated refusal to eat and force-feeding, which may have been a factor in his death. The outcome of his post-mortem is not stated, but post-mortems often did not take place because relatives were more concerned about post-mortem procedures than with establishing a patient's cause of death. At the funeral of C.B.T., for example, the chaplain reported that

> one of the relatives asserted that the coffin was empty and no corpse was buried. I assured this was not so and I would never be party to a mock funeral . . . Evidently his idea was that the Hospital had kept back the corpse for anatomical purposes.[61]

The Emergency section, 1940–47

Until Dr T.D. Brown became its first resident medical officer the Emergency section relied upon visits from Norfolk and Norwich Hospital doctors and a largely temporary nursing staff. A.M. Phillips, the sister in charge, became matron in June 1940, aided by assistant matron Rutherford.[62] In contrast with the mental hospital wards there was a considerable turnover of medical personnel, suggesting that the post was not considered sufficiently well paid or attractive. When the acting medical officer joined the forces in June 1941 Connell was authorised to find a house surgeon and house physician to provide cover.[63] The envisaged salary of £150 plus board and lodging attracted no applicants; it was raised to £200 but even then the new house surgeon left after a month. With eighteen medical officers employed at different times before Drs Kaufman and Jellinek provided some stability, the medical superintendent's roll of honour evidently found 'the succession of medical and surgical officers' too extensive for other individuals to be named.[64] Nurses were recruited temporarily for the section on different pay scales. Male nurses' pay was initially fixed at 50 shillings per week, but rose to 70 shillings in April 1942 and 78s 6d by 1945.[65]

Approximately 1,700 patients were treated in the first two years of the war. Most of these were servicemen, known as 'blue boys' because of their uniforms, who were admitted directly from units based in or around Norfolk

---

[61] Case Books, SAH 591 (C.C., F.H.); Chaplain, 3 Feb. 1940 (C.B.T.). The man thought that the bearers handled the coffin as if it were empty and was handed one of the ropes during the burial.

[62] CVIS, 6 June 1940.

[63] CVIS, 5 June 1941.

[64] AR, 1948, MS, p. 14. Others included Drs Laudernach and Spatz, who may have been American volunteers (CVIS, 7 Aug. 1941).

[65] CVIS, 5 Oct. 1939, 5 Feb. 1942 and 4 Jan. 1945. By 1945 this exceeded the 76/– corresponding point on Rushcliffe scales.

with minor ailments. As the army had no military base hospital north of Colchester, more serious or acute cases were sent to the Norfolk and Norwich and then transferred to satellite emergency hospitals, including Thorpe St Andrew's. Services personnel generally spent a few days or weeks there and almost half recovered to return directly to their units. A similar portion, not yet recovered, was transferred on to convalescent homes for additional rest, therapy or rehabilitation. This arrangement followed precedents established in 1915 and the list of country houses again made available for such purposes included Denton Hall (Harleston), Cranmer Hall (Fakenham), Felthorpe Hall and Wroxham Hall. Some 34 deaths were recorded among 12,802 services cases in all. Over 570 UK personnel were discharged by medical boards as permanently unfit, with some transferred to mental hospital wards. At least 490 injured German and Italian prisoners of war were treated, along with US, Canadian and Polish troops, with more Poles coming from displacement camps immediately after the war.[66]

In the first months there were very few civilian patients; just six at the lowest point in April 1940.[67] A number of 'tip and run' air raids on Norwich in July and August 1940 caused over forty deaths but the Emergency section was not required to deal with serious casualties until better facilities elsewhere in Norwich became fully stretched. On 3 October the hospital was prepared 'for the reception of mothers and children from bombarded areas in London'. Soon afterwards Rev. George Cockin, the hospital chaplain, 'took the funeral of B.D., an evacuee from Stepney . . . this child was 3½ months old and died from pneumonia . . . the first death we have had in this hospital of an evacuee'.[68] His reports covered regular visits to military casualties in ward D and to the evacuees, who were accommodated on wards C, C2 and G at least until early April 1941, when he was prevented by difficulties with petrol rations. Fortunately, there were no other deaths among the 608 evacuees who passed through the hospital.

In the same period there were just thirteen new civilian patients, seven women and six men, with three deaths. A man of 51 and a woman aged 40 died within days of admission on 9 May: these were the only fatalities among forty-three air-raid casualties treated at the Norfolk and Norwich and then transferred to the Emergency section. For example, a husband and wife and three women were discharged after periods varying from two days to three weeks after all were admitted during or just after Baedekker raids on Norwich between 28 and 30 April.[69] More raids on 27–28 June produced further

---

[66] I wish to thank Mr Edward Middleton, senior administrative assistant, for making this information available from his private papers, interview, 2 March 2001.

[67] CVIS, 4 April 1940.

[68] CVIS, 3 Oct. 1940; Chaplain, 30 Oct. 1940.

[69] Register of Casualties 1941–2, SAH 1943. All these cases were numbered within 3445–55. The third death was of an 81-year-old man, who had been in hospital for over six months.

casualties, who were visited by the Rev. Cockin on 30 June. After the Norfolk and Norwich Hospital obtained direct control of fifty beds in the section the workload increased; in all 1,505 civilians were treated, with 51 deaths.

Generally conditions remained much less crowded than in the mental hospital wards and visitors' reports had a more optimistic tone. Patients were often 'particularly cheerful and friendly' and they regularly 'expressed the opinion that everything was very efficient'.[70] However, it was not possible to isolate infectious cases, which led to a request from the hospital committee that fever cases or patients affected by venereal diseases, scabies and impetigo should not be admitted to the section.[71] Correspondence with regional officers of the Ministry of Health suggests that they were less easily satisfied than Board of Control inspectors with facilities in the section. Although 'there was no question of transferring the management of the unit from the Committee' . . . 'the ministry desire to be assured that the hospital was capable of providing for 250–300 cases and they would look into the question of the water supply, kitchen, laundry and other services being adequate'.[72]

As the threat of air raids and the corresponding need to hold vacant emergency beds diminished, the Committee became increasingly agitated. In June 1943 a letter was sent to the Ministry of Health 'pointing out the serious overcrowding of the wards for mental patients . . . and suggesting that consideration be given by the Ministry to the vacation of the Emergency section'.[73] Informed that the ministry 'had an obligation to keep beds empty', it became less co-operative, repeating the same argument to refuse a request from the Regional Hospitals Officer for fifty beds for use by the Norfolk and Norwich Hospital, as in 1942.[74] After more correspondence the ministry agreed to return 100 EMS beds in wards D, F and G early in 1945, but redecoration and staffing difficulties delayed their usage. Meanwhile, wards which could satisfactorily accommodate 863 mental patients, according to revised Board of Control standards, actually contained 1,073.[75] The envisaged phasing out of the remainder of the Emergency section was further delayed because waiting lists for routine hospital work in the Norwich area had increased considerably and Norfolk and Norwich Hospital medical staff were having to undertake surgery and other treatments away from that hospital.[76] Although this need was genuine, these arrangements again suggested the lower official priority given to the requirements of the mentally ill.

---

[70] Visitors, 18 June 1942; 25 March 1943.
[71] CVIS, 1 Jan. 1942. The committee also requested that mental patients were not to be admitted via the Emergency section.
[72] CVIS, 3 Sept. 1942.
[73] ibid., 3 June 1943.
[74] ibid., 5 Aug. 1943 and 7 Dec. 1944. Further requests, including accommodation for German prisoners of war, were also refused in 1945.
[75] AR, 1945, MS p. 9.
[76] Cherry and Ross, 'Norfolk and Norwich Hospital'.

In 1945 1,848 EMS patients were treated at St Andrew's and male Ward E, with 111 beds, was returned at the end of June. This left the Emergency section with 151 beds, 117 of which were still occupied at the end of December. As there were a further 1,116 admissions in 1946, only the thirteen-bed ward 13 was returned, though the number of EMS patients was reduced to 87 at the year end. With ward E now reoccupied, wards 11 and 12 could be made available to their former women patients. Dr Kaufman then left and Dr Jellinek remained with 44 patients in ward C. After a last few were transferred a total of 14,923 patients had passed through the Emergency section when it finally closed on 30 June 1947.[77]

Finance

The limited information on hospital finances during the war, summarised in Table 8.3, must be treated with caution. Pre-war arrangements for funding the mental hospital wards continued and, after some delay, the committee was reimbursed by the Ministry of Health in connection with goods and services in the Emergency section. Some £8,000 was received annually for the wartime building account and this was used mainly for the wages of maintenance and other personnel and payments to fire-watchers. Almost no building or repair work was carried out, other than for air-raid precautions and minor conversions in EMS wards.[78] Spending increased from £11,600 in 1945 to £17,000 in 1947, largely in connection with very necessary redecoration work. In 1947, for example, over £2,000 went on employer's

Table 8.3 Weekly charges for Norfolk patients and annual spending on maintenance, 1939–45

	Weekly charge (average p.a.)	Annual expenditure	Income from outcounty patients, etc.
Late 1939	23s 11d	£73,908	£694
1940	29s 9d	£94,176	£804
1941	30s 4d	£106,404	£682
1942	33s 5d	£123,328	£1,361
1943	33s 10d	£121,188	£997
1944	35s	£126,713	£1,004
1945	35s	£115,289	£782

Source: Based on monthly returns in Committee of Visitors, 1939–48

[77] AR, 1945, MS p. 11; 1946 MS, p. 12; 1947 MS, p. 14.
[78] CVIS, 2 April 1942. With air-raid shelters, etc. completed for £1,717 in 1941, related spending was approximately £200 p. a.

contributions to relevant staff pensions, with wages amounting to £7,500 and repairs, carriage and materials costing a similar amount.[79]

Building accounts continued to be bolstered by surpluses from the hospital farm and service or outcounty patients. In wartime the farm was essentially a source of food rather than of supplementary income and one effect of rationing and price controls was to limit farm earnings, in comparison with levels achieved in the First World War. Its obvious utility was confirmed by the £1,250 purchase of 32 acres of previously rented land on the adjacent Postwick estate in October 1945 and indicated in immediate post-war accounts. Annual farm sales then averaged £11,400, £2,000 of which was from outsales, the remainder representing almost 37 per cent of the hospital's provisions bill in value terms. Over 50 per cent of farm income was spent on additional livestock, but between 25 and 30 per cent was paid in wages to the farm manager and stockman and, appropriately, in allowances to patients. Annual farm profits averaging £1,300 were transferred to the building account.[80]

Estimates of annual expenditure on the maintenance account are compiled from the monthly figures approved at committee meetings. These suggest that spending increased rapidly in the first three years of the war, reflecting increased prices and the additional demands of the Emergency section, but then levelled off and fell slightly in 1945. Information on expenditure items, based on hospital ledgers, is limited but that shown in Table 8.4 confirms the control of wages and salaries. Income totals are not available, but these were boosted by annual earnings of approximately £6,000 on service and outcounty patients, with surpluses averaging £830 transferred to building funds each year. Some forty service patients were joined by an average of twenty outcounty patients, but fluctuations in income from these suggest wartime transfers and some patient mobility. Average weekly costs per patient on mental hospital wards rose sharply, from 25s 8d in the last quarter of 1939 to 31s 1d two years later, and ran ahead of the corresponding charges made upon county authorities until 1942. On occasions price increases caught the committee unprepared; its request for a £10,000 overdraft facility on the monthly maintenance account in June 1942 was out of character.[81] Fortunately, average weekly charges stabilised at 35 shillings by 1944, with quarterly charges varying slightly around this level until 1948.

On behalf of the Ministry of Health, Connell and the committee recruited temporary medical officers, nursing and additional domestic staff for the Emergency section, the ministry also accepting responsibility for the main-tenance of X-ray and other medical apparatus.[82] Initially the committee was

---

[79] AR, 1947, Building and Repairs Fund, pp. 26–7.
[80] CVIS, 4 Oct. 1945; AR, 1945–7, Farm and Garden Accounts.
[81] CVIS, 4 June 1942.
[82] ibid., 7 Nov. 1940, 6 March and 7 Aug. 1941.

Table 8.4 Hospital finances, 1939–48

	1938/9	1939–45 average	1945/6	1946/7	1947/8
All income	£74,799		£122,733	£151,312	£123,767
Norfolk contributions (%)	91.4		74.3	61.3	77.7
Service and outcounty (%)	4.5		5.7	4.9	6.2
Ministry of Health (%)	n/a		17.1	31.6	10.5
Farm surplus (%)	1.5		1.2	1.6	0.3
All expenditure	£73,908	£108, 715	£115,289	£139,730	£165,279
Main items (%)					
Emergency section	n/a		8.1	5.8	1.1
Medical staff	4.1	2.7	2.8	3.2	3.1
Nursing staff	36.1	20.5	23.6	25.1	27.5
Other staff		9.0	12.1	14.5	15.4
Pensions	6.3		6.3	6.0	5.8
Provisions	21.7		20.3	18.7	16.6
(of which farm)	(40.0)		(37.1)	(37.4)	(35.0)
Necessaries	11.7		12.0	11.7	10.5
Furnishings/bedding	2.2		2.8	3.3	3.5
Clothing	3.0		2.5	2.5	2.6
Drugs	1.2	1.0	1.2	1.4	2.0
Rates, taxes, sundries	8.4		6.5	5.8	8.3
Net surplus/deficit on year	+£891		+£7,444	+£11,582	–£41,512

Notes: Individual years based on Annual Reports. Wartime averages for expenditure items from hospital ledgers 1937–41 SAH 371 and 1941–5 SAH 44 and for all spending from Committee of Visitors Monthly Returns 1939–48.

irritated by the 'unnecessarily complicated arrangements' but these were streamlined, with central government payments made for each designated EMS bed whether occupied or not.[83] This was a limited inducement to maintain empty beds for emergencies but any financial advantage arising from the 362 EMS beds was eroded by the high turnover of light casualty patients and had to be weighed against the resultant overcrowding of mental wards. Significantly, the committee was pressing for the return of beds, which implied a smaller EMS grant, from 1943 and the extended phasing-out of the Emergency section probably offered minor financial compensation in view of

[83] ibid., 7 Nov. 1940 and 7 Aug. 1941.

the hospital's problems by 1947. Another central subsidy arose from the 1943 Rushcliffe Inquiry, with grants to assist hospitals paying wages according to recommended scales in an effort to overcome staff shortages. However, some compensation was subject to considerable delay: in 1945, for example, St Andrew's was invited to claim for increases in nurses' pay made since 1943. As repayments on other items were also sometimes necessary, these arrangements complicate the apparent year on year figures and distort trends over time.[84]

The uncertainties of immediate post-war hospital funding are illustrated in Table 8.4. Spending on the Emergency section was running down by 1945 but its earlier significance and the wartime workload can be gauged from the delayed repayment of £34,100, received from the ministry in 1946. Including nursing grants, £13,600 in 1946 for example, short-term central funding featured increasingly in hospital finances and caused wide fluctuations in annual income. Traditional supplements to hospital income now counted for proportionately less. For example, the £1,300 profit from the hospital farm or the £823 surplus on outcounty and service patients made annually between 1945 and 1947 were hard-earned, but together they barely matched the medical superintendent's salary and allowances. Even though most items were restrained, expenditure rose sharply because of rising salaries and pensions contributions for medical, nursing and other staff, almost 52 per cent of all spending in 1947. Some of this was offset by ministry grants but, with additional medical appointments and a shortage of nurses in a competitive labour market, the longer-term position was not encouraging.[85] With maintenance accounts marked by wide fluctuations in the net annual surplus or deficit and underlying rises in spending, with heavy demands on building accounts inevitable if nursing accommodation and admissions facilities were to be improved, St Andrew's required substantial financial help on the eve of the NHS.

Post-war health reforms: crisis management or transition?

Mental illness did not feature prominently in the wartime discourse on future health care, although arrangements separate from other services had been discounted when the coalition government's White Paper, A National Health Service, appeared in 1944. Inter-war ambitions to overcome the separate treatment of mind and body were restated, as was the need to reduce the stigma still associated with former asylums and their patients. The White Paper also highlighted an emerging division between the treatment of

---

[84] e.g. £1,474 was returned on 4 Feb. 1943 for unspecified overcharging.
[85] CVIS Minutes, 3 June 1948, suggest that the salaries of the four medical officers, £4,120 plus emoluments in 1946, rose by 18.3% by 1948.

neuroses, in outpatient clinics, general hospitals and through office-based private practice, and of psychoses (and perhaps the most serious neuroses), for which the mental hospitals would be retained.

The National Health Service Act as presented in 1946 by the new Labour government contained substantial modifications to the 1944 proposals, but there was little detail on mental health care and some ambiguity in the arrangements that were envisaged. Section 51 of the Act continued to allow local authorities to assume responsibilities under the 1890–1930 Lunacy and Mental Treatment Acts and the 1913–30 Mental Deficiency Acts, for example, and section 28 enabled them to provide treatments and aftercare. Yet the new NHS was to be organised essentially as a series of regional hospital-based services for the acute and chronic sick. All but the prestigious teaching hospitals and a few hospitals with religious connections were nationalised and county mental hospitals were brought under the formal control of the Minister of Health. This implied demarcation from routine general practitioner and other primary care arrangements and from residual local authority services.

The NHS embodied a laudable objective, of universalising best-possible health care arrangements. With the poor law formally abolished, there were hopes that the attitudes and stigmatisation formerly associated with it could be ended. These aims were of particular significance to mental health services but, in practice, there were few signs of their fully-resourced integration within the NHS. The previously authoritative Board of Control was subsumed, but as 'an unwilling and inferior partner', according to its official historian.[86] Mental hospitals were to be organised within the network of fourteen Regional Hospital Boards, each with a psychiatrist to oversee them. Such appointments were not compulsory or full time, however, and it appeared that, 'in the arrangements for the new service, psychiatry was very much an add-on'.[87] Below these were more localised sub-groupings of hospital management committees. This arrangement risked the subordination of mental hospitals, either within separate boards that might be isolated, or within more integrated boards dominated by consultants with agendas and priorities linked to general and specialist hospitals. Outcomes could not be predicted with accuracy but, before the Mental Health Standing Advisory Committee was established in 1949, there were few signs of innovative thinking, let alone the capacity to implement any new approach.

Local health committees took over the functions of former public assistance committees and established mental health sub-committees, with

[86] C. Webster, 'Psychiatry and the early NHS: the role of the Mental Health Standing Advisory Committee' in G.E. Berrios and H. Freeman (eds), *150 Years of British Psychiatry 1841–1991*, Gaskell, London, pp. 103–16, 104.
[87] J.V. Pickstone, 'Psychiatry in district general hospitals' in J.V. Pickstone (ed.), *Medical Innovations in Historical Perspective*, Macmillan, Basingstoke, 1992, pp. 185–99, 189.

mental welfare officers developing the old relieving officer's role in certification arrangements or the transfer of patients to and from hospital. Within the Welfare State, other social services and a benefits system were also expected to assume new significance in mental health care; for example, in liaison with general practitioners concerning potential patients or in the organisation of aftercare and support. Again, much depended upon a reforming impetus which, on past experience, was likely to vary considerably from one area to another.[88] Moreover, the rather 'vertical' structural organisation of the NHS, notably the tripartite arrangement of hospital, executive and local authority services, all ultimately accountable to the Minister of Health, did not favour locally based initiatives to provide 'horizontal' integration of services.

What reorganisation was involved for Norfolk and adjacent areas and what were the perceptions and responses at St Andrew's? The striking feature in committee minute books is the limited discussion of potentially momentous issues. In response to streams of minutes, circulars and requests from the Ministry, Regional Hospital Board and Norfolk County Council, the committee took a guarded and pragmatic stance, perhaps aware that alternative scenarios might prove worse than the one emerging. Thus in August 1943 it responded to a Mental Hospitals Association circular on the possible abolition of Committees of Visitors in rather Churchillian fashion. Such issues were best left until after the war, 'when a complete re-cast of the Lunacy and Mental Treatment Acts should be considered under conditions then existing'.[89] Connell was nevertheless part of a delegation to the MHA national conference on the White Paper held on 14 April 1944 and Major Astley attended a local one convened by Norfolk County Council. In both cases, 'in the opinion of this Committee the proposal for such a conference was somewhat premature at this stage'.[90]

During the next few months a reactive stance emerged, based essentially upon the retention of local control over distinct mental health services rather than the regional or integrated models then being developed. This accorded with the committee's predominant Conservatism, although it reflected a pragmatic conservatism: party politics were rarely expressed, 'they had a job to do and did it'.[91] An autonomous position was untenable but, in association with other mental hospitals and their medical staffs, some successes were

---

[88] See Jones, *Asylums and After*, p. 145, for examples of routinism. The lack of relevant GP training features in I. Loudon, J. Horder and C. Webster (eds), *General Practice under the NHS 1948–97*, Oxford, Oxford University Press, 1998.

[89] CVIS, 5 Aug. 1943 (MHA Circular 241).

[90] ibid. Astley was also vice chairman of Norfolk County Council.

[91] ibid., 6 July 1944. The Committee endorsed an agitational circular to this effect from Portsmouth Council, which it sent to the MHA. Comment by Edward Middleton, interview, 2 March 2001.

obtained. A Regional Hospital Board for East Anglia (Region 4), created under the 1946 Act, had major powers concerning the approval of projects and distribution of funds. The Norfolk mental hospitals were grouped separately from other hospitals and, surprisingly, also from each other. Hospital Management Committee (Group 7) assumed the responsibilities of the committee of visitors at St Andrew's.[92] The twenty-one HMC members included medical professionals, including the medical superintendent and the hospital's consulting surgeon, alongside lay representatives with relevant experience, four of them former committee members.[93] Basil Read, hospital secretary at St Andrew's, now became Group 7 HMC secretary and finance officer. It is noteworthy that the HMC also sought to maintain the hospital's influence over patient aftercare, through representation on the RHB mental health sub-committee, rather than leaving this matter to the social services.[94]

Should the immediate post-war years be seen merely as a transitional period, culminating in the advent of the NHS on 5 July 1948? Certainly a combination of problems at the hospital left little time for longer-term policy issues. Between 1945 and 1948 important initiatives were taken, though some represented a false dawn. Yet while the 'Appointed Day' has its own particular symbolism, its significance for mental health policy, mental hospitals and their patients can be exaggerated.[95]

Given the difficulties of attracting medical and nursing staff, it was fortunate that the principal medical officers remained at St Andrew's throughout the war. Connell's tenure as medical superintendent was coming to a close: a student nurse, Mollie Blanchflower, was congratulated by him when she passed her examinations in 1942 and felt 'it was like meeting the King'.[96] Connell submitted his resignation on beginning his twenty-fourth year at the hospital in January 1944, but offered to stay as temporary medical superintendent until the war emergency was over. The committee agreed to this arrangement with effect from 1 April and Major Astley, keen to obtain a suitable replacement before his own retirement as chairman, secured its

---

[92] The City of Norwich Mental Hospital, Hellesdon, was part of Group 8, which absorbed St Andrew's in 1964. Hospitals for the physically sick in Norfolk and north-east Suffolk were covered by the Group 6 HMC. Cherry and Ross, 'Norfolk and Norwich'.

[93] As a consultant at the Norfolk and Norwich Hospital, Noon was a useful link to the Group 6 HMC.

[94] CVIS, 6 Nov. and 4 Dec. 1947, correspondence with Ministry of Health, Norfolk County Council and Regional Hospital Board.

[95] Changing attitudes towards the significance of asylums, the 'pharmaceutical revolution' and the 1959 Mental Health Act were, arguably, of greater importance to patients; see next chapters.

[96] Mollie Middleton interview, 2 March 2001. Mollie Blanchflower later became nurse tutor at St Andrew's and married Edward Middleton, senior administrative assistant, in 1960.

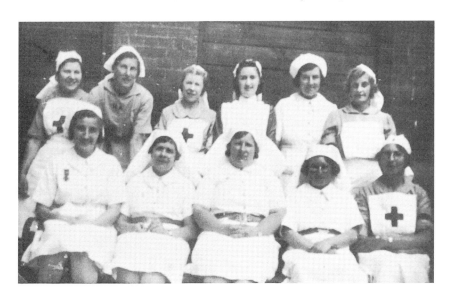

Figure 8.1 Nurses, Red Cross and volunteer nurses c. 1945 (Middleton)

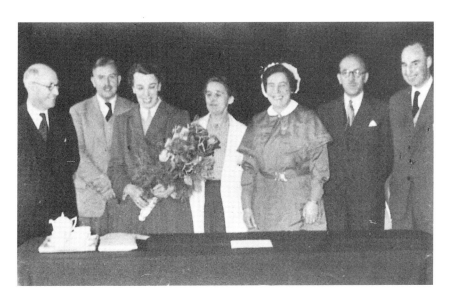

Figure 8.2 Senior personnel at the hospital in 1953 (Drinkwater)
From the left: medical superintendent Dr William McCulley, Dr H.B. Jennings, assistant matron Fawkes, Dr Ruth Meier-Blauw, matron Parry, hospital secretary Basil Read, deputy medical superintendent Dr William Fraser

support for Dr W.J. McCulley as the next medical superintendent.[97] Connell was granted six months' leave in October 1945 so McCulley, then aged 43 years, was effectively in charge and he formally took office on 1 April 1946, supported by Dr. J. Wishart who arrived from the Staffordshire mental hospital.[98] With direct experience of Scottish poor law medicine and of wartime St Andrew's, McCulley was described as 'very focused, a bit Dickensian . . . he came over as a bustling busy little man who didn't have time . . . but he was very committed to the welfare of the residents'.[99] His efforts to modernise and improve conditions for patients were to produce conflicts with the RHB and with Read and HMC.

St Andrew's difficulties in 1945 centred upon the nursing crisis, the need to reopen wards and restore facilities, and to secure improvements, particularly a new admissions hospital. The nursing shortage seemed to defy resolution and its consequences were becoming all too apparent. As the first post-war annual report recognised, this problem was now 'very acute . . . we have endeavoured to obtain applicants but we have not been successful . . . a very difficult and at times anxious year'.[100] Existing staff were expected to work through most of their annual leave entitlement and were paid 'at ordinary rates' for additional days. Overtime payments were introduced in 1946, time and a half rates beginning after 54 hours and later after 48 hours.[101] Red Cross nurses, paid two shillings per hour, were also used. Although 23 student nurses were recruited in 1946, 13 left the hospital within the year. With between 47 and 55 nurses available, 'the care and nursing of female patients was carried on with only 50 per cent of the normal complement of nurses'.[102] Board inspectors noted that for three large and crowded refractory wards, each containing 88 women patients, there were just three day nurses and one night nurse per ward. An increased number of serious incidents in which patients sustained fractures after falls or pushes by other patients was likely to be associated with crowding and insufficient nursing; similarly with 'the abnormally high rate of seclusions on the female side'.[103]

---

[97] CVIS, 6 Jan. 1944. Astley had been a committee member since 1905 and chairman since 1921. With the committee's endorsement McCulley was approached, interviewed and appointed, formally taking over as medical superintendent on 1 April 1946. Connell's wife Mary was in poor health and died early in 1946: he died in 1972, aged 87.

[98] AR, 1946–7, MS, p. 10.

[99] Rita Browne, interview, 9 March 2001. Rita worked in the pathology department from 1960 to 1967.

[100] AR, 1945, Cttee, p. 6.

[101] CVIS, 1 Nov. 1945, 4 April 1946 and 6 Feb. 1947. According to MHIWU Minutes, from 6 Jan. 1946, the union regularly requested meetings over staff shortages. Members still awaited the 96-hour fortnight at the close of 1947.

[102] AR, 1946, Cttee, p. 6. Eight of 19 male student nurses also left. The 1939 nurse complement was 107.

[103] BoC, 5 Feb. 1946, p. 14.

Revised plans for a new nurses' home were submitted to the Board of Control in 1947. Accommodation costing £125,000 for 83 nurses and 22 domestic staff was envisaged, with provision for 54 more nurses in a phased extension.[104] Poor amenities undoubtedly compounded difficulties with recruitment and the committee was left to acknowledge that, 'in comparison with other hospitals, the nurses' quarters are much below standard'. Such deficiencies were cumulative in their effect: as McCulley observed, 'the small number entering upon training shows how little the Rushcliffe scale of salaries has helped to promote the recruitment of nurses for the mental hospital service'.[105] Increasingly, the hospital depended upon the availability of part-time nurses: with 47 part-time and 47 full-time nurses at the end of 1947, what had been regarded as a short-term expedient began to appear as the only long-term option. Future hopes rested upon the training of new staff under the General Nursing Council, which had already inspected relevant hospital provision. With the integration of services under the NHS, a joint preliminary training school was established for St Andrew's, Hellesdon and Little Plumstead hospitals.

McCulley was also attempting to address other priorities. The phased return of Emergency section wards and post-war shortages frustrated his efforts to relieve overcrowding. Wards 11 and 12 were redecorated but could not be reopened in 1946 because of nursing staff shortages and, although there were sufficient male nurses, the redecoration of wards D to G was delayed by licensing problems over the scarce supplies of materials. Early in 1947 there were public indications that this work was under way but visitors' reports in November 1948 were still urging that 'the work of plastering and redecorating all brick walls in the wards should be pressed forward as soon as possible'.[106] McCulley also wished to see the extension of central heating throughout the hospital as part of a general refurbishment. More isolation facilities were to be secured through the construction of a verandah on male ward D and the long overdue division of male ward C was another priority.[107] With the nurses' home now apparently proceeding, the committee took up another familiar theme, acknowledging that 'an admission hospital is a great need and must have preference in any future development schemes'.[108]

A surge in admissions after 1945 demonstrated the need for this facility, but the variable therapeutic responses included a number of measures soon seen to be of doubtful value. In succeeding years there were record inpatient

---

[104] Plans at Drayton Old Lodge indicate a large, functional three-storey brick building, sited across the main road on the north side.

[105] CVIS, 4 July and 7 Aug. 1947; AR, 1946, Cttee, p. 6 and MS, p. 14.

[106] AR, 1946, MS, p. 8 and Visitors, 17 Nov. 1948. St Andrew's medical staff could not reoccupy their living accommodation until Drs Kaufman and Jellinek left in 1947.

[107] AR, 1945, MS, p. 11; AR, 1946, Cttee p. 6 and MS, p. 8; BoC, 23 April 1947, pp. 13–15.

[108] AR, 1947, Cttee, p. 6 (dated 16 March 1948).

admissions, 348 in 1946 and 367 in 1947, three-quarters of which were voluntary patients. The number of new outpatients, one quarter of them seen in King's Lynn, also increased dramatically to 267 in 1947, with weekly clinics introduced in Norwich and further transfers between inpatient and outpatient groups. Consequently, the pressure upon hospital resources and staff was greater than implied in totals for the average number of resident patients, which again exceeded 1,150 in 1947. Until Emergency section wards were reinstated the overcrowding on available accommodation, as defined by Board inspectors, rose to 146. As wards became available this figure was set to fall, but the upward trend in admissions suggested longer-term problems and Board estimates did not sufficiently allow for non-resident users of hospital facilities. Almost one-third of admissions were discharged as recovered and nearly three-quarters were seen as relieved or recovered, although such figures became increasingly unreliable as the proportion of voluntary patients, able to discharge themselves but usually classed as 'relieved', increased.[109]

These trends demonstrated the need for a proper admissions unit and were associated with new treatments and services. Electro-convulsive therapy (ECT) apparatus was purchased at Connell's request in 1942, insulin coma treatment was introduced in 1947 for 'small' numbers of patients, and McCulley announced that the hospital was equipped to carry out pre-frontal leucotomies, using the services of the consultant surgeon.[110] A few general paralysis patients were given malarial therapy with tryparsamide, though no successes were claimed. Limited and vague information concerning the nature, number and outcomes of physical treatments contrasted with the scientific approach conveyed.[111] In 1945 69 patients, including voluntary and outpatients, underwent ECT sessions varying from 'a few' to 'twelve or more'; 47 were discharged and McCulley concluded that the treatment 'continues to give good results'.[112] He urged the provision of theatre facilities within any new admissions unit for more physical treatments. These later became controversial as they involved major risks for doubtful outcomes and suspicions that patients were rarely in a position to give informed consent.[113] Roughly 30 patients had narco-analysis, considered 'very helpful' to the majority who were later discharged. A smaller number underwent

---

[109] AR, 1947, MS, p. 9.

[110] ibid., p. 11 and see Chapter 9.

[111] Eric Browne, the electrician, was asked by one doctor about suitable voltages! Interview, 9 March 2001.

[112] AR, 1945, MS, p. 11.

[113] See Kingsley Jones, 'Insulin coma therapy in schizophrenia', *Journal of the Royal Society of Medicine*, Vol. 93, March 2000, pp. 147–9; 12,000 leucotomies were performed in England and Wales 1945–55 (see Chapter 9 for St Andrew's experience) before the procedure was abandoned. K. Jones, *Asylums and After*, p. 147; P. Fennell, *Treatment without Consent*, Routledge, London, 1996.

continuous narcosis 'where necessary'. However, psychotherapy was 'the method of choice' among voluntary patients and McCulley requested additional medical staff. He also recommended the appointment of a psychiatric social worker to assist outpatients and former inpatients, meanwhile using Cambridge-based helpers from the National Association for Mental Welfare.[114]

The end of the war meant the resumption of full parole status, granted to 67 mainly working patients and increasing to 86 in 1947. More than 160 others had part parole, but this slight improvement on pre-war levels still left three-quarters of patients under very restrictive conditions. Almost two-thirds were 'usefully employed' in 1946 and, with the nursing shortage, they performed a great deal of 'ward work'. Continuing restrictions on suitable materials hampered the resumption of occupational therapy classes, although the appointment of a qualified occupational therapist represented a positive measure and much needed relief for women nurses. Further appointments resulted in bookbinding and rug-making for men patients and leatherwork classes for women, while greater attention to recreation was reflected in the new post of 'occupational and recreational worker'. Innovations in 1946–47 included folk dancing, discussion and practical sessions based around the Red Cross picture scheme, and regular trips to see Norwich City Football Club.[115] Older favourites reappeared, with coast trips for 300 patients and film nights enhanced by new projection equipment costing over £1,400.

As in 1919 a number of key hospital personnel retired, having met wartime obligations to extend their working lives.[116] New staff in place for the inception of the NHS and any necessary adaptation was possibly advantageous, although the loss of experience and sense of discontinuity were heightened. Chief male nurse Percy Keeble retired after 39 years' service and matron Maud Gibbs resigned after 33 years' service: 'she knew every woman patient in that hospital.'[117] Matron Amy Coomber, previously deputy matron at Rampton Hospital, arrived in June 1948 and it was perhaps significant that chief male nurse H. Hutchins, formerly at Winson Green Hospital, Birmingham, held both SRN and RMN qualifications. Yet continuing difficulties over nurse shortages and training were illustrated by the loss of two assistant matrons and of the nurses' home warden and sister tutor in 1946 and 1947.[118]

---

[114] AR, 1945, MS, p. 11. Cecilia Chadwick, Agnes Black and S.B. Jewson successively acted as psychiatric social workers in 1947–8.

[115] CVIS, 7 March 1946; AR, 1947, MS, p. 13.

[116] e.g. Dennis George, general labourer and carter, retired after completing 52 years' service in Nov. 1944. He was then aged 77 years. CVIS, 2 Nov. 1944.

[117] Edward Middleton, interview, 2 March 2001. The son of John Middleton, the former clerk and steward, Edward began as a junior clerk in 1941 and retired as senior administrative assistant in 1981.

[118] AR, 1947–8, pp. 3–4.

Disruption also occurred among the medical staff. Dr J. Wishart left in 1947 to become medical superintendent at Jersey mental hospital. Remarkably, he took with him as nursemaid Lily H—, a middle-aged epileptic patient who had become devoted to his two sons and was treated as one of the family.[119] Dr S.M. Rayner was appointed deputy superintendent with effect from the beginning of 1949 but Dr Crossley, now senior assistant medical officer, was called up for national service in July 1947. This left the hospital short of senior medical staff, although the notional complement was increased from three to four with the arrival of Dr. H.S. Capoore in June 1948.[120] One junior assistant, Dr Colville, stayed only briefly and was replaced by Dr F. Blake in 1947; meanwhile a succession of temporary officers occupied vacant posts, these including Dr A.L. Smith and the first women doctors, Cecilia Chadwick and Agnes Black. Other new posts reflected wider services for patients. A part-time physiotherapist was appointed in 1947 and in April 1948 Miss S.B. Jewson became the hospital's first full-time qualified social worker and, for some patients, a link to new social services and aftercare which were to become increasingly important.

Conclusions

Accepting that source materials on hospital finances and the Emergency section are less full between 1940 and 1945 than in other periods examined, a summary can still be offered. St Andrew's did not undergo the transformation to war hospital seen in 1915 and its residents were spared the excesses of evacuation and the high mortality levels seen in the First World War. Services were better maintained and food rationing may have been a critical feature in saving life. Yet weight loss, the incidence of TB and various forms of intestinal disorders were all indicators of hard lives under very restrictive conditions, and of privations held to be endurable if they were not manifested in the form of increased mortality. The burden of additional stresses arising from the part-adaptation to EMS hospital fell disproportionately upon patients crowded into the remaining mental hospital wards. Whether conditions deteriorated quite so badly as alleged in Parliament on 25 November 1945 is debatable. Considering this question, the committee at St Andrew's concluded that deficiencies were 'greatly exaggerated . . . a recovery rate of about 50% on the admissions at Thorpe is a clear indication that good work is being carried out'.[121] Although that claim actually rested

---

[119] Middleton, interview 13 March 2001. For other instances of retiring staff accommodating patients, see Chapter 10.

[120] Dr Crossley returned in August 1949 but Dr Capoore left that November, creating a new shortage. AR, 1949, MS, p. 16.

[121] CVIS, 3 Jan. 1946.

upon a liberal interpretation of cases 'relieved', admissions and recoveries are not the best guide to the health of long-term patients. Board inspectors and others noted poor conditions, some breakdown in standards of classification and evidence of disorder on big and crowded wards. Nursing shortages compounded these problems and may explain the higher levels of seclusion also recorded.

The extent of wartime disruption, aggravated by post-war restrictions, diminished the prospects of rapid improvement after 1945. Overcrowding was inevitable while the Emergency section continued and, for all its valuable work, the latter exemplified the lower priority given to mental patients when difficult choices were necessary. For the hospital to achieve some stability was a relative accomplishment but not an adequate description of the situation. Wartime problems overlay a pre-war hospital environment which was in many ways outmoded and defective admissions facilities and nursing accommodation went unremedied through eight more years' wear and tear. Without new buildings, overcrowding could only be resolved in the context of more recoveries on increased admissions and 'crisis', rather than stability, was the term officially used to convey the nursing shortage.

Thus, between 1945 and 1948 the hospital was not so much in transition between a peacetime restoration and the advent of the NHS as in a state of flux, arising from growing deficiencies in the 1930s, further disoriented in wartime and, in 1948, with no clear view of the future. Given the political outlook of a majority of its members, the committee's preference for the status quo and its reactive stance on health reform were more predictable. These rested upon the assumption, questionable on the immediate pre-war record, that left to local control, secure foundations for new treatments and measures could be developed. If this position was flawed, how did the alternative appear? The NHS embodied high ideals and was a cause for optimism, but the view from mental hospitals was less rosy and additional resources could not be seen. It was later appreciated that the people's health service had few structures to suggest democratic accountability and, while the primacy of an optimum and equalised service was asserted, resources were all too finite and subject to a priority system which would not favour St Andrew's and similar hospitals. Of course, the full significance of this was not apparent in 1948 and the possibility remained that a lesser share of larger resources might yet exceed tightly managed localised funding. However, the committee as then constituted was always likely to opt for the latter scenario.

As the reorganisation associated with the NHS removed this option, an influential role and the maintenance of some familiarities became paramount. There was scope for both, in that the Regional Health Board had no precise blueprints of its own. For example, it requested Read's views concerning the role and operation of the Group 7 Hospital Management Committee. He responded: 'provided the Management Committee proceeds, at the outset, on similar lines to the present Visitors' Committee as to frequency of meetings, statutory visits, and functions of sub-committees, there should be no serious difficulty in carrying on from the appointed day.'[122] Other requests included a touching letter from J.B.W., formerly a patient and now employed as a stores assistant at St Andrew's, 'asking that his services be not terminated on account of the transfer of the hospital'. He received the personal reassurance, symbolic of wider aims, that 'the Visiting Committee have no intention of altering the existing arrangements'.[123] A sense of continuity also underlay McCulley's remarks early in 1948 that, 'As part of a wider mental health service this hospital will continue to serve the people of Norfolk and will remain a living memorial to the work of successive generations of the Committee of Visitors'.[124] The hospital, officially designated 'St Andrew's Hospital, Thorpe, Norwich', occupied a position within an NHS area structure that looked considerably more familiar than might have been anticipated. There remained the far greater problem of ensuring sympathetic audiences at regional and national levels for problems no less real or persistent after the Appointed Day.

---

[122] CVIS, 3 June 1948.
[123] ibid., 3 June 1948.
[124] AR, 1947, MS, p. 16.

9

'Modern treatment carried out under difficulty', 1948–64

Few people with direct experience of mental hospitals expected a bright new dawn on the Appointed Day, 5 July 1948, but they can hardly have envisaged the nature of developments over the next decades. Overcrowding in mental hospitals nationally was estimated at 14 per cent in 1950; there was an acute shortage of nursing staff and, with an increasing proportion of elderly patients, some form of expansion was seen as a priority.[1] Yet annual spending on mental hospitals averaged only £1 million between 1948 and 1954, compared with £2.3 millions in 1938–9. More invasive physical and electric treatments were used before the pharmacological revolution began, but renewed attention was also paid to occupational and recreational therapies, psychopathology and behavioural training. If the role of mental hospitals was not yet controversial, their modernisation or replacement costs already occupied Ministry and Regional Board officials and hospital administrators and soon became a public issue. Therapeutic and economic considerations assumed additional significance after the 1959 Mental Health Act, which superseded previous legislation and related arrangements and specified informal treatments without stigma in district general hospitals or under new community agencies.

One emerging certainty in this vague future was the running down of mental hospitals, which featured prominently in the 1962 Hospital Plan.[2] Wholesale closures and a halving of the sector's bed capacity was envisaged by 1975, ensuring that further spending upon target institutions would be minimal. St Andrew's, with accommodation dating from 1814, carrying deficiencies acknowledged in the 1930s and compounded by wartime experiences, inevitably came under scrutiny. Until then the hospital offered a range of treatments and good standards of care in rather outmoded conditions and within financial limits suggestive of indifference at regional and ministerial levels. Meanwhile, admissions, readmissions and the proportion of the elderly long-term residents all increased.

---

[1] C. Webster, 'Psychiatry and the early NHS: the role of the Mental Health Standing Advisory Committee' in G.E. Berrios and H. Freeman (eds), *150 Years of British Psychiatry, 1841–1991*, Gaskell, London, 1991, pp. 103–16. 9,000–14,000 extra beds were envisaged by the middle 1950s, though more hostel-style accommodation and greater co-ordination with social services were suggested.
[2] *A Hospital Plan for England and Wales*, Cmnd 1604, HMSO, London, 1962.

By the early 1960s St Andrew's had completed a merger with the former naval institution at Yarmouth, renamed St Nicholas' Hospital. The 1959 Act was operative and the Regional Hospital Board had responded to the Hospital Plan by incorporating both hospitals within an enlarged Group 8 in 1964. Hospital annual reports, already less informative, then changed radically and coverage of St Andrew's diminished. Board inspectors' reports ceased with the abolition of the Board of Control under the 1959 Act but medical superintendent's reports continued beyond the regrouping and McCulley's own resignation through ill-health in 1964, as did visitors' reports.[3] Regrouping also coincided with the sale of the hospital farm and the abandonment of an undervalued but previously essential part of hospital life.

The pressure of numbers

On the first anniversary of the NHS, Board of Control inspectors summarised the situation at St Andrew's in blunt fashion:

> the handicap of lack of facilities, shortage of nursing staff on the female side and overcrowding has stood out. This hospital has no admission unit, no isolation hospital, no modern treatment centre and no convalescent villas. All forms of modern treatment, however, are carried out under difficulty.[4]

They also specified defective heating arrangements, more ward redecoration and refurbishment, and patient-centred improvements from clothing to the provision of hot food at the table and a wider range of occupational therapies. Yet the Hospital Management Committee faced restricted supplies of materials, staff shortages and a Regional Hospital Board which provided insufficient notice of available funds but criticised HMC provisional spending. Within months McCulley protested that 'a feeling of frustration was developing, caused by delay in obtaining decisions on various matters and the realisation that there was now little scope or encouragement for local initiative'. He recognised the constraints upon the RHB but the fact that 'little has been done to upgrade the hospital as advised' probably determined his resignation from the HMC.[5]

---

[3] Medical Superintendent's Journal Aug. 1955–April 1971 (at Drayton Old Lodge), 1 Oct. 1964. McCulley was not expected to return to work for at least six months. He recovered sufficiently to act as a part-time consultant later on and his deputy, H.E. Fraser, became medical, later physician, superintendent at St Andrew's.

[4] Board of Control, Inspectors Reports 1929–59 (BoC), SAH 142; 19 July 1949.

[5] Annual Reports, 1949–63, SAH 35; 1950 Hospital Management Committee (HMC), p. 7, MS, p. 15. McCulley clashed with HMC Secretary Basil Read over hospital funding requirements.

Although the long-awaited admission hospital reached the planning stage in 1954 and pre-NHS hospital managers were committed to a new nurses' home, there was no 'landmark' building project which significantly changed hospital work or life, beyond the introduction of oil-fired central heating in 1961. Instead, piecemeal improvements and attempts by an increasingly frustrated HMC to recycle its stock of ageing buildings provided the immediate context for care and therapy.

An increasing workload pressurised inadequate hospital facilities still further. Record admissions in 1939 represented only half the 592 annual average for the 1948–57 period, with 1,830 patients then under treatment each year, and Table 9.1 shows their continuing rise. According to Board of Control recommendations for the spacing of beds, accommodation for male and female patients was respectively 12 and 30 per cent deficient in 1948. These figures exceeded national averages for mental hospitals (respectively 8 and 17 per cent), and the local situation then deteriorated faster and further. Between 1951 and 1957 the average overcrowding on women's wards was roughly 50 per cent and on men's wards almost 25 per cent, perhaps double the national average.[6] A related problem was the steady increase in the proportion of elderly patients, one quarter of admissions and one-third of all residents by 1954, very few of whom could be treated on a short-term basis. Recovery rates on admissions averaged 20 per cent, but discharge rates rose from 75 per cent towards 90 per cent as the hospital sought to clear beds. In turn, these produced higher readmission rates – over 40 per cent in the early 1950s – and the proportion of resident patients aged over 65 years rose inexorably towards the 40 per cent attained in 1960.

The Committee regularly warned the Regional Board of a 'dangerously high percentage of overcrowding ... it is essential that alternative accommodation be found for those of advanced years ... in order to free beds for earlier cases in need of specialised care and treatment'.[7] In 1952 the RHB revised patient catchment areas so that Group 8 hospitals admitted west Norfolk patients and a few St Andrew's residents were also transferred, but this had only marginal effects on overcrowding. Building improvements included the verandah extension for male ward D tuberculosis patients, completed in 1952, and the division of male ward C into self-contained wards, the upper floor forming a new ward J, in 1953. The phased construction of sanitary annexes began with wards 5 and 6 in 1954 and wards A, B and H in 1956 but at least three wards, F, G and 4, remained unimproved in

---

[6] Based on ARs, 1951–6. Overcrowding in mental hospitals nationally averaged 12% for men and 19% for women in 1953.

[7] AR, 1949, HMC, p. 6. The Committee, chafing at 'the constant pressure of financial limitation', warned that 'unless relief is forthcoming in the near future, it will be necessary to refuse admission to new cases ... normally received on a voluntary basis'.

Table 9.1 Average annual totals for patients, treatments and overcrowding, 1948–63

| | Admissions | | | Under treatment | Average resident | Overcrowding | | New outpatients | Discharge rate (%) |
	No.	% vol.	(% re-adm.)			M (%)	F (%)		
1948–52	507	75		1,729	1,184	19	42	507	78
1953–57	663	86	(43)	1,929	1,203	25	50	602	85
(including St Nicholas' Hospital)									
1958–60	876	92*	(46)	2,274	1,343	13	17	726	80
1961–63	1,051	95*	(44)	2,476	1,360	10	14	778	82

Notes: Compiled from Annual Reports, percentages rounded to nearest whole number. Voluntary admissions (* informal status from 1959) are based on year end classification. Overcrowding data does not allow for patients on leave. Roughly 8% of the patients discharged were 'not improved'.

December 1964.[8] Nursing and domestic staff obtained little more than refurbishment of basic accommodation, some of it once considered temporary in 1915, and the planned nurses' home never materialised.

Heating arrangements were 'a grave defect' and many rooms 'very cold and uncomfortable', according to Board inspectors and visitors. A four-year programme to install central heating, announced in 1949, was completed only in 1958. Temporary appliances were required in at least six wards, including ward 15 for elderly women patients, where 'conditions were such as to cause anxiety during the winter months'.[9] Visitors noted that 'patients in wards 5 and 6 have shown improved behaviour with the extra warmth', but many male wards remained 'inadequately heated . . . the temperature in C ward is 52 degrees Fahrenheit and, we understand, has been as low as 42 degrees'.[10]

Ward redecoration and refurbishment also took several years to complete. Essential comforts were lacking: new visitors to F ward day rooms 'were shocked to see some of these people sitting uncomfortably on hard wooden chairs', and older hands suggested that 'a list of "needs" be compiled and submitted' to the voluntary Norfolk Hospitals Contributors Association.[11] Elementary work was overtaken by renovations which involved the variable colouring of walls, bedspreads and curtains to produce a more cheerful atmosphere, but the modernisation of ward kitchens and sanitary facilities was still incomplete. Although the committee announced the completion of the backlog of work in 1957 and visitors noted improvements, references to 'dingy and drab' or 'very shabby' wards, damp ceilings and the absence of redecoration for ten or even twelve years in areas of patient accommodation persisted. Such comments almost always produced remedial action but the hospital was seemingly unable to manage a systematic programme of redecoration to maintain standards.[12]

Overcrowding persisted as 'many dormitories have three, even four rows of beds and movement about the wards is difficult'. Record admissions in 1956

---

[8] New sanitary blocks were completed for wards 9,10, 13 and 14 (1957), 11 and 12 (1960) and 2, 7 and 8 (1963) covering most of the women's side. On the men's side, wards D and E were also equipped in 1963, leaving F, G and 4. MS Journal, 3 Dec. 1964. The nurses' home was modernised with central heating and additional bathrooms, etc. in 1953, but domestic staff still lived in modified hutments.

[9] BoC, 10 Feb. 1948, p. 17; St Andrew's Hospital Visitors Book (Visitors), 1955–70 (at Drayton Old Lodge), 6 Dec. 1955, 23 April and 26 Nov. 1956; AR, 1953, HMC, p. 9; 1955, HMC, p. 8.

[10] Visiting Justices Report Book (Visitors), 1903–55, SAH 140; 16 Dec. 1952; 16 Feb. 1954.

[11] Visitors, 17 May 1951; 26 Oct. 1949. This rather shaming experience for an NHS hospital was followed by use of £500 of endowment moneys for armchairs in 1951.

[12] Comments, in order, from AR, 1957, HMC, p. 7; Visitors, 22 April 1958, 14 Sept. 1959, 22 Dec. 1960, 20 March 1961, 24 Feb. 1960.

badly affected designated wards and the classification of patients, notably on women's wards 3 and 15, was now 'really poor'.[13] With Ministry of Health officials refusing to sanction extensions to mental hospitals, the RHB excluded St Andrew's from its capital works programme, a decision which the HMC found 'disturbing'. Board of Control inspectors urged the hospital to board out, under section 57 of the 1890 Act, those patients 'who have really no psychosis but are merely old but ambulant', but suitable accommodation was unavailable in Norfolk.[14] Inadequate provision for tuberculous and typhoid-carrier patients at St Andrew's was also highlighted.

In 1957 the Yarmouth Naval Hospital Transfer Act placed this institution, dating back to the eighteenth century, under the control of the Regional Hospital Board and offered an unexpected source of relief. Although in need of considerable modernisation and restricted to male patients, the hospital contained 236 beds, 151 of which were in use at the time of transfer, raising the rare prospect of spare capacity. It was attached to Group 7 HMC on 1 April 1958 and renamed St Nicholas' Hospital after the patron saint of sailors. As its separate status restricted inter-hospital patient transfers and generated administrative workloads, this was removed and St Nicholas' became part of the St Andrew's group a month later. Centralised records facilitated patient transfers and 67 St Andrew's male patients, previously from east Norfolk or Great Yarmouth, were moved to St Nicholas', which had 218 patients at the year end.[15]

Approximately seventy St Andrew's patients were on leave at any one time in the mid-1950s.[16] Desirable from therapeutic considerations, this arrangement was the more necessary since the average number of 1,200 residents greatly exceeded the statutory night accommodation for 919 and approached the total of 1,256 available beds. Such forms of leave and the availability of St Nicholas' allowed McCulley to manoeuvre resources within St Andrew's. Male ward 16 was cleared, redecorated and reopened to accommodate fifty women and reduce their overcrowding. The ward 15 verandah for TB patients was extended and a modest day room and sanitary annexe were added to the building converted from glasshouses in 1927, now known as Orchard Ward, which provided isolation facilities for women typhoid carriers. Arrangements were then made for St Andrew's to receive

---

[13] BoC, 27 April 1955, p. 20; 24 May 1956, p. 23; Visitors, 17 Nov. 1955.

[14] BoC, 24 May 1956, p. 24. Over 1,000 St Andrew's patients had leave at some point that year, not least to relieve overcrowding. BoC inspectors felt that many could advantageously be boarded out for less than £5 per week, compared with the average inpatient weekly cost of £5 6s 6d in 1955–6.

[15] AR, 1957, HMC, p. 7; 1958, HMC, pp. 7–8. St Nicholas' hosted two HMC meetings each year and had bimonthly visitors' inspections. It had two resident medical officers and, initially, its own male nurses.

[16] AR, 1956, MS, p. 14; 1962, MS, p. 17. New drug treatments allowed more patients to take leave.

similar patients from Fulbourn Mental Hospital, Cambridgeshire and to transfer active TB cases there.[17]

Increasingly frustrated by the postponement of new facilities, the HMC determined on 'utilising to the full all available space not required for other or more pressing needs'.[18] In 1959 small rooms were converted as bedrooms for twelve patients and a residential unit for six women patients 'who look after themselves with the minimum of supervision'. A former tailor's shop and linen store became a 24-bed dormitory, extended in 1960 as 36-bed male ward K; 'designed and supervised by the hospital's own officers, without architectural help'.[19] Additional nursing staff at St Nicholas' hospital would enable fifty more patients to be transferred but, even then, there would be overcrowding. Consequently, the RHB was publicly invited to take initiatives, as 'it must now be accepted that the Management Committee cannot take any further action to improve conditions as St Andrew's'.[20] For example, women patients were placed in the former male ward J but the reduced overall figure of 12 per cent masked levels of 50 per cent on male wards E and H and 30 per cent on ward C, where 'the majority of patients . . . are infirm and many have been ill in recent weeks'.[21]

The final Board of Control inspectors' report reiterated, 'both admissions wards are very antiquated . . . overcrowding on the female side of the hospital is severe and . . . classification is poor'. McCulley also continued to urge 'the need for more modern accommodation, for all are agreed on the beneficial effect on patients and staff of the enhanced amenities provided in modern hospital planning'.[22] Yet the post-1959 legislative focus upon community care and special units attached to general hospitals necessarily meant a reduced emphasis upon psychiatric hospitals. In 1961 it appeared that inadequate day accommodation and amenities at St Nicholas' would not be addressed as the hospital was scheduled for closure by 1975. News that 'it is contemplated that St Andrew's may also be taken out of service at some future date' had the HMC simultaneously expressing confidence in the 'fullest consultation' before any final decision, whilst attempting to safeguard the hospital's future. Yet following efforts 'to acquaint the Board of our misgivings and to put forward certain alternative suggestions . . . the Board informed us that . . . it was out of the question to make any fundamental changes'.[23] In October 1963

---

[17] AR, 1958, MS, p. 15; BoC, 1 Oct. 1958, p. 27.

[18] AR, 1959, HMC, p. 8.

[19] AR, 1959, MS, p. 16; 1960, HMC, p. 8.

[20] AR, 1960, HMC, p. 8. Centralised kitchens and new cafeteria were planned to release ward dining rooms, accommodating 50 extra beds, but general stores were converted into new kitchens at lower cost in 1962 and male ward J was cleared for 46 women patients to reduce their overcrowding.

[21] MS Journal, 4 April 1963.

[22] AR, 1959, MS, p. 17; BoC, 3 Sept. 1959, p. 28.

[23] AR, 1961, HMC, 'The Hospital Plan', p. 14; 1962, HMC, p. 14.

the RHB announced the incorporation of St Andrew's and St Nicholas' within Group 8 mental hospitals from 1 April 1964. The subdivision of larger wards, building of sanitary annexes and the centralisation of kitchens would be completed but future developments were to centre upon Hellesdon Hospital.

Nursing staff shortages

Psychiatric nursing was not considered the most desirable of occupations in an era of full employment and conditions at St Andrew's did not enhance this perspective. Nationally, the increase in full-time nurses was fractional and there were fewer student nurses.[24] Some twenty-five Polish nursing orderlies were hastily recruited in 1949 but not all these could be accommodated even in the hospital's stock of hutments.[25] Meanwhile, staff shortages delayed a planned 48-hour working week until 1949 for men and beyond for full-time women nurses, who worked around a 52-hour pattern. By 1951 'a disturbing drop in the number of female nurses' had occurred and Board inspectors considered nursing on the women's side to be 'gravely insufficient'.[26] Full-time qualified women nurses could not adequately be replaced by nursing assistants or by students and part-time staff were less likely to provide nursing cover for early mornings, nights and weekends. In 1956 there were actually ten fewer full-time and six fewer part-time nurses than in 1949. Continuing financial restrictions also dictated a short-term policy of filling casual vacancies as they arose, rather than developing staff skills. French and Spanish nurses, employed from the mid-1950s, often left after one year. Board inspectors still regarded the female nursing resources as 'slender' in 1959. They noted, for example, that admission ward 10 was under-staffed yet its nurses were also expected to supervise convalescent patients on the adjacent ward 9.[27]

As Table 9.2 shows, the number of male nurse orderlies and assistants also increased, although the male nursing staff appeared better qualified and more settled, with students more likely to enrol and complete their training. At St Nicholas' staffing problems were met by the extension of male nurse training to this site from 1961 and the recruitment of male nursing assistants and orderlies. At least two male nurses worked on the women's side at

---

[24] Nationally, full-time general nurses increased by 25% in 1948–51 and mental nurses by just 2.6%. A 38% rise in part-time general nurses compared with 29% for psychiatric nursing and student nurses in mental hospitals fell by 10%.

[25] St Andrew's Polish emigré and ex-servicemen patients were assisted by Dr B. Pietocha throughout this period.

[26] AR, 1949, MS, p. 14 ; 1951 HMC, p. 7 and BoC, 18 Oct.

[27] BoC, 3 Sept. 1959, p. 28; AR, 1961, HMC, p. 13.

Table 9.2 Nursing and other staff, 1948–63, average per annum (part-time in parenthesis)

	Women Registered	Student	Assistant	Orderly	Men Registered	Student	Assistant	Orderly
1948–52	28 (11)	11	11 (48)	21 (1)	62	19	8	1
1953–58	24 (12)	14	19 (50)	7 (2)	72	17	8	8
1959–63	25 (7)	20	26 (59)	4	82	16	28	14

Notes: From Annual Reports; 1959–63 figure for male staff includes 35–40 at St Nicholas' Hospital.

St Andrew's from the early 1950s; a male night nurse supervisor was appointed in 1960 in the absence of qualified female applicants, as was a male assistant matron in 1962. Women student nurses were hard to find and more difficult to retain, with very few proceeding to the General Nursing Council's final examination for mental nurses.[28] Attempts to utilise generic elements of GNC nurse training and exchanges with local hospitals to attract recruits were not helped by the poor accommodation offered at St Andrew's. The employment of school leavers as cadet nurses also foundered upon lack of interest and the two-year wait before full training commenced at the age of 18 years. There was no new nurses' home and a new social club was provided in 1962 only after the exhaustion of the hospital's amenities fund and the receipt of a special RHB grant.

Nurses' pay did not increase significantly in the 1950s despite full employment. It was determined through a system of 'functional councils' which replaced the Rushcliffe Committee in 1948 and there was considerable resentment that COHSE, the main trade union for psychiatric hospital nurses, had only four of the forty-one 'staff' seats available. Following an overtime ban, the standard working week was reduced to 46 hours in 1956 and 44 hours in 1958.[29] Allowing also for night- and shift-working, it is unlikely that patients to nursing staff ratios were significantly reduced at St Andrew's by 1963. On the women's side there was growing dependence upon unqualified personnel and younger women likely to marry were less interested in training for what could be a short, regimented and not very lucrative career.[30] Table 9.2 suggests that the proportion of nurses who were formally qualified fell from 30 per cent in 1948 to 23 per cent by 1963, their actual numbers also declining. As male nurses were more likely to obtain hospital housing and to think in career terms, the qualified male staff were broadly maintained, though additional demands at St Nicholas' hospital had resulted in greater use of male assistants and orderlies.

Although St Andrew's was only able to manage rather than overcome nursing staff shortages by the early 1960s, still more worrying problems emerged. As the HMC reported:

---

[28] McCulley repeatedly drew attention to this problem; e.g. AR, 1951, MS, p. 16. In 1952 eight charge nurses or ward sisters, each with more than 30 years' experience, retired or left the hospital.

[29] MHIWU Norfolk Branch Minutes 1941–58, 18 Dec. 1953, 2 March 1955, 13 March 1956. The Confederation of Health Service Employees originated in a merger of the MHIWU and Hospital and Welfare Services Union in 1946. W. Hamish Fraser, A History of British Trade Unionism 1700–1998, Macmillan, Basingstoke, 1999, pp. 221–3. There was some improvement in pay in 1959.

[30] The hospital was not seen as a model employer: according to COHSE (MHIWU) Minutes, 24 April 1952, a member of the laundry staff had her pay deducted for attending a blood donor session.

repeated references to the eventual closing of both hospitals . . . may have created an impression that psychiatric nursing in the St Andrew's group does not offer a permanent and worthwhile career. Uncertainty about their future has also become evident amongst the [existing] staff for similar reasons.[31]

In October 1963, for example, there were vacancies for four of the five occupational therapists normally in post. Increased professional mobility within the NHS and frustration with local conditions also affected senior staff, who stayed for shorter periods than previously. Thus matron Coomber left after five years to marry in 1953, matron Parry took up another appointment in Chester after three years at St Andrew's, and matron Nelson went to Garlands Hospital, Carlisle in 1962. H.D. Myles, who then became matron, had been deputy matron for just one year: it was ten months before that post was filled by Miss Hannigan, who left a year later.[32]

Under the NHS the junior hospital medical staff increased but theirs was not a prestigious branch of medicine, particularly before the development of drug treatments. Hospital-centred career opportunities were limited; a rigid medical hierarchy remained and accommodation was poor. Construction work on medical officers' houses, planned in 1950, did not commence until 1959 and the hospital was restricted in its purchase or conversion of other properties. In December 1962, for example, junior doctors required to sleep in for night duty refused the house room allocated because it was so cold.[33] More senior staff included Dr A.J. Crossley, who remained at St Andrew's throughout this period, and Dr G.C. Rae, who arrived in 1956 following the sudden death of Dr Ruth Meier-Blaauw. The advantages of medical continuity and experienced staff may have lessened as medical changes quickened but a core staff was surely desirable. Fewer changes occurred among those doctors who had consultant status; McCulley, Dr James Fraser, who became deputy medical superintendent when Dr Rayner left in 1950, and visiting specialists. A third consultant post was successively held by Dr R.J. Rosie, who joined the Board of Control in 1952, then by Dr H.B. Jennings until 1957, and Dr E.R. Mellon, who arrived from Severalls Hospital, Essex. This expansion in the medical staff suggested an increasing commitment to treatments, even though nurses were responsible for constant attention and other health professionals began to feature.

[31] AR, 1963, HMC, p. 13.
[32] MS Journal, 5 July and 4 Oct. 1962; 3 Oct. 1963. On 9 Oct. 1964 Miss Murray declined her appointment as deputy matron.
[33] MS Journal, 5 Dec. 1962.

New treatments for old?

Bounded by the World Health Organisation statement on mental health and Mental Health Year, the 1950s saw new forms of medication and the more effective management of mental illness.[34] A positive interest in community care was reflected in the 1954–57 Royal Commission on Mental Illness and Mental Deficiency and the ensuing 1959 Act suggested new directions. Features such as psychosurgery and physical treatments have subsequently been marginalised and the claimed successes of medication revised to cover illness management or behavioural control, rather than cure or resolution. This section examines how such developments were interpreted at St Andrew's, using case notes, published reports, medical and visitors' journals and the personal recollections of former staff.

Even by the standards of the early 1950s St Andrew's was big, old and overcrowded and McCulley recognised that 'treatment cannot be regarded as satisfactory when judged by that of hospitals with better facilities'.[35] Nevertheless, he was commited to 'modern treatments': they were important to the status of psychiatric medicine and its practitioners within the medical community and he possibly saw them as the means to additional RHB funding. Some treatments revisited nineteenth-century brain doctoring, targeting sites within the brain for surgical intervention or the psychiatric equivalent of magic bullets in an assault upon chronic illness or very disturbed behaviour.[36] They were valued as medical science, with results presented in positive but curiously vague fashion.

New drug treatments were introduced quickly but selectively. Cost considerations, a preference for earlier methods and some suspicion concerning manufacturers' and research claims led McCulley to adopt a cautious approach. He favoured the development of psychotherapy supported by group sessions, occupational and recreational activities, although this was constrained by staff shortages and poor facilities. Until 1956 the hospital had a part-time rather than full-time clinical psychologist and from 1961 it had to rely upon staff from Little Plumstead Hospital for the specialist investigation

---

[34] The WHO sought 'the incorporation into public health work of the responsibility for promoting the mental as well as the physical health of the community'. Technical Report No.9, WHO Expert Committee on Mental Health, 1950, cited by Webster, 'Psychiatry', pp. 109–10.

[35] The Mental Health Standing Advisory Committee opposed hospitals exceeding 1,000 beds. It regarded ex-asylum buildings as inappropriate for treatment and felt that most were starved of resources. National nurse shortages, overcrowding (14%) and elderly residents (then 20%) compounded their difficulties. Webster, 'Psychiatry', pp. 103–16. St Andrew's in 1950 had 1,207 resident patients, 26% aged over 65 years, some in wards dating from 1814. It was 33% overcrowded and had a major nursing crisis.

[36] A. Dally, 'Psychiatric treatment in the twentieth century', Social History of Medicine, 13, 2000, 3, pp. 547–54.

of patient behaviour.[37] Health care appropriate to an ageing resident population, from chiropody to physiotherapy to dentistry, also improved but was limited to basic services. Conservative dentistry, for example, was still not available in the early 1950s.

Although leucotomy procedure was discredited in the 1960s, its publicised introduction at St Andrew's in 1948 confirmed the use of consultant neurosurgeon services on site. Earlier, patient M.W. had been treated at Runwell Hospital and was then discharged 'recovered' from St Andrew's in July 1948.[38] Although M.B.'s husband was 'definitely not willing to give permission' for the procedure, discussion concerning its possible usage apparently triggered a rapid improvement in her condition and she was pronounced 'recovered' in February 1949.[39] Five leucotomies were carried out in 1948 and 81 altogether by 1953, with two deaths and six patients discharged, although their condition was not elaborated upon. Almost all the patients had long-term or intractable conditions, yet optimistic if limited general comments were made. Thus, between 1948 and 1951, 'it is to be expected that results will improve as the series of cases extends'; 'in a number of other [cases] . . . some improvement resulted sufficient to justify the treatment', and 'most . . . showed improved behaviour'.

No subsequent references occurred until 1956, when a 'marked decline in the use of leucotomy' was explained in terms of new drug treatments and the 'increasing number of undesirable results of the standard operation'.[40] Eric Browne, who cleaned surgical drills and instruments following these operations, recalled that patient E.M., who had taken Dr Crossley's car on a jaunt to Yarmouth, was 'subdued' after his leucotomy. To McCulley's great embarrassment, this did not pre-empt his bogus telephone call claiming to have shot a policeman, which resulted in a major police swoop on St Andrew's.[41] No more operations were reported and, by 1958, any possibilities were 'restricted to a few cases of severe obsessional neurosis or cases of schizophrenia with persistent disturbance of behaviour not yielding to new drugs'.[42] If not a miracle cure, leucotomy was presented initially as a

---

[37] AR, 1962, MS, p. 18. Music therapy and psychodrama sessions had insufficient qualified staff. Dr Rafi undertook 200–300 assessments per year and was an active researcher but left in 1961.

[38] Case Books, SAH 741. M.W. was admitted following a suicide attempt in 1946 and had remained depressed, despite home leave alternated with ECT sessions for two years before the leucotomy.

[39] Case Books, SAH 741, M.B., 1945–9.

[40] AR, 1948, MS, p. 10 ; 1949 MS, p. 11; 1950, MS, p. 18; 1956, MS, p. 15.

[41] Eric Browne interview, 19 February 2001. The first part of this story has parallels with an episode in Ken Kesey's novel *One Flew Over the Cuckoo's Nest*.

[42] AR, 1958, MS, p. 16. Michael Glasheen, at the hospital from 1960, recalled the previous apprentice fitter cleaning and sharpening drills used in the procedure. Interview (Plackett), 20 April 1988.

justifiable response, producing benefit in all barring long-term cases but, a decade later, was a measure of last resort.

Insulin coma treatment for schizophrenia had a similar history. Introduced at St Andrew's in 1947, it was still comparatively new and a possible replacement for a previous treatment using cardiazol to induce convulsions. At the neighbouring Hellesdon Hospital, medical superintendent F.H. Healey had already discontinued that practice 'because cardiazol treatment is very terrifying to the patient . . . several . . . have implored me not to give them such treatment'.[43] Insulin treatment rested upon a presumed antagonism between epilepsy and schizophrenia and dosages appear to have been a matter of trial and error: similarly with 'modified' treatments which aimed to stop just short of producing seizures in the patient. 'Small' numbers were initially involved and results were 'both encouraging and disappointing since the cases chosen have been of varying severity'.[44] An average of fifty treatments was reported annually until 1953, with 60 per cent of patients 'greatly improved', and that year ten had 'recovered'. However, at least one woman, aged 18 years, had died from heart failure under treatment. Treatments continued on a reduced scale and without further details until they were abandoned in 1958, because of their expense, intensive staffing requirements and the availability of phenothiazine drug therapy.[45]

Much greater success was claimed for ECT which, from 1942, was 'extensively used in cases of depression', patients undergoing 'a few' to 'twelve or more' sessions.[46] Thus N.A., a previous St Andrew's patient readmitted after a suicide attempt, was required to give consent, with her husband, to her course of twelve ECT sessions. She was taken off the 'red card' and, following a successful fortnight's leave, was discharged 'recovered' with no further consultation necessary.[47] More than 230 patients were treated annually to 1951, nearly two-thirds of them improved or recovered. With the use of Flaxedil and other muscle relaxants over 350 patients were treated by 1953, one-third of them as outpatients. Facilities were basic and the use of a ward 9 dormitory for ECT clinics led to complaints from resident patients and visiting committee members prior to the conversion of a staff mess room in 1958. Sister Olive Clarke recalled that 'straight' ECT, 'frightening when you first saw it', was still used after 1958 but that it 'worked well' for some

---

[43] AR, City of Norwich Mental Hospital, Hellesdon (at Drayton), 1940, MS, p. 9.
[44] AR, 1947, MS, p. 11. Kingsley Jones, 'Insulin coma treatment in schizophrenia', *Journal of the Royal Society of Medicine*, 93, March 2000, pp. 147–9. Dr Isabel Wilson, a Board inspector who visited St Andrew's on several occasions, heavily promoted this treatment.
[45] Based on ARs, 1948–58 and BoC report on inquest, 17 July 1952. See also Kingsley Jones, 'Insulin coma', pp 147–9. Phenothiazine was one early replacement.
[46] CVIS Minutes, 2 Aug. 1942; AR, 1945, MS, p. 9; 1947, MS, p. 10.
[47] Case Books, SAH 607 (NA).

patients.[48] However, outpatient treatments were discontinued as side effects, such as hearing impairment and memory loss, were noted.

McCulley's views on new drug therapies changed slowly. Cost considerations, a preference for earlier methods and suspicions about manufacturers' and research claims informed his cautious approach. Old standbys such as paraldehyde had variable but usually brief effects but the introduction of chlorpromazine (Largactil) in 1954 promised to control the behaviour of many schizophrenic patients. It was also tried in a number of other cases. Early in 1957 McCulley wrote to Runwell Hospital concerning patient M.M., sent there in 1946 for a leucotomy. The operation was unsuccessful and she had continued 'resistive, impulsive and faulty in habits' for ten years at St Andrew's before she was started on Largactil in October 1956. She 'quickly improved' and had remained 'quiet in her behaviour, fairly cheerful and able to converse coherently and occupy herself usefully, although somewhat simple and childish'. There had been help from occupational therapy staff and others, 'but the improvement, I think, must be attributed . . . partly to the Largactil rather than the leucotomy'.[49] This and other successes constituted a 'notable advance . . . the results justify the additional expenditure', which was followed by other ataractic drugs, including Triflupromazine from 1958. More extensive use of 'tranquillising' drugs in the treatment of depression or anxiety was also reported.[50]

The consequences included fewer ward disturbances, particularly at night, and a dramatic increase in patients on part parole, from 139 in 1956 to 757 in 1958. Only male ward A and female ward 3 at St Andrew's then remained subject to locked-door arrangements. These were entirely withdrawn on the women's side in 1962, though 'strong and experienced staff' were used on these wards. Visitors' reports increasingly assumed that the wards would be orderly, despite overcrowding and nurse shortages, since 'owing to the new drugs there were no noisy patients'.[51] Unpredictable patient behaviour still resulted in 'wandering off' and suicide attempts: coming to work, Eric Browne gave a lift 'home' to one woman patient and once retrieved a male patient who had 'gone in the river'.[52] Olive Clarke recalled the continuation of

[48] Visitors, 11 July 1957; AR, 1958, MS, p. 15. Sister Olive Clark, a student nurse in 1958, interview (Plackett), 3 May 1988.

[49] Case Books, SAH 741. Letter 4 Feb. 1957 re: M.M. found in case file for M.W.

[50] AR, 1954, MS, p. 13; 1956, MS p. 14; 1959, MS, p. 17. 'Depression' was a relatively new term, much publicised by drug companies offering products for the particular types delineated. D. Healy, The Antidepressant Era, Cambridge, Mass., Harvard University Press, 1997. The RMPA Handbook for Mental Nurses (8th edn revised 1960) listed endogenous, organic, neurotic, psychogenic and reactive depression.

[51] Visitors, 6 Dec. 1955.

[52] Eric Browne, interview, 19 February 2001. On another occasion he witnessed a ward 10 woman patient, out in her night-dress, given a late-night lift to Yarmouth by a helpful member of the public.

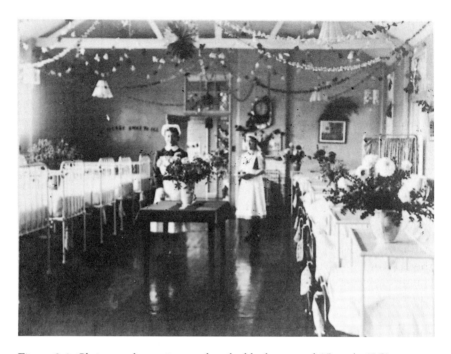

Figure 9.1 Christmas decorations and packed beds on ward 15, early 1950s (Drinkwater)

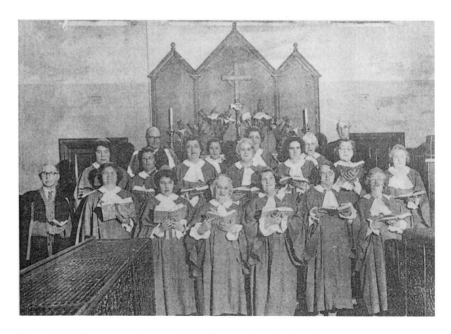

Figure 9.2 The patients' choir, 1964 (*Eastern Evening News*)

patient seclusion on refractory ward 6 alongside the regular use of sodium amytal, Soneryl, and medinal. Some drugs had side-effects which were rarely recorded and may have affected patients' immunity systems. Largactil made patients very sensitive to sunlight, which led to the general issuing of sun-hats. This may have contributed to the 'holiday camp' analogy drawn by some writers on mental hospitals at this time, usually in connection with the occupation and organisation of patients' time.[53] Nursing staff who distributed Largactil in tablet form complained of eye irritations and facial swelling: at least one ward sister developed 'sensitisation' to chlorpromazine and had to be transferred to a 'Largactil-free ward'.[54]

Older approaches revisited

Although the use of patients' medicine cards confirmed the growth of drug therapies by the early 1960s, their case notes increasingly contained comments by nurses and social workers as well as medical officers, suggesting wider staff involvement in therapy. Psychotherapeutic approaches had initially relied largely upon narco-analysis and abreaction in attempts to rediscover patients' forgotten experiences and to release repressed emotions. Up to fifty patients were treated annually, the majority later discharged, although there were insufficient resources or time available for wide-scale use of these or newer analytic methods. Basic prolonged narcosis or 'sleep therapy' using somnifane or pentothol was also used to counter the sleep-deprivation associated with states of anxiety or agitation, the patient awoken after three to five days, hopefully refreshed and more amenable to other therapy. McCulley favoured psychotherapy supported by group sessions, occupational and recreational activities, but these also were constrained by staff shortages and poor facilities. Until 1956 St Andrew's had only a part-time clinical psychologist and in 1961 it relied upon staff from Little Plumstead for the specialist investigation of patient behaviour.[55]

In 1954 Board inspectors noted too many patients 'completely idle, sitting about in their ward or wandering aimlessly about the courts. The attendant evils are readily apparent. Noise, turbulence and violence, degraded habits and extensive use of sedative drugs and exclusion'.[56] This led to occupational and recreational therapy classes, held in three improvised centres for recent male and female patients and long-term women patients. Almost 500 new

---

[53] Olive Clark, interview. On the sun-hat story see also Jones, *Asylums*, pp. 145–6.

[54] She had to avoid contact with the drug and its users. MS Journal, 7 May, 4 June and 2 July 1959. Eric Browne remembers carrying an affected patient from ward D verandah and some nurses 'looking a bit like rabbits with myxomatosis'.

[55] AR, 1962, MS, p. 18.

[56] BoC, 8 April 1954.

patients attended, with 750 by 1960, most having daily PT sessions followed by therapy, with a social club afternoon at least once a week. Exercise classes for older male patients on C and D wards also improved after the appointment of a PT instructor in 1954. Habit training classes were also introduced once staff had trained at other hospitals, though accommodation was again improvised using a corridor in male ward A.

Occupational therapy was underdeveloped and initially restricted to the able-bodied. Three teams of male patients provided farm labour, working for 7s 6d per week or a tobacco allowance, but the development of orchards and market gardening meant seasonal work for women patients, notably fruit picking. McCulley remained convinced that 'the farm and gardens give ample scope for employment of a more healthy kind than the type of factory work which is now being provided in some hospitals'.[57] Pilot schemes for fruit canning and the manufacture of wire netting were tried but did not lead to sustained commercial production, though paper recycling developed and paper bag-making was retained for the hospital stores. With the introduction of full central heating the hand carting of coal came to an end but floor-cleaning teams, with three patients knelt either side of a nurse or assistant, still featured. Clothing, footwear and furniture repairs also continued and upholstery work still included the production of the two-inch thick horsehair and hesian-covered panels for padded rooms. Roughly 1,200 bedsteads were repainted to brighten up the hospital and male patients worked on the conversion of outbuildings into male ward K and occupational therapy rooms in 1961.[58]

Since the early 1950s long-stay male patients on ward 16 had individual garden plots and sold produce to staff, and women patients developed and managed the laundry ward, garden and pets' corner.[59] Older ones had a pocket money allowance from their pensions and shopping evenings, held at the hospital from 1949, or shopping trips supplemented the usual canteens.[60] Younger patients were involved in kitchen and homecraft classes, which also included gardening and the refurbishment of garden seats and shelters. Attempts to rehabilitate patients by improving their interactive and other skills, rather than merely absorbing their time, were probably enhanced by drug therapies. With occupational therapy 'at full stretch', McCulley proposed further appointments and was 'particularly anxious to do more for the large numbers of elderly patients . . . to get these people mobile and active

---

[57] AR, 1956, MS, p. 17. Jones, *Asylums*, p. 151, holds trade unions responsible for the limited 'hospital work' available. Their attitude was not considered at St Andrew's.

[58] Olive Clarke and Mr Alan Adcock, gardener from 1950, interview (Plackett), 20 April 1988, recalled patients buried in double graves and funeral arrangements contracted out from 1950.

[59] BoC, 5 May 1953, Almost all wards had cats, partly to contain the mouse population.

[60] St Andrew's was ahead of Severalls Hospital in such respects. D. Gittins, *Madness in its Place*, Routledge, London, 1998, pp. 134–7.

as quickly as possible'.[61] Basic PT, relaxation, beauty and music sessions were held; some patients attended classes in Norwich or heard visiting speakers; there were more shopping trips and women patients visited male convalescent wards for club and games afternoons. Curiously, the hospital *Newsletter*, which patients helped to write and produce from 1952, was abandoned 'owing to lack of material' in 1960.[62] Such engineered socialisation might be interpreted as ideologically driven or as the reinforcement of gender stereotyping, but Cicely McCall, alert to these issues, felt them to be well-meaning, if somewhat unimaginative.[63]

She was surprised at the number of friends and relatives who visited. In addition to monthly HMC visits, official inspections were carried out by the ministries of Health and Pensions, the RHB, and the General Nursing Council. Visitors came from a range of voluntary agencies, including the Mental Welfare Society and the Association of Friends of Polish Patients. Following the Mental Health Exhibition, attended by 5,000 people in Norwich in 1956, the hospital held an Open Day to celebrate the tenth anniversary of the NHS. However, 'the attendance of members of the public was disappointingly small. We understand that this has been the experience at similar hospitals in various parts of the country'.[64] A similar event for the 1960 Mental Health Year fared better and a special *Newsletter* ran features on the hospital, the 1959 Act, social clubs for outpatients and former patients and on the range of staff occupations. 'The better understanding of psychiatric hospitals, their patients and their staff' was not easily achieved but greater outside contacts produced further benefits.[65] One visitor noted, rather revealingly, that 'the patients themselves were at their ease; due no doubt to the number of visitors they see . . . I found those I spoke to no more inhibited than the average patient in a general hospital'.[66]

From 1953 a recreation officer increased usage of the recreation hall, providing patients and staff with some relief from overcrowded wards. Large numbers attended films, concerts, cards and games evenings and an internal broadcast system relayed performances to all wards, as with church services, football commentaries and pantomimes from local theatres. Eric Browne, electrician and also projectionist, remembers audiences of 600–700 for

---

[61] MS Journal, 2 July 1959.

[62] AR, 1961, MS, p. 20. The *Newsletter* was first edited by an occupational therapist, then a chaplain.

[63] Viz. men growing vegetables for sale and women having make-overs and hairdos. The essential point was to encourage patients' interests and to socialise. Lack of resources powerfully restrains expressions of imagination.

[64] AR, 1956, HMC, p. 10; 1958, HMC, p. 11.

[65] Draft *Newsletter* 1960 (at Drayton Old Lodge). Foreword by F.H. Easton, HMC Chairman.

[66] Visitors, 13 Feb. 1963. At St Nicholas' there were still 'many patients . . . standing about looking lost'. 11 Nov. 1964.

Tuesday afternoon films, previewed so that references to suicide could be masked, with women sitting on the right and men on the left. Free Monday evening staff shows were eventually curtailed because excessive numbers of 'guests' attended. Recreation hall and ward-based film-shows were eclipsed by the installation of television on all wards in 1956. The ability of certain patients to aim chairs at rented TV sets, mounted upon wall brackets, required too many repairs for the company concerned and the hospital later relied upon outright purchases or donations.[67]

In 1957, a typical year in his journal, McCulley reported on performances by two visiting groups of players, two choirs, three variety nights, a dance troupe and the staging of two pantomimes, plus the hospital's own talents. Christmas parties and a bonfire night with fireworks for each side of the hospital were augmented by fancy dress events. Patients could mix freely at monthly Friday evening dances, without being confined to 'their' side.[68] Lectures and talks included travelogues with slides, a 'History through costume', and there was a Chopin recital. The Friends of Norwich Hospitals and the Norfolk Hospitals Contributors Association presented TV sets, radios and gramophones but also provided visitors and penfriends for lonely patients and helped with outings to shops and Women's Institutes.

Summer excursions in 1957 took over 200 patients to the Yarmouth Hippodrome circus and 100 more to the Marina. Multiple coach trips involved visits to the Sandringham estate, the Lincolnshire tulip fields or to the sea; and the combination of river trip and picnic remained popular with older patients.[69] In addition to the annual sports days, patients' cricket and football teams played inter-ward and inter-hospital matches and similar fixtures for darts and bowls included women's teams. Then aged 17, Michael Glasheen played football against a patients' team equipped with hospital hob-nail boots 'made to outlast the patient . . . it was terrifying to have a mental patient run up behind you in boots like that'.[70] Groups of patients also regularly attended 'away' fixtures to support hospital staff teams, winners of the regional mental hospitals' football and inter-hospitals' cricket cups between 1960 and 1963.[71] Exhibition cricket matches between visiting teams became major events for spectators and provided occasional opportunities for enthusiasts of more personal associations.

Participant observers covered other aspects of hospital life. One male nurse, effectively recruited by his father-in-law who was already a charge

---

[67] Eric Browne, interview, 19 Feb. 2001.

[68] MS Journal, 3 Jan.–25 Dec. 1957; Browne, interview, c.f. Gittins' account of dances at Severalls.

[69] As a student nurse in 1958 Olive Clark remembered 'crocodiles' of patients being led down to the 'Regal Lady', which was still in service in the 1970s. Interview, 20 April 1988.

[70] Glasheen, interview, 20 April 1988.

[71] AR, 1963, MS, p. 20. K ward dominated the bowls competition, ward E the darts. McCall, Browne interviews.

nurse, recalled his first impressions of the 'barn like' male ward C before its subdivision. He soon saw the hospital as more than a workplace, got to know patients and to accept some 'odd' behaviour. He felt that the quite voluntary efforts made by many patients in the wards and grounds showed that the hospital 'really was their home'.[72] Some male wards had a rougher edge, but contemporary childhood, education, work or national service were rarely without this. Eric Browne recalled male patients crossing the grounds to talk with him in his garden, particularly F.H., who regularly came to help. As an electrician, he worked on women's wards with the permission of the sister or charge nurse and became the favourite of patient G.L. in ward 11, who was greatly impressed by his additional work in winding up all the clocks.[73]

Cicely McCall detected 'an atmosphere of therapy' at St Andrew's, and felt that 'a big proportion' of the nursing staff was helpful, even if pessimistic about patients' prospects of recovery. She recognised many close attachments between nurses and patients and long-term male patients and the more settled male nursing staff also formed these. Men had a 'rather austere' environment but the greater mobility and variety in their hospital lives were not to be equated with prisons. More women patients seemed less aware of life outside the hospital and were over-restricted because of crowding, safety or risk considerations.[74] Many were institutionalised but may have compared favourably a rather stifling environment with experiences of sexual abuse, domestic violence or upsets in the outside world.

With some appreciation, however momentary, of the nurses' working conditions, Board inspectors and visiting HMC members almost invariably praised the attitude of the St Andrew's staff and the quality of care provided. Staff shortages had adverse consequences for patients, however. In 1952, for example, there were just seven recorded instances of seclusion totalling 27 hours among male patients, compared with 70 seclusions amounting to 15,948 hours on the women's side, where the nursing shortage was severe.[75] 'Serious incidents' of patients injured following falls or pushes more than doubled between 1948 and 1963; a worrying trend even allowing for the increased patient population, the proportion of elderly or frail patients, and the defective and uneven flooring in many wards.[76] Patients whose advanced

[72] Mr K. Roberts, interview, 20 May 1999. His sympathies were very much with long-standing patients with nowhere else to go on ward 16 and he was not impressed with ideas of community care in this respect.

[73] Eric Browne, interview, 19 Feb. 2001. G.L. sent him Christmas cards; he visited her and helped generally on ward 11 and Orchard ward on Christmas Day.

[74] Cicely McCall, psychiatric social worker, 1953–7, interview, 19 March 1999. Having been in the prison service (Holloway) she was definite on this point. She was a keen advocate of Group Homes.

[75] BoC, 17 July 1952. This represents an average of 228 hours for each woman patient secluded.

[76] These averaged annually 17, 1948–52; 26, 1953–7 and 36, 1958–63. Based on annual reports.

age or ill-health led to their immobilisation often died some time after their immediate condition was reported as 'fair' or 'feeble'. Even as wards were reported more quiet and staff congratulated, McCulley remained concerned. Over a twelve-month period from August 1956 he recorded seven suicides and two deaths after falls, one involving septic pressure sores after the patient had been confined to bed.[77]

Instances between 1955 and 1963 where the nursing staff came under suspicion involved escape attempts or alleged pilfering by patients. Allegations after one patient had a fall led McCulley to defend the hospital's reputation in the press.[78] Staff tended to receive the benefit of the doubt after a warning, but one male nurse was dismissed for writing 'an offensive letter' to a male patient and another after he was convicted for stealing from the staff social club.[79] Other incidents were no doubt resolved by ward sisters and charge nurses or at more senior levels in the staff hierarchy. Cecily McCall remembered women patients being roughly handled, particularly when nurses were rushed and overworked, but this took the form of hurrying or pulling along, not hitting or slapping. The former actions were virtually unavoidable with as many as seventy patients on some wards and sisters had their own procedures. Olive Clarke worked on refractory ward 6, which had a padded room: if a particular patient had a sudden violent outburst, 'two of you used to arm them up right quick and run them in there and shut the door so they could throw themselves about as much as they liked without doing any physical damage to themselves'.[80]

Costs and calculations

Hospital finances were not discussed in the annual reports of the 1950s and no overall records are available, so only a brief commentary can be offered. Annual hospital expenditure at St Andrew's on the eve of the NHS averaged £140,100, excluding maintenance and repairs. Rising wage and salary costs, then 49 per cent of annual spending, increased further with the combination of shift working, shorter hours and overtime, though the use of part-time and

---

[77] MS Journal, August 1956–7. One man threw himself under a train, one hanged himself in a linen cupboard, another from a tree in the hospital grounds. Two women from the laundry ward drowned in the river the same day and two others committed suicide during time on leave.

[78] MS Journal, 5 Dec. 1963. A patient sustained a broken leg after a push or fall. She was X-rayed, her leg supported and she was seen by the Norfolk and Norwich Hospital orthopaedic registrar that day. She was transferred to that hospital after four days but died a month later. The *Eastern Daily Press* suggested that 'no one in authority seemed to have taken the slightest trouble to ascertain what happened'.

[79] ibid., 7 April 1960; 15 Jan. 1961.

[80] McCall, Clark interviews.

unqualified staff restricted this increase. Provisions costs, then 19 per cent of the total, fell in proportionate terms, with necessaries (fuel etc.) steady at around 12 per cent and spending on clothing and furnishings (6 per cent) roughly the same as on administration and sundries. These were the main expenditure items, although spending on drugs and medicines increased. The NHS brought two unwelcome features: 'general uncertainty as to funds' because precise spending targets were not set in advance and 'the constant pressure of financial limitation', which 'had a discouraging effect upon all concerned'.[81] Hospital funding was largely based upon bed and patient numbers and annual budgets often produced short-term waste and discouraged medium-term thinking because 'you had to spend it because if not you'd get less the next year'.[82] Within the HMC, the secretary's financial prudence further curtailed McCulley's modernisation plans.

At St Andrew's the average cost per patient per week was £1 15s 0d in 1947–8, slightly less than the national figure for mental hospitals. The national average rose by roughly 50 per cent to £3 9s 0d in 1951–2 and again to £5 6s 6d by 1955–6. This reflected the inflation associated with the Korean war and also hospital refurbishment, even as government and ministerial economy drives curtailed capital expenditure. St Andrew's had the one dubious benefit of hospital overcrowding, its deflationary effect upon average patient costs, although its older buildings and the physical division of the hospital worked against such advantage. The full significance of suggestions in 1956 that overcrowding might be relieved by boarding out suitable patients for less than £5 per week was not grasped locally but it indicated trends of thought at higher levels.[83]

In 1958–9 weekly patient costs of £6 4s 8d at St Andrew's remained 3 per cent below the sector average. Regional comparisons were less encouraging but may have been equally misleading. The St Andrew's figure passed a psychologically important £10 benchmark in 1964–5 because of general price increases and as there was now some spare capacity following transfers of patients to St Nicholas' hospital. It remained lower than at Hellesdon hospital, which offered a full range of services, but exceeded the £7 15s 0d recorded at St Nicholas', which was now completely full, or the £7 13s 0d at the Vale hospital, which offered basic facilities for geriatric patients.[84] Such comparisons ignored hospital functions but furbished powerful economic arguments in regard to future sites of care. St Andrew's had not been rendered obsolete by new drug therapies, for the number of patients and residents

---

[81] AR, 1950 HMC, pp. 6–7; MS, p. 15.

[82] Eric Browne, interview.

[83] BoC, 24 May 1956, p. 24. A scheme at Exminster Hospital, Devon was cited in illustration.

[84] BoC, 1 Oct. 1958, p. 28; AR, 1962, HMC, p. 9; Annual Report of the St Andrew's and Hellesdon Hospitals Management Committee (Group 8), 1965–6, p. 11.

continued to increase. Rather, its need of capital spending became more pressing, but its continued use was necessary until cheaper alternative accommodation became available.

Annual gross hospital revenue for the years 1959–63 averaged £615,487. This included average income of £70,025 from trading services, which rose by 20 per cent over the four years. The main spending items in annual net hospital maintenance expenditure of £546,100 can be identified but are not strictly comparable with the pre-1948 figures. Salaries and wages now accounted for 64 per cent of spending, although this higher proportion included some maintenance and administrative staff whose remuneration would have featured in pre-1948 capital accounts. Provisions costs declined from 19 per cent of all spending in 1948 to 17 per cent in 1954 and to 15 per cent a decade later. Hospital farm supplies remained an important benefit as food prices steadily increased. Roughly 7 per cent of hospital spending was on general services, a figure maintained by the more economic regional purchasing of fuel oil, bedding and clothing and the organisation of services, St Andrew's laundry providing for St Nicholas, for example. Repairs and general maintenance came to a similar amount, with drugs and medicines now representing 3 per cent of all spending. Slightly less went on hospital administration, though items involving central administration were separately charged to exchequer funds.[85]

Although the hospital farm remained a major source of provisions and income it was later regarded as an inappropriate feature in hospital life. Growing proportions of elderly and female patients at St Andrew's and the higher rate of discharge among younger voluntary patients reduced the potential farm labour force. Changing attitudes to farm work as suitable therapy and a reluctance at higher and more removed levels to commit financial resources to projects which carried risks and were not directly concerned with health care also took their toll. Locally the farm was seen more positively and staff did not feel that patients were exploited. Farm gangs started work relatively late, had breaks and a full lunch hour, and finished early. Moreover, 'we all worked harder in those days and accepted it' and 'The men loved it and enjoyed being outside'.[86] Detailed accounts were no longer provided, though the available evidence was favourable and F.H. Easton, chairman of the HMC, took a particular interest in developing the farm. By 1950 an excellent herd of dairy cattle guaranteed the hospital's milk supply throughout the year and beef and pork surpluses were sufficient to sustain contracts with Group 8 mental hospitals.[87] Their value was not disclosed but

---

[85] Based on ARs, 1960–3, HMC 'Finance'.

[86] Browne, Adcock, Clark interviews.

[87] Annual averages for the 1950s included 155 tons of potatoes, 27 tons of beef, 8 tons of pork, over 30,000 gallons of milk and 40,000 eggs. Based on ARs, 1948–60, HMC Farm sub-committee.

additional sales of fruit and vegetables averaged £2,800, sugar beet £1,500 and further sales of pigs £3,250 per year in the 1950s.

Ministry and RHB consideration of the future of hospital farms included the interim conclusion that St Andrew's possessed an economic asset, which was also of value to patients.[88] Further diversification into market gardening was announced in 1959 but an outbreak of fowl pest compounded problems with commercial egg production. The RHB refused to provide additional funds for this or, in 1961, improvements necessary for the hospital slaughter house to meet more stringent food regulations. As a result, the HMC was instructed to reduce its farm livestock; only live animals were sold and meat supply contracts were lost. New records for sugar beet production, sales of over 100 tons of potatoes to other local hospitals and milk yields sufficient also for St Nicholas' were achieved in 1961–2. However, the 1959 Act forced the substitution of paid agricultural workers for patient labour and production costs increased to the point that the hospital catering officer looked to cheaper sources.[89] Further investigations by RHB officials brought a visit from Dr P.C. Clarke, who doubted the value of the farm or gardens as a form of occupational therapy. Instructions to sell the dairy herd, farm and 43 acres, to dispose of a further 100 acres of arable land and to 'reduce considerably all other farming activities', rapidly followed. These changes were rather tamely regretted as 'particularly unfortunate' by the St Andrew's HMC.[90]

With the new focus upon informal patients and the future of psychiatric hospitals under debate, the liquidation of farm assets reflected new policy-making but questionable economic sense and it showed little appreciation of rural lifestyles. Perhaps the latter were also regarded as outmoded and patients were sufficiently served by television and drug therapy. As the farm and land to the south and west of the hospital were auctioned on 20 March 1964, still leaving approximately 90 acres for market gardening, a major part of hospital and community life at St Andrew's was brought to a end.

The 1959 Act and the local setting

During the first decade of the NHS the proportion of voluntary patients within admissions at St Andrew's rose from 72 per cent to 90 per cent. Roughly 20 per cent of outpatients became voluntary inpatients. An upward trend in discharge rates (see Tables 9.1 and 9.3) reflected overcrowding and hospital assent to voluntary patients' requests. As some patients were

---

[88] AR, 1954, HMC, p. 9.
[89] Clifford Graveling, interview, 30 March 2001. His father Fred was farm manager until 1962. He recalled that a number of patients were formerly trusted to work on their own.
[90] MS Journal, 22 May 1962; AR, 1962, HMC, p. 13. RHB pressure had already closed other hospital farms, overriding local opposition; Gittins, Madness, p. 163.

sectioned and others had nowhere else to go, this does not suggest a repressive regime by the late 1950s. To secure support for new patients and aftercare for those discharged, McCulley employed a full-time hospital psychiatric social worker in 1948. Her follow-up visits indicated that recovering patients were being undermined; 'house proud' A.W. by her daughter's own family and friends and K.M. by her husband's domineering mother.[91] McCulley criticised the RHB for its cheaper and ad-hoc use of welfare officers from public health departments in 1951 and he re-emphasised the need for regular and close liaison of staff and patients. These officers were also granted considerable scope. For example, one visited P.W., who was recovering after an overdose and living with her uncle, to ascertain whether her schizophrenic feature was 'pronounced'. She was not required to 'return here for further treatment' but regular domiciliary visits were made to her for a further eighteen months.[92]

On her appointment, Cicely McCall found that medical staff usually had only ten minutes or so for an initial assessment during the admission process, although the patient's own account was considered, especially when general practitioners' notes were unhelpful. She encountered greatest professional difficulty when patients had no family support. Many became plaintive, blamed themselves or made considerable but one-way emotional efforts.[93] Occasional successes included the woman patient who recovered after ten years and became a hospital cook, but most ex-patients obtained only seasonal or temporary work. With no equivalent of sheltered housing, the high cost of continuing hospital accommodation forced many patients prematurely into private lodgings. Long waiting lists for homes for the elderly were also discouraging.[94] Six women patients already lived with minimal supervision in 'the cottage' at St Andrew's but a lack of resources frustrated the development of villa-style residences within hospital grounds. McCall's interest in Group Homes, a modest and voluntarist version of community care, initially drew little support from medical staff apart from Dr Ruth Meier-Blaauw.[95]

---

[91] Case Books, SAH 741 (A.W.); 700, (K.M.). Their own accommodation aided recovery in both cases.

[92] AR, 1951, MS, p. 16. Case Books SAH 741 (P.W.). Monthly visits continued until May 1952.

[93] G.P. was admitted from an approved school in the late 1930s. His father, a doctor, disowned him. He acquired an extensive knowledge of birds and plants and later obtained work as an assistant forester, travelling on a large tricycle from St Andrew's, where he was required to pay a considerable rent by the Ministry of Health. He survived discovery in flagrante delicto with a woman patient in the medical superintendent's garden. He was later discharged and readmitted and died roughly 50 years after his first admission. McCall, Browne interviews.

[94] AR, 1960, Social Worker, p. 28.

[95] C. McCall, Looking Back from the Nineties: An Autobiography, Gliddon, Norwich, 1994, pp. 99–102. These plans were revived in 1965, see Chapter 10.

'Informal' patients were admitted from 6 October 1959 and these could discharge themselves at any time. Current voluntary patients were also given this status before the 1959 Act became fully operational in November 1960 and over 80 per cent of admissions in the early 1960s were informal. Nearly 11 per cent were admitted under an emergency order (section 29), based on a medical certificate and application from a relative or a mental welfare officer. This lasted for 72 hours, after which half these patients were discharged. Less than 7 per cent had an observation order (section 25), which required two medical certificates and lasted for 28 days. Treatment orders (section 26), which required medical certificates but lasted for one year and were renewable, applied to less than 2 per cent of new patients.[96] The transfer process, notably of emergency patients to other status, stimulated weekly case discussions with the appropriate ward sister, doctor, social worker and occupational therapist from 1961. The equivalent of 95 per cent of hospital admissions were discharged by the end of each hospital year, mostly patients 'relieved' but with some recoveries, others 'not improved' and deaths.

If the 1959 Act reduced the stigma attached to treatments and fears of restraint for most patients, increasing readmission rates and the need for alternative sites of treatment, particularly for the elderly, went unresolved. McCulley acknowledged that 'the replacement of the so-called physical treatment by medication has certainly been more effective and labour saving' and that 'considerable overspending on the drug account' was justified in terms of results and less toxic treatments. However, he interpreted low recovery rates as 'a sobering reminder that the complexity of mental illness still largely defies the ingenuity of the bio-chemist'.[97]

Published information on recoveries, summarised in Table 9.3, expressed these as a percentage of admissions and was inevitably affected as the latter increased rapidly. However, the hospital claimed that roughly three-quarters of admissions were discharged 'relieved' if not recovered. More than one-third of new patients left within one month and nearly two-thirds within two months. A steady accumulation of elderly and incapacitated patients continued and this may explain the threefold increase in hospital deaths during the period. Other information also suggests this: heart and circulatory

---

[96] Patient H.A. was admitted from Norwich prison under Section 60 of the new Act following offences committed whilst an undischarged bankrupt. Psychological measurement indicated that 'a defect in retention does exist', whilst other tests suggested brain damage linked with alcohol abuse. He was reviewed and detained annually, but his regular appeals to Mental Health Tribunals culminated in a re-grade to informal status and assistance from psychiatric social workers in finding accommodation and a job. An industrial injury later produced cash benefits considerably better than his wages. Following his hernia repair H.A. returned to St Andrew's but his complaints, 'obviously prolonged by the wish to gain further compensation', went unattended and he discharged himself. Case Books, SAH 607 (H.A.).

[97] AR, 1959, MS, p. 17; 1960, MS, p. 17.

Table 9.3 Admissions, recoveries, discharge and deaths, 1948–63

	Annual admissions			Recovered %			Relieved %	Discharged %	Died %		
	Total	M	F	Total	M	F	Total	Total	Total	M	F
1948–52	507	217	290	26.9	22.4	30.4	47.2	78	6.2	7.3	5.3
1953–57	663	275	388	19.0	18.5	19.6	56.4	83	8.9	10.3	7.8
1958–63	963	374	589	15.8	19.3	13.5	59.3	81	13.7	13.5	14.0

diseases produced almost one half of deaths and respiratory illnesses roughly one-third, with cerebral haemorrhage or thrombosis and cancers also prominent. Nearly three-quarters of those who died in St Andrew's in the early 1950s were aged over 65 years and four-fifths of all deaths occurred in this age group a decade later. In 1960, for example, one-third of all patients who died were actually aged over 80 years.[98]

With more patients and shorter treatments, the 'revolving door' analogy became commonplace in 1960s mental hospitals. It derived also from an increasing proportion of readmissions, from nearly 40 per cent in the early 1950s to 45 per cent or more by the early 1960s at St Andrew's. This represented 'a persisting challenge and it is hoped to reduce the figure by increasing the degree and scope of aftercare provided . . . under the Mental Health Act of 1959'.[99] Earlier indications were that this process had previously featured at St Andrew's, but its modern form also suggested the underdevelopment or ineffectiveness of social services in averting relapses among recovering patients. Medication could not ignore economic and social contexts, let alone overcome these, even in years of full employment and apparently expanding welfare services. A marked excess of female admissions and discharges probably arose because more women received medication for depression and were then discharged 'relieved', although overcrowding was more serious among women patients. The availability of additional male accommodation at St Nicholas' produced a rapid reduction in the gender imbalance among resident patients, but not in admissions.[100]

[98] MS Journal 1960. Of 140 deaths reported that year, 4 patients were aged under 50 years; 10 were 50–59 years; 15 were 60–65 years. 101 were over 65 years old, including 51 aged over 80 years.

[99] AR, 1963, MS, p. 18.

[100] viz. only 40% of admissions 1948–63 were male. Though the hospital population aged and life expectancy among women was greater, men comprised 40% of residents in 1948 and 48% in 1958–63.

Endings and beginnings

Reviewing his chairmanship of the Group 7 HMC, F.H. Easton concluded: 'the outlook on mental illness has undergone a complete transformation . . . advances in medical science, methods of treatment and nursing techniques have resulted in a rate of progress far outstripping that . . . in former years'.[101] He also acknowledged the 'formidable task' of modernising the hospital, given the problems inherited in 1948 and encountered subsequently. Hopes expressed that St Andrew's 'should provide adequately for some years to come' indicated the shortfall from ambitions in 1948 to universalise the best and the diminished role envisaged for the hospital.

Comparison with a theoretical 'best-possible' scenario is unfair, but there were official yardsticks. New admissions facilities and nurses' residences, planned before 1939 and considered overdue by Board of Control inspectors in 1948, had not materialised. Board inspectors later noted that essential central heating was the only major structural improvement at St Andrew's.[102] Meanwhile, hospital treatments had risen by two-thirds between 1948 and 1963. Gross overcrowding was relieved only by transfers to St Nicholas' hospital, some rather desperate conversion work to supplement ward accommodation, and an increase in the proportion of patients discharged. This last feature suggested an improved therapeutic approach but was accompanied by increased readmission rates. Criticisms by hospital visitors were addressed wherever possible but, despite attempts to produce a lighter atmosphere, some wards remained in poor condition until the early 1960s. The hospital still led a hand-to-mouth existence, with increasingly outmoded facilities requiring additional maintenance and repair.[103]

McCulley had far less influence upon the RHB than his predecessors had on the former hospital committee and his resignation from the HMC shows some independence of approach. He provided 'modern' treatments, including those later discredited, and remained attached to psychotherapy even as new drug therapies became prevalent. Psychotherapy was under-resourced but gave scope to other health care professionals which, on balance, represented a positive contribution to patients' lives. Case notes suggest that voluntary patients did consent to particular treatments and that McCulley acquiesced when close relatives objected, for example, to leucotomy procedure. Patients were given limited recognition as individuals; inventories were taken of their personal effects and clothing on admission and personal lockers were gradually introduced. Insistent patients such as K.M. were allowed to wear

---

[101] AR, 1963, HMC, 'Conclusion', p. 14.

[102] BoC Report, 30 Oct. 1957.

[103] Visitors' comments on ward 15 included a patient bitten by a rat (27 Feb. 1958); crowded (26 Feb. 1959, 25 April 1962); poor sanitary arrangements (20 Dec. 1961); defective (27 Sept. 1962) and 'redecorated' (22 Oct. 1963).

their own clothes from 1948. McCulley himself was formal, 'very vigilant; he walked around a lot' and apt to make a beeline for the sister or nurse in charge. He was open to new ideas, conscientious on his rounds and took a keen interest in particular patients, though he maintained face-to-face contacts generally in the form of a rather awkward shaking of hands with every patient on Christmas Day. Medical superintendents were not generally noted for these qualities and some in the East Anglia region were better known for their interest in golf or an ingrained tendency to 'wait and see'.[104]

Appreciative comments concerning the nursing staff frequently acknowledged their poor working conditions but the absence of criticism is noticeable. Nurses and assistants were over-stretched and sisters imposed their own routines, including patient seclusion on difficult wards, simply in order to cope. Male staff were more settled, although this might preserve older attitudes and routines. Whether new medications or more amenities improved ward life, a better and even friendly atmosphere was noted by 1960. Cecily McCall felt that staff were sometimes too closely involved with patients to have the time or imagination to consider alternatives, but she was a reforming spirit and they were not encouraged to instigate change. A therapeutic regime probably coexisted with tendencies to treat patients as children but also to form genuine friendships as well as working relationships. Analogies with home or even family life provided for longer-term patients were sometimes tenuous and sat less comfortably alongside the modern revolving door approach to informal patients.

Yet the separate status, social relationships and economic activities which made St Andrew's a community were undermined, ironically, in the name of community care. When Board inspectors suggested the boarding out of patients to offset overcrowding in 1956 they also noted the shortage of suitable accommodation for the elderly, chronic sick and infirm in Norfolk. This was both an antecedent and an ill omen for community care. Institutions such as St Nicholas' and the Vale offered short-term relief but no future model and regional experiments had not progressed beyond the reduced supervision of tiny groups of patients within hospital grounds. The 1959 Act produced meetings of medical superintendents and health officers at county and regional levels but no details, other than the eventuality of hospital closures, were announced. For example, after a conference at St Andrew's in January 1962, McCulley provided only standard euphemisms concerning the 'very useful exchange of views' and 'suggestions for improving after-care'.[105]

In 1963 *Health and Welfare: The Development of Community Care* introduced local authority responses to the 1962 Hospital Plan; 'the more timely as whole new fields of prevention and community care, above all in relation

---

[104] Based on interviews. McCall contrasted his interest in Group Homes with responses at Hellesdon.
[105] MS Journal, 11 Jan. and 1 Feb. 1962.

to mental disorder, were coming into view'.[106] Initial comments also noted great variation in local provision and that 'about half' of those leaving mental hospitals in 1961 had arrangements for further treatment. Moreover, the number of available social workers, of which psychiatric social workers constituted a fraction, was itself only half that envisaged by the 1954–7 Royal Commission prior to the 1959 Act.[107] Returns for Norfolk indicated above-average provision of homes for the elderly, but so was the proportion of 65-year-olds; 14 per cent compared with 12 per cent nationally. Some 350 additional places in homes for the elderly, including those discharged from mental hospitals, were envisaged by 1967 but, apart from a hostel with fifteen places in Norwich, there were no centres for the mentally ill.[108] Such plans hardly embodied McCulley's hopes for the 1959 Act. They suggested that St Andrew's would continue, as economically as possible and less prominently than Hellesdon hospital, in the dual role of psychiatric hospital for short stay, younger and informal patients and as the provider of comprehensive care for an ageing group of long-term residents.

[106] *Health and Welfare: The Development of Community Care*, Cmd 1973, HMSO, London, 1963, p. 1.
[107] ibid., pp. 23, 25. The 1954–7 Royal Commission on the law relating to mental illness and mental deficiency estimated that 2,269 social workers were needed. Less than half that number were available in 1961 (1,128) before the question of appropriate training was considered.
[108] ibid., Norfolk, pp. 146–7; Great Yarmouth, pp. 148–9; Norwich, pp. 150–1. Facilities for the mentally subnormal included junior training and adult training centres in Norwich, Great Yarmouth and Norfolk.

10

Community care and the end of a community, 1964–98

By the time James Fraser was formally appointed medical superintendent in August 1965 St Andrew's was earmarked for a reduced role within Norfolk Group 8 hospitals and the closure of the satellite St Nicholas' hospital was under active consideration.[1] Fraser was the last medical superintendent – the post was abolished in 1971 – and the closure of the hospital was a recurring issue over almost four decades. Care in the community proved to be a controversial subject and its development was slower and less extensive than originally envisaged. The national and county context, surveyed briefly below, involved the closure of psychiatric hospitals with gathering momentum: almost seventy had gone before the demise of St Andrew's in 1998.[2] Yet the local story was of a protracted and uneven decline which included a changed role from the mid-1980s and more than one glimpse of a very different future. Such possibilities depended upon a succession of plans for general NHS hospital services in and around Norwich and the emergence of a local strategy for relevant community care services, examined in a second section. This particular narrative can be traced from several sources and within the hospital there were differing interpretations and experiences of unfolding events, as is clear from interviews with staff personnel.

National and local developments

A national reorientation of mental health services away from large psychiatric hospitals was already envisaged and ostensibly under way by the mid-1960s. Beyond this broad objective, details on suitable forms of community care, the requisite resources and the timetable involved in this transformation remained unclear, however. The desirability of hostel-style accommodation, day-hospitals, short- and longer-stay annexes to general hospitals and co-ordination with the social services had been

[1] As deputy medical superintendent since 1950 Fraser was already acting medical superintendent during McCulley's illness in 1964. E.R. Mellon became the new deputy. Medical Superintendent's Journal (at Drayton Old Lodge), 4 March and 6 May 1965.
[2] P. Barham, *Closing the Asylum*, Penguin, Harmondsworth, 1992, p. 20.

expressed well in advance of the 1959 Mental Health Act and the preceding Royal Commission within the psychiatric profession.[3] Most of Fraser's colleagues acknowledged that new medications allowed forms of mental illness to be managed, rather than cured outright. The prospect of more people receiving treatment and living outside traditional mental hospitals was enhanced, but few considered such institutions to be wholly obsolete.[4] Nor did the advent of new medications sufficiently explain the development of community care, as this was not the predominant influence in parallel proposals for care of the mentally handicapped, the very elderly and chronic mentally ill.[5]

The practice of long-term institutional care attracted growing criticism within and beyond the psychiatric profession as repressive, self-defeating or the cause of further disorders. Figures such as Russell Barton, medical superintendent at Severalls hospital, Essex from 1960, focused upon institutionalisation as 'a man made disease caused by lack of contact with the outside world', producing in patients 'the mental bedsore . . . lack of interest . . . loss of individuality' and similarly affecting staff.[6] He described Severalls as 'a grim institution' and influential studies suggested more extreme examples, if not necessarily typical of practice in Britain.[7] Alternative provision outside the psychiatric hospital might involve a diminution in professional control or even liberation from harmful environments, but others saw in such diversification signs that professional influence was actually extending beyond hospital boundaries.[8] Either way, a professional

[3] C. Webster, 'Psychiatry and the early NHS: the role of the Mental Health Standing Advisory Committee' in G.E. Berrios and H. Freeman (eds), *150 Years of British Psychiatry 1841–1991*, Vol. 1, Gaskell, London, 1991, pp. 103–16.

[4] S. Goodwin, 'Community care for the mentally ill in England and Wales: myths, assumptions and reality', *Journal of Social Policy*, 18, 1989, pp. 27–52.

[5] L. Prior, *The Social Organisation of Mental Illness*, Sage, London, 1993, pp. 37–42.

[6] R. Barton, *Institutional Neurosis*, Wright, Bristol, 1959, p. 12. He was interviewed in a radio broadcast featuring Roy Porter and Dianne Gittins (date unknown). See D. Gittins, *Madness in its Place: Narratives of Severalls Hospital 1913–1997*, Routledge, London, 1998, pp. 67–75.

[7] E. Goffman, *Asylums*, Penguin, Harmondsworth, 1961. Goffman's study used a harsh American example, St Elizabeth's Hospital, Washington, DC. B. Robb (ed.), *Sans Everything: A Case to Answer*, 1967, detailed neglect and abuse of elderly long-term patients in Britain.

[8] Barham, *Asylum*, p. 12. M. Foucault, *Madness and Civilisation*, Tavistock, London, 1967, provided blanket criticism of institutions and professional personnel as agencies of social control wherever they operated. T. Szaz, *The Myth of Mental Illness*, 1961, and R.D. Laing, *The Politics of Experience and the Bird of Paradise*, 1967, also featured in the disparate 'anti-psychiatry' movement, though Szaz had no difficulties with fees for counselling in the 'problems of living'. ('For Szaz the only legitimate psychiatry is contractual', according to W.F. Bynum, R. Porter and M. Shepherd (eds), *The Anatomy of Madness*, Tavistock, London, 1985, Vol. 2, Institutions and Society, pp. 1–16, 2.)

and reform ethos which had formerly emphasised the prompt admission of patients to asylums in order to maximise their prospects of recovery was transformed into the view that their rapid de-institutionalisation was essential to that objective.[9]

Still more noteworthy, one reduction in the number of mental hospital patients had already occurred, in the Second World War (see Chapter 8), and an upward trend in hospital admissions during the late 1940s and early 1950s had not been accompanied by new hospital building. This reflects views, at the heart of the political establishment, that mental hospitals were costly to maintain and prohibitively expensive to replace. Consequently, these hospitals became a particular target in the 1962 Hospital Plan, which simply projected the decline in mental hospital bed numbers from 1954 to 1959 to produce the objective of a near-50 per cent reduction over the ensuing ten years. Currently increasing admissions rates or the ageing population and its likely care needs were insufficiently considered. Further, the emphasis upon expenditure curbs meant that wider issues involving economic prospects, opportunities for former psychiatric hospital patients and their possible impact upon community tolerance of such patients were not allowed for. Nor was the likelihood that core groups of psychiatric hospital patients with severe difficulties might, at best, be reduced only at decelerating rates.[10]

Early measures associated with community care were reactive to institutional problems and closures and were facilitated by improving drug treatments, but there were few signs of an underlying proactive approach or political leadership at central or local levels. Thus in 1963 Health and Welfare: The Development of Community Care was presented as complementary to the 1962 Hospital Plan but, even after revisions, the appended proposals from local authorities remained variable and piecemeal.[11] In Norfolk the number of mental hostel places was planned to double, but only to 30, between 1967 and 1972, and the overall expenditure target was already being revised downwards. Vague references to 'special housing' accompanied proposals for 411 additional residential places, intended to suffice for everyone in the county aged over 65 years.[12]

These arrangements implied no psychiatric hospital closures and little perception of mental health care in community settings. Transitional measures, such as group homes for ex-hospital patients and suitable work in anticipation of full-time employment, remained experimental in nature. When the Norfolk branch of the National Association for Mental Health

[9] There were always forms of 'non-asylum' care. See P. Bartlett and D. Wright (eds), *Outside the Walls of the Asylum*, Athlone, London, 1999.

[10] K. Jones, *Asylums and After*, Athlone, London, 1993, p. 162; Barham, *Asylum*, p. 11.

[11] *Health and Welfare: The Development of Community Care*, Cmnd 1973, HMSO, London, 1963.

[12] ibid., 1963, pp. 100–1. Norfolk's forecasted spending was reduced from £1.25 million to £1.12 million.

purchased a house in Norwich for use as a group home in 1966, for example, Fraser was invited to select suitable patients. Five women aged between 58 and 75 years were helped to live independently on a weekly allowance of 30 shillings prior to their discharge.[13] Fraser was unable to convert cottages at St Nicholas' hospital as a holiday home for suitable patients but 'Highfield' house at St Andrew's became a training centre for small groups of patients in anticipation of more group homes.[14]

Any extension of mental health care beyond hospitals required co-ordination within and between the social and health services, particularly at local levels. The 1968 Seebohm Committee, which endorsed the rational-isation of social services under managerial control, noted the 'sad illusion' of community care for mental patients in many areas.[15] Psychiatric hospitals remained the poor relations within the NHS hospital sector and local authority health provision was neglected in comparison with hospital and primary care provision. New regional and area health authorities offered district, rather than hospital or individual practitioner, focuses for services under the 1974 NHS reorganisation, achieved in conjunction with the 1970 Local Authority Social Services Act.[16] Yet community mental health occupied a low priority under this potentially favourable development, even though there were 5,000 fewer psychiatric hospital beds in 1974–5 alone (see Table 10.1).[17]

A more positive strategy emerged in the 1975 White Paper, *Better Services for the Mentally Ill*. Integration rather than isolation was emphasised, notably in the concept of 'normalisation', helping those with dependency to lead ordinary lives.[18] Combinations of local psychiatric units in general hospitals, day inpatient services, and primary care with psychiatric and therapeutic help in the patient's home setting were to be offered, supported by the social services. Doubts that all patients could be cared for under these arrangements persisted. The approach presupposed an accepting and tolerant community and the social processes whereby the mentally ill might be marginalised or isolated were not widely anticipated. Although resources were increased they

[13] Inspired by a pioneer scheme at Severalls Hospital, Edith Botting (St Andrew's psychiatric social worker), George Brown (county welfare officer) and Dr D.H. Neale were actively involved with hospital occupational therapy staff. MS Journal, 6 Oct. 1966; McCall, *Looking Back from the Nineties*, p. 99. Patients were then supported by national assistance, later supplementary benefit.

[14] MS Journal, 3 Nov. 1966; 14 Dec. 1967. With the first group patients doing 'fairly well', Fraser considered the money well spent; 2 Feb. 1967.

[15] *Report of the Committee on Local Authority and Allied Personal Social Services*, Cmd. 3703, HMSO, London, 1968, para. 339.

[16] C. Webster, *The National Health Service: A Political History*, Oxford University Press, 1998, pp. 108–9, 118–20.

[17] Jones, *Asylums*, pp. 186–7.

[18] *Better Services for the Mentally Ill*, Cmd 6233, HMSO, London, 1975.

Table 10.1 Psychiatric hospital beds and patients 1961–93

	Available beds (000)	Resident population (000)	Residents per 1000 of whole population	Admissions (000s)
1961	155	135.4	3.0	
1965		123.6	2.6	
1970		103.3	2.1	
1975	97	83.3	1.8	179
1980	87	74.8	1.6	174
1985	76	64.0	1.5	204
1990	55			219
1993	47			

Sources: Jones, *Asylums and After*, pp. 187, 243–4; J. Raftery, 'The decline of the asylum', p. 19.
* includes limited amount of accommodation in other hospitals.

remained inadequate for the tasks envisaged, for older mental hospitals still contained the great majority of places for the mentally ill and half of these residents were aged over 65 years.[19] It was estimated that only one-fifth of the day centre provision and one-third of the residential places envisaged for mental patients had been completed nationally by 1979.[20]

Table 10.1 suggests that the halving of mental hospital beds envisaged in 1961 occurred not within a decade but during the early 1980s. There was a corresponding reduction in resident populations, numerically and as a proportion per 1,000 of the whole population. It is less clear whether alternative accommodation was found, as a major feature in the long-term decline in resident populations was death. Between 1964 and 1984 mental hospital residents of one year or more were as likely to be discharged dead as alive; among residents of at least five years the ratio of dead to living within 'deaths and discharges' was three to two.[21] Such figures reflected the elderly age composition of resident populations and suggest the importance of continuing care provision rather than successful new medication or therapies, even though the latter may have improved the quality of patients' lives. By the mid-1990s there were signs of a further halving in bed provision and an

[19] MIND *Mental Health Yearbook*, 1981–2, pp. 405, 527–9. Capital spending on accommodation, etc. outside the former asylums averaged £25 million annually 1975–9 compared with the mental hospitals' budget of roughly £485 millions. A decade later more than half the £1.4 billion NHS mental health budget was spent on 40,000 psychiatric hospital patients, most of them elderly. G. Thornicroft and G. Strathdee, 'Mental health' in *British Medical Journal*, 303, 1991, pp. 410–12.
[20] Webster, *NHS*, p. 126.
[21] J. Raftery, 'The decline of the asylum or the poverty of a concept' in D. Tomlinson and J. Carrier, *Asylum in the Community*, Routledge, London, 1996, pp. 18–30, 25.

upward trend in hospital admissions: there were two admissions per bed in 1980 but four by 1990. If most beds were still occupied by elderly patients, this suggests greater emphasis upon short admissions to the remainder, a speeding up of the 'revolving door', and growing reliance upon delivery of care in the community.

How did experiences in Norfolk compare? Shortly before the 1974 NHS reorganisation the Group 8 Hospital Management Committee reviewed progress towards objectives set in the early 1960s and considered future developments. Increased numbers of hospital patients were discharged or had been found alternative accommodation, almost 150 since the beginning of 1972. Nearly 200 more, including 75 at St Andrew's, were considered for discharge by May 1974. However, it was openly recognised that 'a number . . . will undoubtedly die or become too ill for discharge as a high proportion of those involved are over 70 years of age'.[22] Separate district health authorities centred upon King's Lynn and Great Yarmouth were created in 1974, each with a psychiatric team. Norfolk and Norwich were divided into three sectors, each with consultant-led services. The David Rice Hospital, adjacent to Hellesdon, served north Norfolk, the Yare clinic was for central Norfolk and the Waveney clinic at Hellesdon for south Norfolk. County mental hospitals remained under a single management team but envisaged developments at King's Lynn and for Yarmouth and Lowestoft would mean reduced patient numbers at Hellesdon and St Andrew's hospitals respectively, with the latter scheduled for 'eventual rundown'.[23] Some patients were already transferring between hospitals or to the fifty-bed Yare clinic, an important facility operating in temporary buildings attached to West Norwich general hospital.

Details concerning private residential care or 'informal' care by patients' relatives were not given but local authority provision remained meagre. In 1980 the county offered just 29 places in seven unstaffed group homes, although 68 more were available under voluntary sector provision. Hospital day-centres included Hellesdon and the flat-roofed, unprepossessing facility which had opened at St Andrew's in 1972 on a site adjacent to the hospital chapel. Former inpatients, including a number at work, attended for general assessment and medication and were offered meals, craft therapy and cookery classes, with reminiscence therapy for the very elderly. Hostels had not developed beyond those at King's Lynn and Norwich and hospital accommodation still predominated. St Andrew's retained 600 beds, mainly for psycho-geriatric patients, though at least 30 residents were working at or outside the hospital. Hellesdon, with 450 beds, had a greater proportion

[22] Group Eight Mental Hospitals HMC Minutes 1972–3, SAH 509, 8 June 1972 and 17 May 1973.
[23] '1974 NHS Reorganisation, Norfolk Area Joint Liaison Committee' (LS c362.1), 1974, p. 11.

of admissions and acute patients but 120 elderly patients remained in rather depressing conditions at the Vale hospital. St Nicholas', earmarked for closure in 1962, had obtained a new lease of life with its day-hospital and admissions ward and 190 beds there were fully used.[24]

Long after 1980 broad agreement on the issue of de-institutionalisation was insufficient to identify alternative providers or suitable forms of care. Plans to disperse mental health care services in 1983 were still predicated upon 'the general run-down of large hospitals over a period of ten years . . . the resources released and deployed to fund the new pattern of services'.[25] In part, the situation in Norfolk reflected national experience: some patients were simply too dependent to move. Although bed numbers were reduced and older psychiatric hospitals were less exclusively used for the purpose, nationally about 30 per cent of psychiatric patients had been in hospital for at least five years at the end of the 1980s and had long-term conditions.[26] New health authority facilities in Norfolk included the elderly severely mentally ill unit at King's Lynn, opened in 1987 to provide residential, respite and day care. This offered a model for informal, individual care but the initial cost was £2.5 million and others were needed. Meanwhile, ward closures at St Andrew's and other hospitals meant rising unit costs and efforts by health authorities to discharge or transfer patients increased problems for social services, not least because local authorities were reluctant to provide more expensive residential accommodation.

These difficulties were compounded as successive Conservative governments emphasised private and voluntary effort, with or without public subsidy, rather than public sector provision within the mixed economy of health care. Even as NHS spending on mental health care declined after 1980, authorities at the local level were invited to take initiatives but also left with the responsibility for continued shortcomings.[27] From 1982 area health authorities were replaced by district and unit management structures. These operated initially on a consensual team basis, reducing traditional medical influence, but their managers were increasingly able to determine reform agendas. Although the 1983 Mental Health Act restricted compulsory admission procedures and extended provisions for discharge and the frequency of patients' right of appeal to Mental Health Review Tribunals,

---

[24] MIND *Yearbook*, 1981–2, pp. 34, 184. 150 places in homes for the mentally handicapped compared with 694 beds at Little Plumstead.

[25] Interim report, Working group on services for the mentally ill, 6 September 1983 (at Hellesdon Hospital Library). This document referred to the acute admission unit for elderly patients at St Andrew's and to the regional secure unit to be opened north of the hospital site.

[26] J. Allsop, *Health Policy and the NHS*, Longman, London, 1995, pp. 98–9; J. and D. Taylor, *Mental Health in the 1990s: From Custody to Care*, London, 1989.

[27] NHS spending on mental health care peaked at 20% in 1980. MIND *Yearbook*, 1981–2; *The Observer Review*, 25 Feb. 2001.

these safeguards were incomplete. Nor did they guarantee adequate care, particularly for the larger numbers of informal patients.[28] The concept of individual guardianship of vulnerable patients under the 1983 Act was re-worked in the 1989 White Paper *Caring for People* and under the 1990 Community Care Act, effective from 1993. Local authorities were now formally responsible for this form of community care, with care managers acting for patients.[29] Operating within financial limitations, the latter were to purchase services for their patients within the mixed economy of care. Nursing and community-orientated mental health teams also featured more prominently in service provision.

If statements that 'the number of hospital beds should be reduced only as a consequence of the development of new services' imply recognition of previous failings, these were not fully remedied.[30] Efforts to distinguish 'social' from 'health' care appear to reflect the structure and funding of services rather than the variable needs covered by the collective term mental illness. At the individual level, the same person may have very differing needs at different times. In aggregate terms, up to 5 million people reported forms of depression, anxiety or 'mental stress' to their general practitioners annually in the late 1990s. At least 5 per cent of all those aged over 65 – 18 per cent of those aged 80 or more – had moderate to severe dementing illnesses. While many of the latter required continuing care, hospital closures and the cost of alternative residential facilities have, in conjunction with all too finite resources, inevitably resulted in the focus of care shifting to families, relatives and their homes or to forms of private rented accommodation. It is currently estimated that 1.3 million people are directly involved in caring for someone with a mental illness, but neither they nor professional teams can ensure that former patients continue with any necessary medication or even remain in contact.[31] Consequently, unknown numbers of people are as likely to experience community neglect as forms of care.

What role for St Andrew's?

Discussions concerning the reorganisation of mental health care in the early 1960s did not envisage the early closure of St Andrew's. Although new drug therapies were regarded as a considerable success, the hospital was still

[28] Sectioned patients could have three months' compulsory treatment. Jones, *Asylums*, pp. 206–13.
[29] *Caring for People, Community Care in the Next Decade and Beyond*, Cmd 849, 1989, HMSO, London, paras 7.1–7.23.
[30] ibid., para. 7.5.
[31] National Schizophrenia Fellowship, 'Forgotten army', *Guardian Society*, 6 June 2001, p. 119.

heavily used: there were over 1,460 patients on New Year's Eve 1960 and annual admissions exceeded 1,000 for the next three years. Nearly 2,500 people received inpatient treatment or care each year and there were roughly 700 outpatients. All voluntary patients admitted before the 1959 Mental Health Act became effective were asked whether they wished to be discharged but most opted to stay, under 'informal' status.[32] Such decisions may reflect medical influence and the process of institutionalisation, but few patients had real choice when alternative accommodation was lacking. Voluntary group homes were not yet established and public spending in this area was unlikely without a successful and economical model, as Norfolk plans in 1962 and 1963 confirmed. Hospital ground staffs were meanwhile informed of an RHB work-study that doubted the therapeutic or economic efficiency of the farm and gardens. Yet the retention of roughly 140 acres of land, to avoid commercial or housing encroachment upon the hospital site after the farm was sold, suggests that the closure of St Andrew's was not imminent.[33]

In other respects the hospital's position seemed less assured. From April 1964 it was one of five hospitals within the enlarged Group 8, controlled by an unwieldy 29-member bimonthly committee. With the adoption of joint purchasing schemes and centralisation of Group resources the laundry and bakery at St Andrew's were closed.[34] Planned improvements included the subdivision of male ward A and extensions to wards 9, 10, 13 and 14 and to Orchard ward, now the regional centre for typhoid carriers, but overcrowding at the Vale and St Nicholas' hospitals was the immediate concern.[35] St Andrew's briefly had a house committee but the group secretary's department transferred to Hellesdon in February 1966 and a streamlined monthly HMC, meeting around the various hospitals, replaced all other bodies. This was subsumed within the Norwich district and area health authorities under the 1974 NHS reorganisation, coincident with a period of retrenchment following the 1974 oil crisis.

With minimum education standards required for psychiatric nurses under the 1964 Nurses Act, the completion of a nurse training school at Hellesdon in May 1966 was timely but symbolic of the shifting focus within Group 8 hospitals.[36] More laboratory work was diverted to the Norfolk and Norwich hospital, not least because St Andrew's facilities were inadequate by 1960s

---

[32] Mollie Middleton (nurse tutor), interview, 2 March 2001.

[33] In 1962 or 1963. Reference from Alan Adcock, a gardener in 1950 and gardening manager, interviewed (Plackett), 20 April 1988.

[34] Group 8 St Andrew's and Hellesdon HMC Annual Report 1965–6 (at Drayton). Staff shortages prevented full utilisation of the bakery at St Andrew's.

[35] Ibid., HMC, p. 7; MS Journal, 4 Nov. 1965.

[36] The General Nursing Council supervised training along with courses for state-enrolled and pupil nurses. Mollie Middleton, interview, 2 March 2001. She was nurse tutor but did not wish to go to Hellesdon so was back night nursing at St Andrew's in the mid-1960s.

standards and could not attract suitable staff, resulting in closure of the pathology laboratory.[37] St Andrew's did have an increased complement of medical posts yet it seemed permanently understaffed. In 1965, for example, Drs Castell and Neale were appointed as consultants but the shortage of registrars obliged Fraser to engage a retired consultant on a part-time basis. Dr Crossley, who had been at St Andrew's since January 1939, retired in 1966 and Dr McCulley briefly reappeared on a part-time basis in 1968.[38]

To encourage younger doctors Fraser linked the hospital to the new Norfolk and Norwich Institute for Medical Education and established a medical library, though neither measure had an appreciable effect on staff turnover. Without a senior house officer for two years, he acknowledged that staff were under-strength and overworked.[39] Yet Fraser himself had less direct influence within the wider hospital group and his post, re-titled physician superintendent in 1969, was abolished in 1971. He then joined other consultants, already appointed to the group rather than to a particular hospital, within a larger and less closely knit medical team. One of the consultants acted as convenor to the group but each was responsible for his or her own patients, drawn from particular areas of Norfolk but often placed in different hospitals or clinics.[40]

These new arrangements marked the demise of the traditional authorities speaking or acting for St Andrew's and further increased staff concern over job security, working conditions and changes within the hospital. At a special meeting in March 1965 staff expressed 'great anxiety about the increasing number of elderly patients . . . in looking after these with the shortage of staff, and stated that they were unable to give their time adequately to the younger and recoverable patient'.[41] During the next month Fraser recorded twelve deaths from pneumonia and, in June, three accidents in which the average age of patients was 90 years. July saw the substitution of a garden fête for the traditional sports day, much appreciated by elderly women patients, although 'some of the men have told me that they prefer the old fashioned sports'.[42] Quiet rooms were introduced as 'we have now reached the stage where many people find the television rather noisy and . . . wish that there was somewhere . . . to get away from it'.[43] Although patient numbers began to decline, the combination of staff shortages, ward closures and insufficient accommodation outside the hospital meant that wards again became overcrowded. Meetings

---

[37] MS Journal, 5 Feb. 1970.

[38] ibid., 7 April 1966; 4 April 1968.

[39] ibid., 2 Sept. and 2 Dec. 1965; 4 April 1968.

[40] Consultant psychiatrist Dr Ted Olive had 200 patients in 1979, nearly half of them at Hellesdon or at the Yare clinic, West Norwich hospital. Interview, 27 Feb. 2001.

[41] MS Journal, 1 April 1965.

[42] ibid., respectively 6 May, 3 June and 1 July 1965.

[43] ibid., 3 Nov. 1966.

with Group 8 medical staff, the RHB and local authorities on this question featured prominently among Fraser's last notes as physician superintendent.[44]

Group 8 hospitals' annual reports, published until 1967, provide few details on St Andrew's. With more readmissions and attendance by former inpatients at day-centres, historic categories of 'recovery' or 'relieved' were probably considered inappropriate, although there was surely some merit in differentiating between patients discharged alive or dead. Fraser's monthly returns to 1971 suggest 973 patients in December 1970, roughly 150 less than in the mid-1960s. St Nicholas' meanwhile maintained an average of 260 male patients throughout. Over 60 per cent of St Andrew's patients were women, producing a rough gender balance in the two hospitals. More than 95 per cent had informal status and almost 100 were on leave at any time, Christmas peaks suggesting that others were received by relatives at least for a short period. A yearly average of 276 deaths and a 20 per cent mortality rate reflected the elderly hospital population. Available information from the mid-1960s is summarised in Table 10.2.

The run-down pending eventual closure of St Andrew's can be traced from several sources and reveals a process subject to very different interpretations and one which produced contrasting experiences. In the late 1960s the improved assessment of patients of working age had already resulted in some leaving hospital. For example, wards A1 and 2 together had by then approximately thirty-five patients, less than half the former ward A complement. However, the discharge of elderly patients was restricted by the limited places available within the county's generic accommodation and two registered mental nursing homes.[45] There were no indications that Fraser ever retained patients to maintain the psychiatric community under his control and no individual could wield such influence after 1971. Subsequent health authority returns did not refer directly to patients but indicate a sharp reduction of beds in use, from 925 to 561, in the three years to 1974. The number of patients 'discharged or died' also fell dramatically, from 1,032 in 1971 to 622 in 1973 and to just 215 by 1974. Given previous mortality rates and the ageing hospital population, this suggests a surge in patients discharged at the beginning of the 1970s which could not be sustained.

Health authority efforts to comply with earlier planning targets were thus obstructed by a still considerable core of elderly and chronic inpatients and insufficient alternative accommodation. Returns for the mid-1970s referred to inpatient waiting lists and the retention of a group of twenty 'sick beds' in

---

[44] ibid., 7 May 1970. Fraser's notes were increasingly brief and apparently evoked little response, although the arrival of the Hospital Advisory Service Team in June may have been connected with this overcrowding; 3 July 1970.

[45] Kevin Long (interview, 4 April 2001) was a nurse cadet in 1962 and trained 1964–7. He returned in 1986 and is now Director of Nursing Practice. Only ward 16, an isolated north-side ward successively used by TB, elderly male and female patients, had closed.

Table 10.2 Beds, inpatients and outpatients at St Andrew's, 1965–86

	Av. beds available	Av. daily occupied	Patients discharged or died	(died)	New outpatients	Outpatient attendances	Outpatient clinics
1965–69	1,117	1,008	1,138		189	2,898	n/a
1970–74	805	718	786		248	2,902	226
1975–79	611	564	200		37	1,076	179
1980–84	557	497	269	(102)	53	421	97
1985–86	461	390	444	(103)	51	520	80
1985–89				(98)			
1990–94				(81)			
1995–98				(45)			

Source: Norwich Health Authority SH3 Hospital Returns for DSS 1965–86; East Anglia Regional Health Authority, NHA Mortality Database 382/1/24 1979–98.

the hospital.[46] St Andrew's became increasingly a residual institution. The day-centre was used primarily by former inpatients, returning for occupational therapy and limited treatments, including ECT. Outpatient clinics and attendances continued to fall but the number of new outpatients declined most, from 345 in 1972 to just 47 in 1974. Bed numbers were reduced from 700 in 1974 to 600 in 1980, although there were still over 500 inpatients, more than 60 per cent of them female. In line with national trends there were as many deaths as patients discharged alive in the early 1980s, the combined total exceeding elderly and chronic inpatient admissions, which varied between 150 and 200 annually.[47] According to 1980s mortality returns, few patients went back to their own homes and 80 per cent of those who died at St Andrew's had no other address. Thus, elderly and chronic patients spent their last years at the hospital: even in 1993 more than half of the 107 who died there had no other address.[48]

Yet the hospital's last years were not to be a story of quiet decline. They were marked by a change of role and increasingly influenced by the search for a new strategy in health care provision; first in the context of wider hospital services, then with a more positive emphasis upon community services. An old age psychiatry unit, established at St Andrew's in 1983 under Dr Elizabeth Taws, was supported by the NHS 'Rising Tide Initiative' for three years and then received additional financial support from the area health authority as it developed into a county-wide service.[49] This aimed to upgrade standards of provision for elderly patients, so often the last to be considered and frequently dispersed around hospital back wards, and acute services for those aged over 65 years were reintroduced. Patients were assessed at home and acute cases were admitted to wards 2, 13 and 14 at St Andrew's, along with wards at the Norfolk and Norwich and, later, Hellesdon hospitals. The emphasis was upon hospital treatments, discharge and the development of community nursing, rather than long-term residence.[50] With additional staff appointments this 'deprived specialty' developed a range of services which, although geographically dispersed, were focused upon the requirements of elderly patients. Dr Taws felt that 'the people and the style of

---

[46] Norwich Health Authority SH3 Hospital Returns for DSS 1965–86, 1974–80 inclusive (at NHA offices, Northside, Thorpe St Andrew's). It is unclear whether sick beds were retained for readmissions or current inpatients with physical illnesses.

[47] Patient Daily Numbers 1974–80, SAH 585; Register of Admissions, Discharge and Deaths, 1980–1990, SAH 563.

[48] East Anglia Regional Health Authority, NHA Mortality Database 382/1/24 1979–98 (NHA, Northside).

[49] Dr Elizabeth Taws, interview, 30 October 2001. Almost £500,000 was secured for services focused upon Norwich for a three-year period.

[50] This relatively new sub-specialism attracted 'demonstration services' money from the RHA, initially for Norwich and widened to Norfolk. Glanford ward at the Norfolk and Norwich was used.

service' were critical for future arrangements that might extend beyond the existing hospitals.[51]

Meanwhile, greater numbers of patients were discharged from St Andrew's and the transfer of younger and rehabilitation patients to Hellesdon in 1985–6 (see Table 10.2) reflected this new demarcation of workloads between the psychiatric hospitals. Some older patients who required continuing care had also been transferred to the Vale hospital but a fire there served to emphasise the shortfall in social service residential care and community nursing in the county and necessitated some returns to St Andrew's.[52] Admissions rose appreciably, beyond 300 from 1984, and remained at this level well into the 1990s. A considerable number of readmissions also indicated the use of respite care, first as a stopgap measure but increasingly as part of efforts to offset or delay long-term or hospice-style care.[53] In the early 1990s south side wards 7a and 7b were used for these purposes, wards 9 and 10 offered continuing care, and day-hospital facilities were supplemented by the addition of the Octagon Centre in buildings formerly used as a social club. North side wards E, G, and J had closed by 1986 and first floor accommodation on wards B and H was converted into offices for the Norwich Health Authority, the hospital retaining the ground floor facilities more suitable for elderly patients.

As continuing care facilities for elderly and dementing patients were developed at Great Yarmouth, further rationalisation of wards at St Andrew's helped to improve standards and the effectiveness of nursing, with A1 the last north side ward to close in 1993.[54] There was some reduction in staff, particularly as support services were contracted out in line with government policy, and the trade unions concerned reluctantly had to accept transfers and natural wastage among staff members.[55] Short-term spending focused upon the south side, where wards were typically reduced to 18–20 beds although wards 7a and 7b had just ten each. Some of these had also closed: the success of rehabilitation ward 6 meant that it had virtually emptied and long-term ward 5 patients aged under 65 years had moved to Hellesdon. Wards 8–14 were still open in 1993, however, as were wards 2, 7a and 7b, which received acute cases.

Surviving nurses' day and night reports for mixed sex, ten-bed ward 7a give some indication of ward life at this time. In a six-month period 51 patients were admitted; 18 from their own homes, 26 from residential or local

---

[51] Dr Elizabeth Taws, interview, 30 October 2001.

[52] Dr Chris Reynolds (Medical Director NMHC), interview, 30 April 2001.

[53] Deaths among elderly people reduced waiting lists, even after the Vale hospital closed.

[54] Hospital plans for 1990 show that north-side wards A1, 2, C, D, F and K were still available, if not in use.

[55] These were COHSE, NUPE, NALGO and the RCN. COHSE, with a 75% female membership in the early 1980s, was disproportionately affected by the contraction and closure of its psychiatric hospital base.

authority homes and 7 directly from Norwich hospitals. Some came for observation or cognitive assessment, others for prescribed periods of respite care, but most patients suffered from memory loss, self-neglect, or were confused and occasionally aggressive. All were very elderly; where mentioned, their ages were from 77 to 90 years. Nurses appear to have explained procedures and their rights to the six patients who were sectioned and four section orders were later allowed to lapse. Patients' anxieties, the incidence of pushes and falls, the snatching of personal effects, wandering and the odd escape attempt were carefully monitored, with 'active listening techniques and reassurance' based on one-to-one nursing logged as frequently as medication. Those patients in reasonable health had trips out with occupational therapy and other staff, often for assessment pending their relocation. Altogether, 38 patients were discharged; 10 to close relatives or their own homes and 28 to local authority or private residential homes.[56]

St Andrew's had gained a new lease of life but strategic considerations affecting general hospital and mental health care in Norfolk ultimately produced its closure. Until the 1980s successive NHS reorganisations kept the psychiatric hospitals together and retained the hospital model as a template. St Andrew's and Hellesdon were shrinking and each required a considerable upgrade, yet hospitals were increasingly regarded as unsuitable sites for rehabilitation or long-term care. Rationalisation implied the development of only one hospital, but its selection was caught up in another issue: the perceived need for 'Norwich II', a second district general hospital which would include psychiatric wards and services. Local implementation of the 1962 Hospital Plan had stalled with the failure to establish a medical school at the new University of East Anglia but proposals for 'Norwich II' were revived in 1981.

A large number of potential sites for the new hospital were identified but St Andrew's and Hellesdon were actively considered. The ageing infrastructure at St Andrew's and its dependence upon a Norwich outer relief road yet to be constructed possibly decided the issue in favour of Hellesdon.[57] This apparently final choice, made by Norwich Health Authority in 1984, was resisted by a number of acute services consultants whose lobbying persuaded Tony Newton, then Minister of Health, to reopen the matter in 1986. Amid some controversy, a site adjacent to the University of East Anglia at Colney was eventually selected in 1989.[58] The first phase of the new hospital's

[56] Nurses' Day and Night Report Books, ward 7b, Sept.–Dec. 1991 and March–June 1992. Held privately to be deposited at NRO.
[57] Had Hellesdon become Norwich II without mental health facilities, further development rather than closure of St Andrew's might have occurred.
[58] Michael Falcon and David Walker, respectively Chairman of the Health Authority from 1988 and its Chief Executive from 1989, were evidently more appreciative of the need for revision than their predecessors. See also Norwich Health Authority, A New District General Hospital for Norwich, 1992, pp. 4, 23.

development centred upon 140 beds for acute psychiatric treatments, intended to replace services at Hellesdon and the Yare clinic.[59] Meanwhile, a detailed review of services for old age patients pointed to the closure of St Andrew's, now regarded as outmoded and prohibitively expensive to refurbish. It was envisaged that resident patients would be transferred to four new 24-bed units, which would be built across the county using funds realised from the sale of the St Andrew's site.[60]

These developments were portentous but neither went according to plan. The construction of Norwich II was delayed but building costs were rising, as were the likely operational costs, and the concept of two general hospitals for Norwich was criticised. Rationalisation seemed all the more appropriate in the light of advances in hospital treatments, particularly in keyhole surgery, which suggested that fewer acute beds were necessary. By 1990 central government policy was to establish NHS Trusts for operational purposes and, though Norfolk Health Authority was slow and possibly reluctant to consider the form these might take, further reorganisation was inevitable. Not until 1993 were separate Trusts envisaged for mental health services (excluding learning disabilities), acute medical and surgical services, and community health services. By then consultant staff central to the organisation of acute services were expressing a desire for the complete relocation of the Norfolk and Norwich hospital to the Colney site.[61] As a reduced number of beds would be available, previous arguments that the shortage of general hospital accommodation allowed little or no room for psychiatric services at the Norfolk and Norwich hospital were repeated.

Fortunately, there were also proactive features in the reorganisation of mental health care. Within the Mental Health Division of the NHA a General Management Board had replaced the consensus management team responsible for services and was developing its own strategy by 1990.[62] Aware of a history of relative neglect at the hands of the RHA before 1986, it concluded that mental health issues were again being relegated in discussions

---

[59] At this point the acute psychiatric units for those aged under 65 were at Hellesdon (for east Norfolk and north-east Suffolk); the David Rice clinic (central and north Norfolk) and the West Norwich hospital (Norwich and south Norfolk).

[60] Interview, Prof. Frank Curtis, 14 Sept. 2001. Prof. Curtis chaired the Norwich Health Authority Working Party referred to, which reported in 1991.

[61] N&N Health Care NHS Trust, 'Outline business case for acute services in Norfolk and Norwich', 1994, p. 6 (at NLS). The cramped N&N site; proximity to the private BUPA hospital and University, where a medical school had been established; and the trimming of bed requirements were cited.

[62] The 1983 Griffiths Report recommended that General Managers should set objectives and take decisions, arguing that consensus approaches were inconclusive and/or time-consuming. A key figure locally was Graham Shelton, Director of Mental Health Services from 1986 who, as Acting Chief Executive for the Health Authority in 1988, was well aware of the problems surrounding Norwich II.

over proposed acute and general hospital services.[63] The Board had also concluded that the 1960s model of a balanced general hospital with psychiatric services was not sustainable in practice. Psychiatric services located within a high-tech, acute hospital environment were likely to be very expensive, but cost was not the only consideration.[64] While the Board was prepared to make existing hospital wards more patient-centred, it was increasingly focused upon the provision of appropriate services rather than the buildings in which they were accommodated.[65] Hospital environments did not suit patients with delusional states or elderly people confused but aware that they were removed from their domestic setting.[66] Moreover, as the new commissioning system funded locally agreed services, including responses to eating disorders, substance abuse, attempted suicide or need for continuing care, their providers could exercise greater control of resources in meeting these objectives.

Mainly community-based services were envisaged and the status of an independent NHS Trust offered managerial opportunities for radical revision. Some medical staff had reservations over the loss of professional association and control implicit in such a move, feeling that the demarcation of mental health care ran contrary to the 1959 Act and subsequent thinking over two decades. Others looked more confidently towards greater co-operation with social services. Fears that developments might occur over the heads of staff were partly allayed by opportunities for their involvement in planning arrangements and a sense of improvement was later to emerge.[67] A shadow NHS Trust Board, established from November 1993 and formally constituted from 1 April 1994, replaced management by the Health Authority.[68] Almost the first act of the new Trust was to abandon the pursuit of acute psychiatric beds within the new Norfolk and Norwich hospital. A four-year period of intense activity followed, marked by the rationalisation of acute services, centred upon new facilities at Hellesdon, and the development of community services. Even then, the envisaged construction of four 24-bed residential

---

[63] Graham Shelton (General Manager and later Chief Executive to the Norfolk Mental Health Care NHS Trust 1994–9), interview, 1 June 2001. The point was also made by Kevin Long and Chris Reynolds. The Board included Dr Reynolds, medical staff representative, plus others representing mental illness and mental handicap services, occupational therapy and physiotherapy, an accountant and the general manager.

[64] Paul Thain, Director of Strategic Development, interview, 27 Nov. 2001.

[65] Shelton interview. A design team, established for the purpose at St Andrew's, later undertook work for the new Julian hospital and continuing care unit at North Walsham.

[66] ibid. For all its historical significance, Shelton found the Bethel Hospital 'wildly outmoded and inappropriate' for child outpatients with learning disabilities or special needs.

[67] Interviews, Drs Olive and Reynolds, Thain.

[68] Prof. Frank Curtis was Chairman (1994–9) and Graham Shelton the Chief Executive, with four executive and five non-executive directors.

units across the county was only partly implemented, and further revisions were to culminate in the opening of the Julian hospital in west Norwich and the closure of St Andrew's.[69]

All this involved major logistical and financial problems. Although the St Andrew's site was a major economic asset and its sale or leasing might finance new developments, replacement facilities had to be provided before any case for closing the hospital could be made. Moreover, as the site was not owned by the Norfolk Mental Health Care NHS Trust but leased from the Regional Health Authority, there were also risks that income raised from its redevelopment as a business park and residential area might be siphoned into other forms of care. The Trust had obtained an alternative site, adjacent to the West Norwich hospital and partly occupied by the former Norwich Isolation hospital, the Yare clinic and the Bure drug clinic. With the latter relocated in former hotel accommodation specially purchased in Norwich and the Yare clinic transferred to new accommodation at Hellesdon, the new site offered considerable scope for development.[70] Its acquisition proved doubly fortuitous since major expansion at Hellesdon beyond that proposed in 1986 was limited by planning restrictions, somewhat relaxed in later years.

In an optimistic first annual report the Trust outlined new arrangements but made no direct references to St Andrew's or the Julian hospital site. Diversified provision for elderly patients had begun with the opening of Cygnet House, Long Stratton, which offered 24 beds for permanent and respite care, followed by Rebecca House, at North Walsham. Where appropriate, other St Andrew's patients were transferred to accommodation in Northgate hospital, Yarmouth and to long-stay wards at Hellesdon. Alternative premises had been obtained for a new day-centre, used by 66 former St Andrew's patients transferring to social services care in 1994, and additional community mental health teams for north and south west Norfolk were established.[71]

Planning for the new Julian hospital involved considerable input from practising staff, resulting in the more spacious layout of wards and gardens and safe sitting areas for the less mobile patients able to go outdoors. Construction was announced in March 1996 and facilities included three wards offering 100 short-stay beds in single or shared rooms for elderly acute patients under assessment, a 30-place day-centre and an outpatient clinic.[72]

---

[69] Two units were built to high standards at North Walsham and Long Stratton but staff shortages and running costs were higher than anticipated.

[70] Shelton interview. The former hotel was purchased for £400,000 and the new and refurbished facilities at Hellesdon cost approx. £5.5 million.

[71] Norfolk Mental Health Care NHS Trust, *Annual Report*, 1994/5.

[72] *Eastern Daily Press*, 22 March 1996; NMHCT *Report*, 1997/8, p. 5. The wards were intended as replacements for Glandford ward at the Norfolk and Norwich and St Andrew's.

In December 1997 the St Andrew's site was placed on sale and the hospital's Octagon day-centre relocated to the converted ward 16 at Hellesdon. Interim accommodation for the remaining St Andrew's patients was provided on Earlham ward at the West Norwich hospital, pending completion of the Julian hospital in March 1998.[73] Four staff symbolically locked the main entrance door of St Andrew's for the last time in July: the ward pass key used was an original but it did not fit the lock.[74]

Inside stories . . .

What was the atmosphere like at St Andrew's and how were changes affecting the hospital from the 1960s interpreted there? Limited official information provides few insights and is used in this section to connect or augment more direct, subjective accounts provided by former and current hospital personnel. It is apparent that a particular community lifestyle, rural but lacking its former association with farm-work and labour intensive hospital support services, was disappearing. The number of elderly patients with rural backgrounds declined and long-term residents who died in hospital were only partly replaced, by older patients drawn from Norwich as well as the county. A trend towards continuing care was later accompanied by greater emphasis upon the treatment and discharge of such patients and, although there had been earlier developments in rehabilitation therapy, the association with younger patients and with work ceased to apply at St Andrew's by the 1980s.

A former patient, Mrs M—, admitted in 1959 after harrowing domestic experiences, remembered 'looking around at all these people standing around shaking and dribbling and I thought this was hell and I just had to get out and go with my kids'. She had panics when 'I just wanted to end it', but was comforted by nurses and other patients and was 'glad to have someone to look after me'. ECT, valium and lithium were helpful, but she particularly valued the companionship and the space which St Andrew's offered: without these 'I'd probably have jumped off a bridge'. On ward 10 there were other women with postnatal depression and 'a woman I went to school with who'd got housewife's syndrome'. In 1959–60 she spent time sweeping up; her occupational therapy consisted mainly of basket weaving and associated jumble sales. During periods of residence in the late 1960s and early 1980s she did bulb-packing, rather enjoyed the company of mixed nursing staff, and was slightly envious of the growing proportion of patients with single bedrooms.

---

[73] *Eastern Daily Press*, 16 March 1998, NMHCT *Report* 1998/9, p. 2. The Trust now provided 7 community mental health teams, 8 elderly centres, 3 additional outpatient clinics and a mobile day treatment service.

[74] Brian Watling, interviewed 27 November 2001, was one of those involved.

Whether on wards 6 or 10 she spoke of 'feeling happier in there than outside . . . I had companions in there . . . it took a big burden off me'. However, 'there was always space to get away . . . I walked round and round the grounds and up to the river and over to the men's side cricket pitch. No one ever stopped you'.[75]

Another patient, admitted in the late 1970s with Paget's disease and postnatal depression, was more critical. 'None of the drugs ever done me any good'; ECT sessions were 'not much good at first but then you felt wonderful'. St Andrew's 'didn't feel like a prison' and there were no locked doors but she 'wondered why they'd put me in with a lot of old people'. She appreciated being taken for lots of walks by staff and the strong support from her family, although this increased her awareness of the plight of the very elderly patients and those without visitors: 'they never took them poor old dears out at St Andrew's.' Before she was transferred to Hellesdon hospital, her lasting impression was of 'them long corridors – people always walking up and down'.[76]

Hospital staff freely discussed their varying experiences and opinions and, although there is no convenient representative sample or synthesis of views, some features can be noted.[77] Those working at the hospital from the early 1960s inevitably experienced the greatest amount of change. Many, giving their best in difficult circumstances and not wholly aware of wider developments affecting 'their' hospital, working lives and relationships, did not always welcome it. The scale of upheavals from the early 1980s possibly evoked more favourable memories of earlier and more settled times. Other staff moved on, some unhappy in the hospital environment, some for career development. Still others remained and saw change as a prerequisite for patients to realise their potential and improvements in the quality of care, not necessarily confined within St Andrew's. And yet, contrary to presentations of subjection and control of patients by staff, the hospital was generally regarded as a 'kindly' place, even where otherwise contrasting assessments were offered.[78]

Beginning as a hospital gardener in the 1950s, Alan Adcock worked with patients and shared recreation with them in century-old patterns, but he also filled security ditches, dismantled the iron rails dividing off the former airing courts and saw the unlocking of wards. He did not associate the hospital with confinement but with 'looking after mental patients who, given their full

[75] I am particularly grateful to Mrs M—, a former patient who consented to be interviewed by Mary Fisher on 29 August 2001, and I thank Dr Chris Reynolds for facilitating the interview.

[76] Mrs D—, a former patient interviewed by Mary Fisher on 19 September 2001.

[77] Over twenty staff personnel were interviewed, see Acknowledgements, p. xi.

[78] Kevin Long, critical of some aspects of hospital culture was among those using this description.

freedom, were a danger to themselves', and soon came to acknowledge that 'being mentally ill and sane, as far as I'm concerned, that's just a narrow gap'.[79] Clifford Graveling, brought up on the hospital farm before training as a nurse, felt that St Andrew's in the 1960s had 'quite a lot of very contented patients . . . there because they didn't have homes to go back to . . . and I suppose quite a lot of them didn't want to go back'.[80] Rita Thomson, a laboratory assistant from 1961, recalled visits to the still-locked ward A, 'a vestigial feature from how it always had been . . . one accepted there were reasons . . . we were dealing with very unpredictable people'.[81] Generally, she felt that on the wards 'there was no sense of oppression . . . always a feeling of movement . . . there was a sense of interaction', though the atmosphere improved after further new medications and the introduction of mixed-sex wards.

Even after nurse training transferred to Hellesdon and the hospital farm closed, a strong community feeling remained at St Andrew's. Interviews confirm that succeeding generations of families worked at the hospital as nurses, carers, farm-workers, craftsmen and even in senior administration. Male nurse Jimmy Browne felt that male staff 'got on' because qualified men often worked at the hospital for thirty years or more, several had married nurses or other staff, clusters of hospital housing meant that they were close neighbours and many came from rural backgrounds, shared with older patients.[82] The staff social club and trade unionism added to staff solidarity but neither was viewed by those interviewed as antagonistic to patients and analogies with family life were often drawn. Mollie Middleton, a former nurse tutor who preferred to remain at St Andrew's rather than transfer to Hellesdon and switched to night nursing from 1965, recalled that 'it was certainly not unusual to use your half-day off to take patients into Norwich shopping'.[83] Older patients often knocked on the windows of Eric and Rita Browne's house to see the 'St Andrew's babies'. He sometimes took the children on the wards and she felt that 'the ethos at St Andrew's was so positive, so well-balanced, so thought through that you didn't feel insecure . . . We knew the patients; it was just like this huge family'.[84]

---

[79] Alan Adcock, interview, 20 April 1988.

[80] Clifford Graveling was brought up at the hospital farm, worked at St Andrew's 1955–7 and nursed at Hellesdon hospital 1957–91. Interview, 30 March 2001.

[81] Rita Browne, née Thomson, interview, 9 March 2001.

[82] Jimmy Browne, nursing assistant 1957–89, interview, 21 March 2001.

[83] Mollie Middleton, interview, 2 March 2001. Her father-in-law John Middleton, formerly the hospital secretary, had taken patient Billy O— to live with the family as he had no relatives of his own.

[84] Eric and Rita Browne, interview, 9 March 2001. This maintained one tradition: as children, Clifford Graveling, Vivienne Roberts and others had the run of the hospital farms and estate. Sister M.G. maintained another in the 1980s, taking to her home two elderly female patients as companions when she retired. (Middletons, 13 March 2001; Bonds, 23 March 2001, interviews.)

Fraser's innovations as medical superintendent tended to be hesitant, combining useful changes with an almost quaint outlook.[85] Staff and patients still invested considerable time and effort in maintaining sports facilities and coaching in cricket or football often proved critical to increasing patients' confidence. However, an ageing resident population inevitably settled to bowls and putting, with darts, quoits and skittles in the winter, which remained well organised and supported.[86] After visiting hours were extended to three evenings per week in 1966, Fraser had some success in encouraging university and school students 'to bring the mental hospital more in touch with the youthful members of the community'.[87] He also co-operated with the National Association for Mental Health (MIND), which in Norfolk remained a pragmatic rather than a radical campaigning body. A conference at St Andrew's during mental health week in 1967 was the first of several and marked the establishment of the hospital's own League of Friends. This body subsequently organised successful open days and fêtes as well as fund-raising and visiting when, arguably, these might well have collapsed long before the hospital closure.[88]

Although medication and forms of rehabilitation therapy were increasingly understood as essentials in enabling younger patients to leave hospital, the situation in the mid-1960s was not promising. The traditional emphasis was on work, but token payments for patient labour were frowned upon after the 1959 Act and opportunities for paid employment diminished with the closure of the farm and laundry. There was less horticulture and Fraser cancelled the reclamation of paper bags as this posed health risks to patients and smacked of outright exploitation. Attempts to extend occupational therapy at Thorpe End, the former medical superintendent's house, were frustrated by staff shortages and delayed RHB support. 'Incentive money' was paid to patients but was at first limited to those willing to help with ward work.[89] Staff initiatives could produce quite exceptional responses: a sale of work by ward 5 patients financed a London excursion for all 70 of them in 1969, leaving sufficient funds over for a cinema night in Norwich.[90] Yet from different vantage points in hospital administration and maintenance, Edward Middleton and Eric Browne felt that many patients 'were completely lost; they used to go back to the places where they had worked or sit around on the wards'.[91]

---

[85] e.g. his concern that an increase in football fixtures was likely to affect the condition of the cricket square the following season. MS Journal, 1 Dec. 1966.

[86] Trevor Pull (nurse and recreation officer), interview, 4 May 2001.

[87] MS Journal, 4 July 1969. Such visits were sustained into the 1990s.

[88] ibid., 3 Feb. and 3 Oct. 1970, 1 April 1971. Edward Middleton was the chairman in April 1998. Records relating to the League of Friends of St Andrew's 1970–98 are now held at Norfolk County Record Office SO 194.

[89] ibid., 4 March and 1 April 1965.

[90] ibid., 1 Jan. 1970; Dr Olive interview.

[91] Eric Browne, interview. Edward Middleton made the same point.

Better paid and regular 'industrial work' at St Andrew's in the early 1970s included the production of bird boxes and tables, interwoven fence panels, concrete paving slabs, paper shredding and baling and the commercial packing of flower bulbs. The latter began with twenty residents and two former patients and the reversal of these numbers by 1980 indicated one modest success for industrial therapy.[92] Three-quarters of the 600 patients in 1973 had occupational therapy and 100 were paid; 10 already worked outside, 28 doing hospital work and roughly 60 on industrial therapy.[93] Over two decades male patients who had benefited from basic habit training and medication had helped to convert sheds and the hospital ash tip into a landscaped recycling area known as 'the Mount'. This became a depot for parties, including younger day patients, who went out doing gardening and odd jobs at group homes, health centres and parks around Norwich, with the result that 'some wards were empty during the day'.[94] Such activity provided a focal point for patients, enabling some to develop relationships and a social life, before operations and patients were transferred to Hellesdon hospital in 1986.[95]

Most of the staff interviewed felt they had caring relationships with patients and some saw a gulf between medical and nursing staff, rather than between nurses and patients. This originated in the traditional hospital hierarchy, the status and small number of medical staff, and until the late 1960s very few doctors socialised with nurses.[96] The development of ward teams for patient assessment helped to reduce barriers, particularly where junior medical staff were concerned, although the role and responsibilities of consultants was a source of new tensions. They were more likely to make decisions for patients regarding medication and its continuation and acknowledged that this occurred for some time after the 1983 Act. At the same time, their reaffirmation of the hospital as a place of treatment rather than of residence also challenged nurses inclined to operate as a 'benevolent dictatorship'.[97] Improving therapeutic approaches by the early 1980s could not be summarised as a simple division between bio-medical and holistic

---

[92] MS Journal, 7 April 1966; Jimmy Browne, interview, 21 March 2001. Some patients earned £12 per week in 1972.

[93] HMC Minutes, 30 Sept. 1973.

[94] Jimmy Browne, interview, 21 March 2001; Wally Bond, nurse orderly 1956–85, interview, 23 March 2001.

[95] Wally Bond recalled that older patients who preferred a ride out and a drink to shopping often accompanied the younger ones on excursions: he knew every pub from Brandon in west Norfolk to Thorpe Ness on the east coast that would take in parties of mental hospital patients.

[96] Rita Thomson, interview. The long-serving Dr Pietocha (see Chapter 8) was an exception mentioned by male staff: he regularly 'dropped in' on the north-side barbers and was not adverse to the occasional bet.

[97] Long, Olive, Reynolds, interviews.

alternatives, however, or between psychiatrists or therapists and carers. Neuroleptic drugs, for example, helped some longer-term patients to respond to other therapies and the value of rehabilitation for those with severe debilitating illness was more generally recognised.

For decades psychiatric nursing had been undervalued and conditions at St Andrew's were not easy. Nursing had been conducted on a same-sex basis, with largely separated staffs appointed and led by the matron and chief male nurse, who were respected as highly knowledgeable and generally fair in their dealings with staff and patients.[98] In the early 1960s it remained ward-based, with pairs of sisters or charge nurses alternately responsible for their ward, its patients and staff during morning and afternoon shifts. Shift times overlapped to ensure that incoming staff were aware of any developments on their ward and similar procedures operated as the smaller regular night staff came and went.[99] Staff worked a six-day week, the rest day for one nurse requiring his or her opposite on the other shift to work from 7.00 a.m. until 9.00 p.m. until 1968, when a five-day rota system was introduced. Nurses were normally allocated an area to supervise on the ward or outside it and their duties included cleaning work with patients. They were expected to extend their shift as required and overtime, paid at standard rate, had only been reintroduced in 1960 after trade union campaigns.[100] Entitlement to five weeks' holiday, considered a major bonus, was subject to arrangements largely determined by the matron or chief male nurse.

Staff shortages affected morale, undermining the recruitment and retention of new personnel. Turnover was a greater problem among women nurses and the promotion of fully qualified personnel over those who had not enhanced their preliminary training led to some resentment. Mixed-sex nursing was one response to a preponderance of qualified male over female nurses but the reluctance of some men to work under female sisters or charge nurses on women's wards was often reciprocated. Two male volunteers, 'doing very well' by September 1965, were later designated ward sisters but these remained exceptional.[101] Women patients had already been moved to the 'male' north side after wards K and 16 were cleared, but further transfers of elderly women patients created the first mixed-sex geriatric wards in 1970 and a reverse movement extended these to the south side. These changes improved the patients' living environment and undermined resistance to mixed-sex nursing, but coincided with new concern over hospital nursing.

---

[98] None of the nursing staff interviewed, including the trade union activists, expressed a contrary view though many were less impressed with other hospital officials or their nursing officers in later years.

[99] Typically: mornings 7 a.m.–1.30 p.m., afternoons 1–9 p.m., nights 8.30 p.m.–7.30 a.m.

[100] Wally Bond, Molly Bond, née Sexbery (nurse 1951–91), interview, 23 March 2001. Nurses were members of the Confederation of Health Service Employees; other staff were in the National Union of Public Employees.

[101] MS Journal, 6 May and 2 Sept. 1965; 4 Dec. 1968.

A series of open study days at St Andrew's aimed to boost staff morale and persuade other student nurses to take secondments at the hospital. Attempts to safeguard nurses' working conditions included the recruitment of domestic staff, the payment of 'incentive money' to some patients for ward work, and the vacation employment of university students to ease staff shortages because of holidays. School parties were also welcomed to the hospital wards as of interest to patients and for potential nurse recruitment.[102] Limited results in the face of poor pay and conditions and the loneliness of some overseas nurses, upon whom the hospital increasingly relied, posed further problems. Some twenty incidents in which patients sustained fractures after falls or pushes between July and September 1969, although non-slip flooring was generally adopted, suggested insufficient supervision of an ageing patient clientele. Spot checks by Fraser and matron Myles on 20 September 1969 revealed 19 staff nursing 412 male patients on nine wards and 29 staff for 627 female patients on thirteen wards. Not surprisingly, they informed the RHB that 'this nursing staff is dangerously low'.[103]

Local staffing issues were aggravated by national concerns. Influential reports for the Ministry of Health, not primarily concerned with psychiatric hospitals, nonetheless had important implications. One consequence of the 1967 Cogwheel reports on medical work in hospitals was the abolition of the medical superintendent post and the loosening of ties between consultants and particular hospitals. The 1968 Salmon report proposed greater managerial responsibilities for nursing officers under one principal officer, ending the traditional roles of matron and chief male nurse.[104] These recommendations had unsettling and divisive effects upon hospital nursing staff. Senior personnel submitted applications for the post-Salmon version of their posts, some nurses applied for management training courses, and others looked to trade union efforts in relation to discontent over pay restrictions under the Labour government's incomes policies.[105] Some who pursued none of these options nevertheless saw the abolition of matron and chief male

---

[102] ibid., e.g. study days, 10 Nov. 1965, 24 May 1966; patient incentives, 1 April 1965; university students, 4 May 1967; school visit, 6 July and 5 Oct. 1967. Press advertising was followed by a feature article covering a journalist's 'day with a nurse', *Eastern Daily Press*, 16 Oct. 1969.

[103] MS Journal, 30 Sept. 1969.

[104] Webster, *NHS*, p. 94; Jones, *Asylums*, p. 187. The post of matron is currently being reintroduced.

[105] MS Journal, 1 May and 4 Dec. 1969. Ten staff had applied for management training courses. Jack Boddy, HMC chairman and himself a farm-workers' trade union official, may well have instituted the series of open forums in Group 8 hospitals from November 1969 to help defuse this situation. COHSE leaders had misplaced hopes that post-1966 incomes policies implied preferential treatment for their low paid members, repeated with the 'social contract' of 1974–9 before the 'winter of discontent' in the public sector.

nurse posts as another critical event at St Andrew's, after which 'no one accepted responsibility' even for minor decision-making.[106]

After 1968 each nursing officer was in charge of a group of wards and often had another area of responsibility, which meant less involvement in the ward team. Flexibility in nursing areas of the hospital in response to staff shortages increased, but the ending of traditional patterns of working and recruitment caused some resentment. Senior staff emphasised the quality of care required, rather the efforts currently made in difficult circumstances.[107] Others saw them as bureaucratic, preferring 'office work' to direct engagement with patients on the wards. Long-standing administrative staff felt that some newcomers had no feel for the hospital or its patients, lacked the personal touch or 'just came and went'.[108] Later attempts by a nurse manager to focus upon patients as clients were interpreted as proof that informal relationships between staff and patients on first-name terms were being undermined. Similarly the rationalisation of wards, to maintain staffing ratios and raise standards on those remaining, was associated with loss of positions for former charge nurses and ward sisters or attendants. By 1973, for example, the hospital had nine charge nurses, one staff and three enrolled nurses and forty-four nursing assistants, 60 per cent of them part-time.[109] Staff used to taking patients for outdoor work or rehabilitation therapy often had difficulty adjusting as shortages required their presence on the wards caring for 'informal' patients no longer expected to work and often far too old to do so.[110]

Eric Browne remembered 'much more to-and-fro at the hospital' after the day-centre opened in 1970, although there were 'fewer excitements' among the resident patients, noticeably on ward 3. Older long-term patients were dying and he was aware of others discharged to half-way homes; but a dwindling group of regulars who never had visitors seemed more isolated and any younger patient 'really stood out'.[111] Until then the hospital seemed full, even as new medications were introduced, but rumours of closure resurfaced. Most staff remained sceptical, remarking that 'there will always be mad people' or assuming that 'this place will never close', but more sensed that the hospital was in decline, as 'no money was being spent on it' and staff homes on the estate were being neglected or leased out.[112] Feelings that the hospital

---

[106] Eric Browne retired in 1988. After 42 years he was sad to leave but had 'had enough' of 'new systems' and felt that things were falling apart, a process which he dated from the HMC's loss of control. The Middletons expressed similar views.

[107] K. Long (nursing in 1968, later Director of Nursing Practice), interview.

[108] Edward Middleton, interview, recalled one Hospital Secretary who had no knowledge of the whereabouts of ward 12 after two years at St Andrew's.

[109] HMC Minutes 1972–3, SAH 509, 27 Sept. 1973.

[110] Wally Bond, interview.

[111] Eric Browne, interview.

[112] Eric and Rita Browne, interview.

was becoming more like a nursing home for residents in a quiet but decaying atmosphere may also have contributed to a certain lack of vision. Not surprisingly, some staff concentrated upon caring relationships; one felt that most psychiatric hospital patients needed to be there, but that 'the elderly still need warmth, love, care and security; that was what applied at St Andrew's'.[113]

Arriving in December 1977, Dr Chris Reynolds compared St Andrew's favourably with London psychiatric hospitals where he had worked: it was traditional but well run and patients had their personal possessions if not much privacy. He had roughly fifty middle-aged patients on mixed-sex wards 13 and 14 with forty more on segregated wards F9 and M10. In an effort to minimise long-stay patient numbers, he used weekly ward meetings for group therapy but noted that the nursing staff often found such situations more challenging than patients did.[114] Dr Ted Olive also had mixed-sex wards and long-stay psycho-geriatric patients, including some isolated on Orchard ward on the basis of tests conducted years previously. Accommodation for the elderly was reasonable and staff were conscientious in providing basic care, but he felt that some geriatric patients needed greater stimulation. Arguing for the closure of Orchard ward, he attempted to mix patients of differing ages to encourage family-like relationships in association with rehabilitation. Again, some staff were reluctant, preferring a more fixed system based on generations of custom and practice, which had protected their positions and jobs. He believed the area health authority was insufficiently proactive, although problems at St Andrew's were minor when compared with issues in the wider reorganisation of health care.[115]

Mental health nursing had lost many of its former certainties by the 1980s. A growing emphasis upon therapies required new skills with patients and suggested different and uneasy relationships with medical and other professional staff. From 1982 a nationally revised psychiatric nurse-training syllabus emphasised community rather than hospital care. Studies of newly qualified and career-minded nurses suggest that, while few saw role models within hospitals like St Andrew's, they rapidly experienced the uncertainties of community care, of patient behaviour and a gulf between teaching and practice in the treatment of patients.[116] In related areas of hospital life, the introduction of sub-contracted services from 1983, the prospect of hospital closure, and longer-term doubts over the future of a distinct psychiatric nursing service had unsettling effects. Differences between established and

---

[113] Rita Browne, interview.

[114] Chris Reynolds, interview. He acknowledged the influence of Barton's ideas concerning institutionalisation (see note 5).

[115] Ted Olive, interview.

[116] P. Nolan, *A History of Mental Health Nursing*, Chapman & Hall, London, 1993, pp. 143, 146–52.

newly trained staff may be exaggerated and oversimplified, not least because they understate a process of change already under way, but there may be some substance to national research findings that 'allegiance to a particular hospital was no longer fashionable and more nurses . . . lived independently of their place of work'. Such was the rate of change that 'many older staff experienced occupational disorientation and felt forced to take early retirement'.[117]

Trevor Pull's description of rehabilitation procedures at St Andrew's in the early 1980s indicates their improvement over two decades. Patients were assessed and the detailed findings discussed with them, prior to transfer to mixed rehabitation wards. They had periods in a self-contained flat improving their life skills and worked within the hospital while the rehabilitation officer sought half-way accommodation and suitable employment outside.[118] Reminiscence and cognitive therapy were more extensively used to motivate longer-term patients for an active part in hospital life, although it was acknowledged that with 'most of the patients suitable for rehabilitation and return to the community . . . we are left with the hard core . . . who may never leave the hospital'.[119] Elizabeth Taws was supported by a group of enthusiastic nurses, physiotherapists and community practice nurses who volunteered for the old age psychiatry unit in 1983. Kevin Long, whose training at St Andrew's in the 1960s had led him to think beyond long-term institutional care, left to complete general nurse training and post-registration courses as a staff nurse in Nottingham before he returned as nursing services manager in 1986. He found the psychiatric unit already established and a number of younger charge nurses interested in developing services, wherever they might be located, rather than in maintaining St Andrew's as such.[120]

This suggests one key factor in the eventual closure of the hospital: it was overtaken by changes in mental health care. Graham Shelton felt that, in Norfolk, 'we made a quantum leap shift in the space of a decade'.[121] Older concerns over the suitability of psychiatric hospital facilities were replaced by positive emphasis upon user-orientated services provided by teams of professionals in community settings. There was still a place for hospital care but the concentration of facilities at Hellesdon since the 1960s counted heavily in its favour. St Andrew's had an older infrastructure and the high ceilings and windows were less suitable for its largely sedentary psychogeriatric patients who could not easily look outside. The likely modification and upkeep of elderly buildings hardly negated the case for newer, diversified

---

[117] ibid., p. 157.
[118] Trevor Pull, interview. Norwich City Council parks and gardens department was a major employer.
[119] ibid.
[120] Elizabeth Taws, Kevin Long, interviews.
[121] ibid.

or specialist accommodation, provided at the Julian hospital, at continuing care units or at Hellesdon.[122] If the staff culture at St Andrew's had changed, strong emotional attachments to the hospital among former and current staff remained. For some this amounted to a grieving process, recognised in a celebratory service on 9 September 1996, 'letting go' of the hospital in another form of closure.[123]

The rationale of service provision and financial necessity pointed to the closure of St Andrew's and some staff felt that determined efforts were made to secure favourable alternative developments for patients, rather than mere cost-savings. However, other former staff considered that psychiatric hospitals and their patients generally were abandoned by central government and they expressed concerns extending beyond their own attachment to the hospital. These focused upon a gulf between the rhetoric of client choice and the delivery of improved services to all who need them. A former ward sister gave the example of a 97-year-old patient whose habit of hiding food and eating with her fingers caused few problems at St Andrew's but led to her readmission from alternative accommodation. Another patient, admitted in 1918, went on to work at the hospital until her retirement in 1963, after which she was allowed to stay in familiar surroundings and spent much time cleaning the hospital church. Neither had sufficient insight into their illnesses to cope with life outside the hospital.[124] Edward Middleton cited another patient, well provided for in the present-day Julian hospital, who still asked to be taken 'home': 'if somebody has been in a place for forty years and you move them what are they going to do? I know what patients have said to me about this'.[125]

Even though an important feature of community care is to reduce the incidence of institutionalisation, some long-term patients appear to have been disadvantaged under transitory arrangements as the hospital ran down. A related problem is that some patients receive a range of treatments without appreciable results and those with few relationships or contacts outside hospital, who often lived contented if organised lives based around therapy, low levels of supervision and modest entertainment, are particularly vulnerable. Such 'institutionalisation' was, arguably, not unique to hospitals like St Andrew's and patients' choices might not necessarily be more

---

[122] Suspended ceilings, swept upwards to the window tops, were used to reduce heating loss. Dr Olive felt that a blunt choice was necessary: St Andrew's 'had to go' and, with new resources, Hellesdon 'has improved quite dramatically'.

[123] This was appreciated as 'the right way to do it' by several of the staff interviewed but other aspects of closure, for example the disposal of former staff accommodation, were greatly resented by some.

[124] Olive Clarke, interview, Plackett, 3 May 1988.

[125] One patient, readmitted to St Andrew's after three years, declared 'it was lovely to be home'; Middleton, interview.

realisable under community care.[126] The experience of discharged patients barred from return to their private lodgings for much of the day was also cited and the whereabouts, let alone the state of health, of others asked to leave such accommodation were sometimes unknown.[127] Those without informal support might reappear following some transgression and the increased usage of sectioning procedures and secure units is a feature with disturbing echoes of measures for vagrants two centuries earlier.[128] The Norvic Clinic, the regional forensic unit, was constructed in 1983 on the northern edge of the St Andrew's site: its patient rehabilitation services use the former Mount workshops and the hostel accommodation includes Meadowlands, the former nurses' home which was refurbished yet again in April 1998.

As a place for madness for almost two centuries, St Andrew's was considered outmoded by 1998. A late change of role may have delayed the final closure, which was very much connected with the need to provide resources for more appropriate developments. Mental health care had by then been reconstituted as a range of services operating beyond hospitals but the Hellesdon and Julian hospitals, the latter with its St Andrew's Lodge, accommodated some former patients and, along with more dispersed continuing care units, have partly replaced its functions. Yet, aside from alleged shortcomings in community care, doubts remain over the diminution of 'asylum', in its original sense, in mental health care. This is not to idealise the former hospital but to recognise the limitations of some replacement residential settings and, all too often, of wider social tolerance.

Asylums had their own spatial, behavioural and temporal routines, but they offered a protective space in which people were allowed to be 'mad', eccentric or unable to cope. At St Andrew's the hospital estate supported a community in which staff and patients were ordered and separated, but which was not wholly exclusive towards patients. If somewhat crowded and dated, it was usually seen as a 'kindly' place by long-serving staff and newcomers. This sense of community was undermined by the loss of local control over its resources; by the decline of hospital-related occupations in which patient involvement had been prominent; and by engineered changes to the patient clientele in the transition to community care. The therapeutic properties of the wider hospital landscape for patients, particularly from rural environments, may have been neglected in this process. Studies of similar asylums suggest that 'scant regard has been paid to the loss of "a place in the country" and its healing effects . . . the Victorian belief in congenial

---

[126] Ted Olive, interview.

[127] This was identified as among the most glaring of deficiencies in the Middleton, Roberts and Browne interviews.

[128] An analogy highlighted by Michael Glasheen, property management, 1960, (interview, Plackett, 20 April 1988). The Norvic Clinic has four of the six currently locked wards in Norfolk; there had been none in 1979.

countryside settings as therapeutic for patients is as valid today as it was over a century ago'.[129] In another example, a former patient linked her recovery with 'plenty of places to look and come to terms with one's feelings . . . in the grounds, you know, you were safe. It was an asylum and yet you were free'.[130] And as one former St Andrew's patient put it, 'You need to get away from the problem. You need asylum . . . There was always space to get away from anyone if you wanted to'.[131]

[129] J. Pettigrew, R. Reynolds and S. Rouse, *A Place in the Country: Three Counties Asylum 1860–1998*, South Beds Community Health Care Trust, 1998.
[130] Cited in Gittins, *Madness*, p. 9.
[131] Mrs M—, interviewed 29 August 2001, spent periods at St Andrew's from 1959 onwards.

11

Postscript: findings and speculations

The history of St Andrew's Hospital as examined in previous chapters reveals a strong institutional 'storyline' and provides a case example for a wider theme: the rise and fall of the asylum/psychiatric hospital. It has been placed in the contexts of local and national developments in mental health care, drawing particularly upon public statements concerning the hospital and the more private medical observations of its patients. Such information is more extensive and accessible compared with that offering intimate details of hospital life or glimpses of patients when considered essentially as people rather than as cases. It does not guarantee accuracy or objectivity and must remain only a guide to understanding what, over two centuries, could be construed as forms of mental health care. Any sense of social relationships or hospital routine which emerges is impressionistic, though that conveyed is based upon written records, the sometimes contradictory recollections of people working at the hospital or closely connected with it, and of patients' reported experiences.[1] This postscript offers a more personal view of the history of the asylum/hospital in relation to other research and considers briefly what has replaced 'St Andrew's', in terms of services for patients and a new role for some of the former buildings.

At the risk of oversimplification, nineteenth-century asylums have been generally depicted as hierarchical, male-dominated, isolated communities, offering forms of care ranging from custody to cure and involving processes of control. These expanding places for madness became sites of professional power, in which illnesses and therefore patients were segregated and categorised with relatively little success in managed communities offering limited therapy and lots of work. Studies of asylum administration, admission and discharge procedures and institutional connections have tested these broad narratives without resolving more contentious issues.[2] Until recently there has been less research on such features in twentieth-century hospitals, although the 'war neuroses', controversial physical and pharmaceutical treatments, patients' rights and the debate surrounding de-institutionalisation and community care have attracted considerable attention.[3]

---

[1] The interview material is not offered as a representative sample but to illustrate people's own experiences and to supplement limited or sparse official records.

[2] Despite new work, such as J. Melling and B. Forsythe (eds), *Insanity, Institutions and Society 1800–1914*, Routledge, London, 1999; P. Bartlett, *The Poor Law of Lunacy*, Leicester University Press, 1999, the extent to which asylums could simply be 'used' by patients' families or were institutions of social control remains unresolved.

[3] In 1991 Roy Porter felt that 'most asylums await study, the history of the asylum in the

All these features were evident in Norfolk but some can be highlighted, beginning with broad observations. The transformation from asylum to psychiatric hospital suggests a medical approach to mental illness but it is rather less clear how and when this became predominant. For example, almost fifty years elapsed before Norfolk Lunatic Asylum had a medical superintendent, although medical attendance for 'the patients' was provided from the outset and the 1845 legal requirement of a resident medical officer was met. Although the turnover of junior medical staff was high in later years, a number of relatively young men spent good proportions of their careers at the asylum before moving on for promotion. The post of medical superintendent, once attained, represented a professional standing for life and was indeed a lifetime's work. Each holder had a characteristic regime and sought to introduce reform as he felt appropriate, but all were subject to rather variable guidance from external lunacy commissioners or Board inspectors and to the financial and political concerns of the local committee of justices or county councillors. William Hills was abreast of contemporary medical opinion but it is questionable whether the asylum seriously lagged in its treatment, care or provision for patients under non-medical super-intendence prior to his appointment. David Thomson was primarily an influential organiser and manager, as demonstrated in his reorganisations of the asylum and the war hospital. Oliver Connell might have proved a greater mental health care reformer than he was allowed to be. William McCulley found his role increasingly restricted under the National Health Service and James Fraser's position was outmoded in a period of hospital reorganisation and new therapies.

Given the medical superintendent's managerial role, a maximum of two other medical officers in peacetime before the introduction of the NHS suggests that doctors had very little time for individual patients. This practical restriction probably explains the late nineteenth-century focus within the asylum upon treatment for the new admissions and minimal doctoring of chronic or long-term patients, even as a 'scientific rationale' for this approach was being provided nationally.[4] Local medical regimes broadly reflected the conventions of the day, with concern over miasmas, hygiene, senility and hereditary features added to the reconfigured continuities of moral treatment. Junior staff sometimes brought to medical casebooks vogue preoccupations,

---

twentieth century is almost virgin territory', R. Porter, 'History of psychiatry in Britain', *History of Psychiatry*, 2, 1991, 3, pp. 271–9, 276–7. For contrasting approaches to this see D.H. Clark, *The Story of a Mental Hospital. Fulbourn 1858–1983*, Process, London, 1996, and D. Gittins, *Madness in its Place: Narratives of Severalls Hospital 1913–1997*, Routledge, London, 1998.

[4] Viz. that various forms of 'degeneration' placed increasing numbers of patients beyond hope of recovery. R.C. Olby, 'Constitutional and hereditary disorders', in W.F. Bynum and R. Porter (eds), *Companion Encyclopaedia of the History of Medicine*, Routledge, London, 1993, Vol. 1, pp. 412–37.

for example with head shapes, family backgrounds and galvanism, but few of these seem to have been carried to excess in Norfolk. Thus MacKenzie Bacon's war on masturbation was not waged surgically until he had left for another institution and the 1909 public inquiry into alleged abuses may have provided a salutary check on galvanism. Thomson's own interest in sterilisation was either not allowed to develop or was itself cut short by the war emergency.

If the impositions of staffing and overcrowding featured in medical outlooks there is local evidence that insanity might also be 'restructured' in response to external pressures. A rise in NLA admissions coincided with social unrest in the 1840s and further increases followed the opening of the auxiliary asylum, pessimism concerning the proliferation of the chronic insane and a widening of the 'borderlands' of insanity at the end of the nineteenth century. Perhaps these admissions also reflected the transfer of people already regarded insane as the asylum's capacity expanded, reflecting not simply more madness but recognition of the asylum as the appropriate place for madness. Yet it is noteworthy that acute overcrowding and wartime impositions on the asylum/hospital also produced surges in the number of patients discharged as 'relieved' or 'recovered'.

Over the nineteenth century medical claims concerning the cure of insanity were modified to cover its detection, explanation and appropriate management, thereby also helping to safeguard the health of wider society.[5] Pre-war signs of local identification of the asylum and its medical staff with hospital treatments may have been enhanced by its wartime role and later association with voluntary patients, outpatient clinics, the Norfolk and Norwich Hospital and a second wartime spell as an Emergency Hospital. All may have contributed in first steps towards 'community care', perhaps even anticipating the 1930 Mental Treatment Act. Yet this reworking of the therapeutic regime also involved some controversial and dubious physical treatments, encouraged by inspectors of the Board of Control. When resumed after the Second World War these were presented as modernistic and scientific, and it seems fortunate for their exponents that this episode was soon overshadowed from the 1950s by comparatively successful pharmaceutical and therapeutic approaches.

According to a leading exponent, these developments heralded 'a more venturesome and enthusiastic policy of treatment'.[6] If they also served to raise the status of their practitioners, new difficulties for psychiatric hospital medical staff soon emerged. Lay and professional concern with institutionalisation as a contributory feature in mental illness increased over

---

[5] J. Andrews, 'Notes on mental health care and prophylaxis in late 19th century Britain', *Health Care Discussion Papers*, 1, Oxford Brookes University, 1998, pp. 14–34.

[6] A. Lewis, 'The chemical treatment of mental disorder', *Biology of Human Affairs*, 1947, 27, pp. 19–26, 19.

the 1960s. A subsequent revised focus upon patient rehabilitation and discharge was then compromised as the limitations imposed by shortages of time and resources within the hospital had to be balanced against suspicions of inadequate health care and social provision outside it.[7] The need to convince some nursing staff, devoted to earlier perceptions of care, or to work in association with other therapists and to recognise the rights of mental patients also provided challenging circumstances. It appears also, from the complex saga surrounding the 'Norwich II' district general hospital, that professional support or empathy for psychiatric hospital staff and their patients was not a priority for local senior medical staff, despite efforts pre-dating the 1930 Act to place 'mental' on a par with 'physical' illness.

Another theme to emerge from this study is that medical influence did not override economic factors, which were of particular if changing importance throughout. As a county pauper asylum, the NLA received patients who were casualties of economic and social dislocation, disordered by unemployment, emiseration or family breakdown, in addition to those unable to bear emotional traumas or sufferers from conditions such as epilepsy. There was a role for friends and families, particularly those willing to support prospective patients at home or those in hospital but considered fit for discharge, though it was arguably less than some studies imply.[8] In particular, it is questionable how much choice was afforded to the 'clients' of the early nineteenth-century poor law.

For much of the time the role and costs of asylum care, in comparison with poor law alternatives, were justified by demonstrations of industry and self-sufficiency. The asylum operated in close association with the poor law and did not decisively supplant the workhouse as the place for madness until subsidies on asylum treatments became available in the early 1870s.[9] Its reorganisation as a regimented community embodied principles dear to the new poor law: work, sexual segregation and the forfeit of family life. Farmwork and other labour reduced running costs and earnings on out-county, private and later service patients were significant. From the late 1840s until the 1930s it was not unusual to raise 10 to 15 and even 20 per cent of maintenance income by accommodating such patients. As with the asylum farm the effect, one way or another, was to subsidise contributions required from Norfolk ratepayers, an objective also retained during the Norfolk War Hospital period. Direct spending upon patients was closely restricted: this was to be expected within the poor law ethos and it persisted

---

[7] This is to set aside issues such as whether policy objectives (e.g. discharge of patients) impinge upon clinical decisions; whether medical staff are empowered to make decisions for patients; the over-reliance upon medication etc.

[8] Cf. J. Melling, 'Accommodating madness. New research into the social history of insanity and institutions' in Melling and Forsythe, *Insanity, Institutions*, p. 7.

[9] I see this as an important addition to arguments advanced by Bartlett, *Poor Law*, note 2.

between the wars because of the county's concern with economy and developing commitments to 'mental defectives'. A more surprising conclusion is that St Andrew's probably fared still worse under the NHS, as the needs of mental patients were more remotely interpreted through a less sympathetic Regional Hospital Board in the light of centrally determined spending allocations.

The asylum/hospital was also a place of contrasts. Some patients were incarcerated and isolated but others maintained contact with visiting relatives to the point of their release, another feature of asylum life from the very beginning. Regulatory inspections exposed deficiencies, though whether the NLA merits the rather harsh attributes suggested in published historical and contemporary comparisons seems questionable.[10] Inspection led to improvements and patient transfers, probationary leave, discharge and even recovery featured more prominently in asylum routine. If a substantial level of readmissions also occurred, this demonstrated movement in and out of the asylum, at least a century before the 1960s 'revolving door' analogy was drawn.

It is also clear that some people were committed to a lifetime in the asylum as a place of last resort or under the vagaries of moral insanity. Others were admitted in concussion, delirious from fever or childbirth, or as the victims of violence or alcohol. These issues might be compounded for working-class women patients whose experiences were interpreted by male officials and doctors from very different socio-cultural backgrounds. Undoubtedly there were victims, for example the woman not released because of her husband's drinking habits, although others may have considered the asylum a place of refuge and there is little evidence that Norfolk County Asylum had an increasingly disproportionate number of women patients.[11] However, women rarely had outdoor work or recreational opportunities compared with men, raising concerns whether improvements in asylum facilities, therapies and engineered social relations were geared to the reinforcement of gendered social roles or should be seen as progressive measures.

Even by late nineteenth- and early twentieth-century standards the county asylum was, as its senior medical staff recognised, an inappropriate place for children or those handicapped in some way.[12] It provided the equivalent of continuing care for some patients, with a certain amount of freedom for the 'elderly gentlemen' tending their allotments on ward 16 and

---

[10] Viz. J. Conolly, *An Inquiry Concerning the Indications of Insanity, With Suggestions for the Better Protection and Care of the Insane*, Taylor, London, 1830; L.D. Smith, *Cure, Comfort and Safe Custody*, Leicester University Press, 1999.

[11] J. Busfield, 'The female malady? Men, women and madness in nineteenth-century Britain' in *Sociology*, 28, 1994, 1, pp. 259–77. This applies until the 1960s imbalances involving St Nicholas' hospital. It does not invalidate the point that, elsewhere, middle-class women may have been disproportionately affected.

[12] See M. Jackson, *The Borderland of Imbecility*, Manchester University Press, 2000.

for women on ward 15. For others, to live on the 'laundry ward' or to be a 'working patient' spoke volumes about hospital life. Some wards, notably A and 6, remained fearful places well into the era of medication and unlocked doors. However, any speculation concerning serious defects in institutional standards of care, as with the seclusion of women patients in the early 1950s, should also acknowledge the pressures on nursing staff and that not all patients were equipped for predictable or orderly lives. In practice, risks, threat, vulnerability and abuse did not end at the hospital driveway, regardless of the direction of travel.

Standards of care and the tenor of asylum or hospital life were largely determined by the nursing staff. Medical officers were not constantly involved with patients and relied heavily upon the regulation and compliance of nurses. Almost every medical superintendent's regime had instances of patient abuse but the positive influence of informally trained local staff with recognisably similar backgrounds to their patients may have been underestimated.[13] Although in-house training was provided from a comparatively early date at Norfolk County Asylum, staff turnover and shortages were almost constant problems and steadily rising standards cannot always be assumed. Late in the twentieth century, for example, improvement was often considered in terms of looking after patients rather than by engaging or encouraging them. Staff interviews confirm these as real issues and also tensions between new developments and established practices. However, the polarisation of an old guard immersed in hospital culture and new reformers can be overdone; similarly with the blanket attribution of 'kindliness' or 'aloofness' towards patients among these respective groupings.

Let us turn from broad observations to points emerging from particular chapters. Norfolk Lunatic Asylum ranked among the pioneer county asylums. It was built at a time when social elites were concerned with internal as well as external threats to their wealth and property, although it was not simply the direct expression of such fears. Rather, it reflected faith in the reforming capacity of specific institutions and assumptions, encouraged by doctors, that the prospect of cure as well as safe custody could be offered to suitable inmates, significantly referred to as patients. Concepts of 'retreat' implied more than isolation or incarceration, as it was felt that asylum in itself might produce or facilitate a patient's recovery.

As the NLA demonstrates, asylum as a policy initiative was no cheap, stop-gap solution. Its actual costs far exceeded those envisaged, but the asylum was designed to rank among the best of contemporary examples and its first doctors were considered to be the local experts. Patients were differentiated according to their behaviour and prospects but it was possible even for the 'incurable' to obtain release. Early shortfalls in practice stemmed from Thomas Caryl's efforts to punish whatever he regarded as bad behaviour

---

[13] P. Nolan, A History of Mental Health Nursing, Chapman & Hall, London, 1993.

but, although doctors provided him with few alternative guidelines, he used such measures and restraints less frequently by the 1830s. Corrections to unforeseen faults in heating arrangements and water supplies were delayed by economy measures intended to assuage Norfolk ratepayers after the initial asylum costs incurred, and with an eye firmly upon comparative asylum and poor law charges.[14]

With a building plan which facilitated the movement of patients and 'rewarded' the convalescent literally with the prospect of release, the importance of moral treatment and reduced restraint became appreciated at the NLA without direct medical influence as such. Although the medical superintendence of asylums was increasingly accepted as the mid-nineteenth century yardstick of 'progress', this indicates the growth of professional influence rather than more successful treatments.[15] If the NLA failed this particular test in the 1850s, it had a resident medical officer and other wise displayed the conventional signs of improvement. Work therapy had been adopted, there were positive responses to comments by the lunacy commissioners and medical officer, and Ebenezer Owen personally investigated standards at comparable institutions. It appears that the committee of justices willingly accepted central regulation when this corresponded with their own focus upon work, value and economy, the focus of earlier poor law reform. After subsidies on asylum care reduced the sense of competition with poor law provision they became more inclined to expand the asylum, to achieve economies of scale and enhance earning capacity through the acceptance of out-county and other boarders. In part, then, the growth of the NLA reflected transfers of patients rather than 'more' insanity.

The asylum was among the first to adopt probation for patients. Some historians have located the intellectual origins of community care in this system, though it suited the justices' earlier objectives as it offered a practical response to asylum overcrowding, it contributed to longer-term savings and it tested the patient's sense of moral obligation.[16] It is noteworthy that William Hills, the first medical superintendent at the NLA, developed rather than contradicted this strategy. However, he also articulated professional claims to the management of an extended range of illnesses and accentuated divisions between curable and chronic cases, who could be maintained in some productive capacity or nursed at reduced cost in an auxiliary asylum. Consequently new admissions received most of the medical care available and older cases were left to the routine of quarterly inspections, work gangs

---

[14] At least the NLA had the prospect of debt-free expansion, a considerable benefit if the difficulties which beset the Suffolk County Asylum are any guide. M. Fisher, 'Getting out of the asylum: discharge and decarceration issues in asylum history c. 1890–1959'. UEA PhD thesis, 2003.

[15] L.D. Smith, *Cure, Comfort and Safe Custody*, Leicester University Press, 1999.

[16] The justices had stated this position in the 1854 Annual Report.

and organised recreation. With less individual attention and more signs of batch living, one person's therapeutic community might then resemble another's 'warehousing' of the mad. Patients were still discharged, to recover or be readmitted, but it remains questionable how exactly they were cured by virtue of a scientific understanding of insanity, compared with an older process of undergoing the asylum regime for a period of time, which allowed some to recover. It is not implausible that an ordered combination of work, sufficient food, exercise, rest and contact with attendants and nurses leading similar lifestyles served sufficiently to reconnect patients with the normality of rural life that they could be discharged.

David Thomson's arrival broadly coincided with altered asylum management under the 1888 and 1890 Acts, which he used to his advantage. His main innovation was to undo Hills' approach and to expand the asylum on twin sites on the basis of complete sexual segregation. By 1914 considerable physical improvements to the asylum environment coincided with usage of the term 'hospital' long before its requirement under the 1930 Mental Treatment Act, although most patients remained highly organised within the economic community. Staff training was part of Thomson's achievement but there is much less sense of his involvement with patients: his acceptance of blanket theories involving hereditary defect suggested paternalistic management rather than individual attention and may have informed his emphasis upon sexual segregation.

The low status accorded to patients and, despite appearances to the contrary, the flexibility of approaches to insanity and asylum care were vividly demonstrated in the Great War. Thomson's organisational skills were harnessed to the Norfolk War Hospital and most asylum patients were dispersed to other institutions, where their vulnerability in the face of overcrowding, food shortages and deficiencies in nursing care was confirmed by increased mortality rates. This much can be unravelled, but there are no indications that the traumatic and disturbing effects of these events upon patients were seriously considered. Rather surprisingly, given its location and staff, the NWH remained very much a place for physical casualties, with relatively little attention paid to 'war neuroses', although numbers of 'service patients' were to feature on wards long after peacetime re-conversion as Norfolk Mental Hospital.

For all the emphasis upon war as a catalyst for psychiatric treatments and the impact of the 1930 Mental Treatment Act, the inter-war St Andrew's Hospital provided a more relaxed but not dissimilar environment from the Edwardian asylum.[17] Parole became more extensive, voluntary patients and outpatients were admitted and links made with the Norfolk and Norwich Hospital. Yet no attempt was made to develop alleged public interest, arising

---

[17] The therapeutic emphasis and improvement is perhaps overstated in K. Jones, *Asylums and After*, Athlone, London, 1993.

from the hospital's wartime role or from changing attitudes to mental illness, and signs of treatment in the community can be exaggerated. After NWH equipment had been absorbed, spending at St Andrew's was confined to the infrastructure of power generation and sewerage: patients and nurses did not obtain new accommodation and legislative change did not bring appropriate facilities. Extended systems of leave, parole and transfer were in no small measure linked with hospital overcrowding as the committee and county council attempted to make additional provision, notably for the mentally handicapped, in unfavourable economic circumstances. Relations between staff and patients were considered comparatively good, death rates fell and more recoveries were claimed but an overall improvement in standards of care in these circumstances was increasingly difficult to sustain.

When St Andrew's became an Emergency Hospital in 1940 mental patients were again adversely affected but their mass evacuation and its consequences were avoided. Wartime disruptions aggravated the emerging nurse shortage and overcrowding but the ethos of 'make do and mend', familiar at St Andrew's before the war, also became the watchword for mental health care under the National Health Service. Admissions, outpatient attendance, discharges and readmissions all increased, suggesting the growth of active therapy, although staff shortages restricted the rise of physical treatments with the exception of ECT. This was no great disadvantage, for in most mental hospitals 'the new treatments . . . were being administered by staff who were very unsure about what they were doing'.[18] Similar remarks may apply to the introduction of new medications in the 1950s, although McCulley was more cautious in this respect.[19] Only in conjunction with a more therapeutic regime and a sympathetic nursing staff could drug treatments have been responsible for the 'kindly' atmosphere frequently referred to at St Andrew's.

What former staff saw as essential in a caring institution others identified as paternalistic and even disabling, but an alleged 'asylum culture', perhaps founded upon an ageing core of residents rather than upon its 'revolving door' patients, was less recognisable as that of a 'total institution'. Interviews confirm traditions of staff recruitment through particular families as one answer to the perennial problems of turnover and of training geared specifically to the needs of the asylum/hospital. The sustained prominence of farming and the estate in hospital life at St Andrew's may have strengthened affinities between staff and patients, possibly for a longer period than in many other psychiatric hospitals. These traditions were already undermined by the 1960s, however; rural lifestyles and institutional loyalties were less predominant, staff were as much international as local in origin, long spells of farmwork were considered of little therapeutic value in medical models

---

[18] Nolan, *Mental Health Nursing*, p. 99.
[19] As seen in Chapter 9.

of care and inappropriate for short-term patients with informal status. However, St Andrew's still had peak numbers of patients and a large core of long-term residents and, without alternative provision, its closure was not a short-term possibility.

Successive reorganisations and innovations under the NHS stripped away familiar institutional practices and the remaining elements of localised control at the hospital, although it retained a role in continuing care and was capable of some modification, as demonstrated with the elderly acute psychiatric unit. National goals were increasingly expressed in terms of short treatments, rehabilitation and discharge, preludes to care in the community. Yet, as one observer has noted, though

> the asylums and mental hospitals were accused by their critics of embodying a system of oppressive paternalism; it may be argued that the advocates of the community health care movement were equally paternalistic in their unbending conviction that all clients would prefer to be treated outside hospital settings.[20]

The timing and nature of this end-product was imprecise but the closure of old psychiatric hospitals was clearly sign-posted and in that respect a local choice between St Andrew's or Hellesdon hospitals was inevitable. Complicating factors, involving association with general hospital facilities, consideration of the kind of mental health services required, the establishment of a separate NHS Trust and the practicalities of planning permission and logistics, all delayed this eventuality.

The closure of St Andrew's Hospital represented the end of a particular continuity in approaches to madness and in the life of buildings lasting for almost two centuries. It was also an episode in the wider development of a range of services which confirms the shifting boundaries of mental health care. Continuing care facilities for elderly patients have been diversified and these, along with respite care and day-centres, are offered at Rebecca House, North Walsham and Cygnet House, Long Stratton. Refurbished accommodation at Northgate, Yarmouth and at Carlton Court, Lowestoft, provides similar facilities, as do Hellesdon Hospital, which also has long-stay wards, and the Heron Lodge rehabilitation centre. The new Julian Hospital, formally opened on 11 July 1998, consists of three wards with 100 short-stay beds in single or shared rooms for elderly acute patients, a 30-place day-centre and an outpatient clinic.[21] By then the establishment of six community mental health teams for Norfolk and four in Norwich had 'enabled the strategic reduction to 100 inpatient beds to be achieved' and these have been

---

[20] Nolan, *Mental Health Nursing*, p. 191.
[21] *Eastern Daily Press*, 22 March 1996, 16 March 1998. These wards replaced Glandford ward at the Norfolk and Norwich Hospital as well as St Andrew's wards. The Bickley and Albion day hospitals operate at Attleborough and Aylsham respectively.

strengthened subsequently by a psychological therapies team and 24-hour home treatment teams for Norwich and central Norfolk.[22] Additional outpatient clinics and mobile day treatment services have been organised, particularly for north Norfolk.[23] Along with social workers and community nurses the teams visit patients and former patients in local authority, private and voluntary accommodation, including relatively unsupervised group homes.

Current if underdeveloped models of accommodation, as at Oak Street, Norwich, combine flatlets, communal housing and residential staff within mini-settlements, providing a sense of community without institutionalisation. Such purpose-built or refurbished accommodation and greater attention to the rights and needs of clients suggest improving standards of care, but this remains subject to important qualifications. One concerns finite resources, which dictate that better facilities are limited or rationed in some way. This is most obvious with residential provision or services which have a definite physical location, but is no less a problem where care is offered to people in varied 'domestic' settings. The latter raises discomfiting questions concerning wider community toleration and provision, particularly for those who have no family or obvious 'informal' sources of support. No less than in 1814 tensions exist within a rhetoric of care which simultaneously asserts the entitlements of the client but can involve regulation and restriction, particularly of the unresponsive or unco-operative. The same individual may require very different forms of care at different times and, for a variety of reasons, people can miss or avoid medication, advice or supervision. Consequences may include the invoking of custodial approaches and placement in secure accommodation, which echoes the earliest of asylum facilities.[24]

The therapeutic properties formerly attributed to the wider hospital landscape have been discounted, perhaps as an unaffordable objective, in shifting the boundaries of mental heath care. Yet everywhere this feature is highly valued for the purposes of residential redevelopment on former hospital settings. If this suggests the continuing potential of St Andrew's as a site of care, the conversion of many of the former hospital buildings into attractive private residences has confirmed their adaptability and raises the question of what else might have been achieved there. Ironically, the very attractiveness of the St Andrew's site probably determined that a modernised

---

[22] Norfolk Mental Health Care NHS Trust *Annual Reports* 1997–8, p. 6; 2000–1 p. 8; Reynolds interview. Mental health care services of the former Anglian Harbours Trust have been incorporated and similar services developed for the east coast and Waveney Valley areas.

[23] Ibid., 1998–9; Reynolds and Thane interviews.

[24] Such fears are expressed by a former medical superintendent David Clark, *Fulbourn*, p. 243. Several current staff and former staff at St Andrew's made the same point and drew attention to the reliance upon secure units, in the local case the Norvic Clinic.

and improved hospital would not be located there in the twenty-first century. One hospital closure enabled other qualitative improvements in services to be offered. The cost of these services is often seen as problematic and, while questions of standards and adequacy are preoccupations for professionals, patients and their relatives, they should be a cause of sympathetic concern in wider society. It would be a sad social commentary if, over two centuries, buildings at St Andrew's, associated once in the public mind with dread and now with desirability, should be changing more than our perceptions of mental disorders and our willingness to respond positively to those affected by them.

Select bibliography

Primary sources used

At Norfolk County Record Office

Minutes of Committee of Visiting Magistrates, Norfolk Lunatic Asylum
Oct. 1813–July 1890, SAH 2–11
Minutes of Committee of Visitors, Norfolk County Asylum (Mental Hospital)
Aug. 1890–Feb. 1923, SAH 12–15
Minutes of Committee of Visitors, St Andrew's Hospital
March 1923–Nov. 1931, SAH 16

Minutes of Committee of Visitors to consider Special Business
July 1903–Dec. 1931, SAH 19–24

Annual Reports
1844–5, 1850–76 SAH 28; 1877–86, SAH 29; 1887–96, SAH 30;
1897–1905, SAH 31; 1906–21, SAH 32; 1922–33, SAH 33; 1934–8, SAH
34; 1949–63, SAH 35; 1967, SAH 36.

Patients Maintenance Ledgers
May 1814–Oct. 1824, SAH 52.

Wages Books
1854–90, SAH 75; 1910–12, SAH 79.
1940–5 (female), SAH 93.

Master's Journals and Report Books
May 1814–March 1843, SAH 123–127.
Superintendent's Journals
April 1843–June 1861, SAH 128–130.
Medical Superintendent's Journals
July 1861–March 1927, SAH 131–136.

Visiting Justices' Report Books (Committee of Management 1948–)
July 1814–Aug. 1844, SAH 137
Aug. 1844–April 1868, SAH 138
May 1868–Jan. 1903, SAH 139
Jan. 1903–Oct. 1955, SAH 140.

Reports of the Commissioners in Lunacy (after 1914 Board of Control)
1844–1925, SAH 141; 1926–59, SAH 142.

Clerk and Steward's Report Books
72, SAH 143; 1872–83, SAH 144; n/a; 1891–1906, SAH 145;
1906–25, SAH 146.

Physician's Report Books
June 1814–Oct. 1817, SAH 147; Oct. 1817–Oct. 1820, SAH 148; May
    1829–Feb. 1835, SAH 149; Oct. 1843–Feb. 1845, SAH 150.

Visiting Doctor's Journal
Nov. 1814–Jan. 1817, SAH 151.

Chaplain's Report Books
1860–1957, SAH 152–157.

Registers of mechanical restraint and seclusion
1894–1913, SAH 202; 1920–24, SAH 203.

Registers of discharges, departures, transfers and deaths
Discharges 1913–49, SAH 207–209.
Discharges, removals and deaths 1881–1906, SAH 210.
Discharges and deaths 1843–1930, SAH 211–216.

Patient Case Books
Admissions, male and female 1846–88, SAH 259–272.
Admissions, male 1898–1908, SAH 273–277.
Deaths, male 1910–37, SAH 278–281.
Discharges, male 1910–31, SAH 282–284.
Admissions, female 1885–1909, SAH 285–297.
Deaths, male and female 1910–30, SAH 298–301.
Discharges, male and female 1910–34, SAH 302–4.
Chronic, male 1862–1909, SAH 305–306.
Chronic, female1863–87, SAH 307.
Chronic, male and female 1879–1914, SAH 308.
Male alphabetical 1900–47, SAH 587–590.
Deaths, male 1944–7, SAH 591.
Discharges, male 1944–7, SAH 592.
Female alphabetical 1900–47, SAH 593–599.
Deaths, female 1931–47, SAH 600–601.
Discharges, female 1930–47, SAH 602–606.
Case papers, male and female 1900–48, SAH 607–742.
Patient daily numbers books, 1953–80, SAH 583–585.

Miscellaneous
Farm Records 1892–9, SAH 110.
New Buildings Account 1876–1912, SAH 355.
Maintenance Account Books 1921–46, SAH 500.
E. F. Cannell, 'The progress of a century: Norfolk County Mental Hospital Engineering Department', mimeo, 1914, SAH 325.
Particulars of patients transferred to other asylums in order to provide accommodation for sick and wounded soldiers, 1915, SAH 326.
Regulations and orders . . . 1923, SAH 327.
St Andrew's and St Nicholas' Hospitals Newsletter (Special for Mental Health Year 1960), SAH 331.
Photographs relating to St Andrew's, SAH 754–757.

Norfolk War Hospital
War Hospital Orders 1915–19, SAH 335–359.
NWH magazine 1916–17, SAH 340.

Emergency Section
Emergency Hospital Scheme correspondence and patients, SAH 758–779.

St Andrew's/Hellesdon Hospital Management Committee
Minutes 1968–9, SAH 508.
Minutes 1972–3, SAH 509.

Admissions 1980–90, SAH 563.
Discharges 1970–4, SAH 569.
Patient numbers 1974–80, SAH 585.

Norfolk County Council Mental Deficiency Committee Minutes, Oct. 1930–March 1934 C/C/10/370.

At Drayton Old Lodge

(At the time of writing many of these records and architects' drawings, plans, etc. are being transferred to the Norfolk County Record Office.)
CVIS Minutes Dec. 1931–March 1945; April 1945–July 1948.
Group 8 St Andrew's and Hellesdon HMC Annual Report, 1965–6.
Medical Superintendent's Journal; Aug. 1955–April 1971.
Norfolk County Council, Mental Deficiency Committee Minutes 1913–19.
St Andrew's Hospital Visitors Books, 1955–70, 1971–3.
St Andrew's Hospital, *Mental Health Year, 1960: Your Hospital*, 1960.
Norfolk Mental Health Care NHS Trust, Annual Report, 1998–9; 1999–2000; 2000–01.

At Norfolk Local Studies Library

Norfolk Area Joint Liaison Committee '1974 NHS Reorganisation', LS c362.1, 1974.

Norwich Health Authority, 'A New District General Hospital for Norwich', 1992.

Norfolk and Norwich Hospitals Health Care NHS Trust, 'Outline business case for acute services in Norfolk and Norwich', 1994.

Norfolk Mental Health Care NHS Trust, Annual Report 1994–5; 1998–9.

At Norwich Health Authority, Northside, Thorpe St Andrews

SH3 Hospital Returns 1965–86.

NHA Mortality Database 1979–98. 382/1/24.

Material in private possession

Mr T. Pull

MHIWU (COHSE) Norfolk Branch Minutes 1941–58.

'Rehabilitation facilities' (mimeo 1982).

Mrs V. Roberts

Staff Rules and Orders 1893 (hand copied) and photographs.

RMPA Examination papers 1920–2.

Mr and Mrs E. Middleton

Photographs.

Mrs G. Drinkwater

Photographs.

Major Acts of Parliament and official publications referred to in the text

1808 *An Act for the Better Care and Maintenance of Lunatics, being Paupers or Criminals in England*, 48 Geo. III c.96 (Wynn's Act).

1828 *An Act to regulate the Care and Treatment of Insane Persons in England*, 9 Geo. IV c.41.

1845 *An Act for the Regulation of the Care and Treatment of Lunatics*, 8 & 9 Vict. c.100 (Lunatics Act).

1845 *An Act to amend the Laws for the Provision and Regulation of Lunatic Asylums . . .*, 8 & 9 Vict. c.126 (Lunatic Asylums Act).

1853 The Lunatic Asylums Act, 16 & 17 Vict. c.97.

1886 Idiots Act, 49 Vict. c.25.

1888 Local Government Act, 51 & 52 Vict. c.41.

1890 Lunacy Act, 53 Vict. c.65.

1899 Elementary Education (Defective and Epileptic Children) Act, 62 & 63 Vict. c.45.

1909 Asylum Officers Superannuation Act, 9 Edw. VII c.48.

1913 Mental Deficiency Act 3 & 4 Geo. V c.28.

1914 Elementary Education (Defective and Epileptic Children) Act, 4 & 5 Geo. V c.45.

1929 Local Government Act, 19 Geo. V c.17.

1930 Mental Treatment Act, 20 & 21 Geo. V c.23.

1946 National Health Service Act, 9 & 10 Geo. VI c.81.

1959 Mental Health Act, 7 & 8 Eliz. II c.72.

1983 Mental Health Act, c.20.

Report of the Interdepartmental Committee on Physical Deterioration, Cmd 2175, 1904.

Sir Marriot Cooke and H. Bond, *History of the Asylum War Hospitals of England and Wales*, Cmd 899, HMSO, 1920.

Hansard's Parliamentary Debates, 6 Nov. 1945, 'Mental Hospitals' 1188–1204.

A Hospital Plan for England and Wales, Cmd 1604, HMSO, 1962.

Health and Welfare: The Development of Community Care, Cmd 1973, HMSO, 1963.

Report of the Committee on Local Authority and Allied Personal Social Services, Cmd 3703, HMSO, 1968.

Better Services for the Mentally Ill, Cmd 6233, HMSO, 1975.

Caring for People, Community Care in the Next Decade and Beyond, Cmd 849, HMSO, 1989.

Theses and dissertations

H. Bettinson, 'The Norfolk War Hospital: military use of the county asylum, 1915–19', MA, UEA Norwich, 1997.

C. Bowler, 'The importance of architectural and medical theories in the planning and construction of Norfolk County Lunatic Asylum', MA, UEA Norwich, 1997.

M. Fisher, 'Getting out of the asylum: discharge and decarceration issues in asylum history c.1890–1959', PhD thesis (in progress), UEA Norwich, 2003.

Books pre-1948 (place of publication is London except where specified)

F. Bateman and W. Rye, *The History of the Bethel Hospital*, Norwich, 1906.

F. Blomfield, *History of Norfolk* (3 vols), 1806.

G.K. Blyth, *Norwich Directory*, 1842.

British Red Cross and Order of St John, *Joint War Committee and Finance Committee 1914–19*, 1921.

J. Conolly, *An Inquiry Concerning the Indications of Insanity, With Suggestions for the Better Protection and Care of the Insane*, Taylor, 1830.

J. Conolly, *The Construction and Government of Lunatic Asylums*, Churchill, 1847.

Eastern Daily Press, 'Norfolk County Asylum', 18 Sept. 1903.

F.M. Eden, *The State of the Poor*, Warrington, 1797.

A. Halliday, *A General View of the Present State of Lunatics and Lunatic Asylums, in Great Britain and Ireland, and in some other kingdoms*, 1828.

History of the Mental Hospital and Institutional Workers Union 1910–31, Manchester, 1931.

History of Norfolk, Norwich, Yarmouth etc. Or Supplement to Excursions in the County, Norwich, 1825.

J. Howard, *The State of the Prisons*, Warrington, 1778.

Joint War Committee and Finance Committee, British Red Cross and Order of St John 1914–21, HMSO, London, 1921.

H. LeStrange, *Norfolk Official Lists, from the earliest period to the present day*, Norwich, 1890.

C. Mackie, *The Norfolk Annals*, (2 vols), Norwich, 1901.

Royal Medico-Psychological Association, *Handbook for Mental Nurses*, Ballière, Tindall & Cox, 8th edition, 1937.

S. Tuke, *Practical Hints on the Construction and Economy of Pauper Lunatic Asylums*, Alexander, York, 1815.

Articles to 1948

'Misgovernment at the Norfolk County Asylum', *The Asylum Journal*, 7, 15 Aug. 1854, pp. 99–104.

'Inquest at Norfolk County Asylum', *The Asylum Journal*, 9, 15 Oct. 1854, pp. 143–4.

Eastern Daily Press, 'Norfolk County Asylum', 18 Sept. 1903.

A. Lewis, 'The chemical treatment of mental disorder', *Biology of Human Affairs*, 1947, 27, pp. 19–26.

S. MacKenzie, 'The value of Indian hemp', *British Medical Journal*, 15 Jan. 1887, pp. 97–8.

G. MacKenzie Bacon, 'On the treatment of epileptic insanity', *Practitioner*, 1869, 2, pp. 334–6.

H. Maudsley, 'On opium in the treatment of insanity', *Practitioner*, 1869, 2, pp. 1–8.

C. Myers, 'A contribution to the study of shell shock', *The Lancet*, 1, 1915, pp. 316–20.

G.H. Savage, 'The use of sedatives in insanity', *Practitioner*, 1886, 37, pp. 181–5.

D.G. Thomson, correspondence/notes and news, *Journal of Mental Science*, 26, 1890, pp. 154–7.

D.G. Thomson, 'Presidential address on the progress of psychiatry during the past hundred years', *Journal of Mental Science*, 60, 1914, pp. 541–72.

D.G. Thomson, 'Norfolk War Hospital', *Eastern Daily Press*, Part 1, 4 June 1919; Part 2, 5 June 1919.

(Obituary, D.G. Thomson), *Journal of Mental Science*, 69, 1923, pp. 259–60.

Books from 1948

B. Abel-Smith, *The Hospitals 1800–1948*, Heinemann, London, 1964.

J. Allsop, *Health Policy and the NHS*, Longman, London, 1995.

A. Armstrong, *The Population of Victorian and Edwardian Norfolk*, Centre of East Anglia Studies, UEA Norwich, 2000.

P. Barham, *Closing the Asylum*, Penguin, Harmondsworth, 1992.

P. Bartlett, *The Poor Law of Lunacy*, Leicester University Press, 1999.

P. Bartlett and D. Wright (eds), *Outside the Walls of the Asylum: The History of Care in the Community 1750–2000*, Athlone, London. 1999.

R. Barton, *Institutional Neurosis*, Wright, Bristol, 1959.

G.E. Berrios and H. Freeman (eds), *150 Years of British Psychiatry 1841–1991*, Gaskell, London, Vol. 1, 1991, Vol. 2, 1996.

J. Busfield, *Men, Women and Madness – Understanding Gender and Mental Disorder*, Macmillan, Basingstoke, 1996.

W.F. Bynum and R. Porter (eds), *Companion Encyclopaedia of the History of Medicine*, Routledge, London, Vols 1, 2, 1993.

W.F. Bynum, R. Porter and M. Shepherd (eds), *The Anatomy of Madness: Essays in the History of Psychiatry*, Tavistock, London, Vols 1, 2, 1985, Vol. 3, 1988.

B. Cashman, *A Proper House. Bedford Lunatic Asylum 1812–60*, North Beds. Health Authority, 1992.

S. Cherry, *Doing Different? Politics and the Labour Movement in Norwich 1880–1914*, Centre of East Anglia Studies, UEA Norwich, 1989.

D.H. Clark, *The Story of a Mental Hospital. Fulbourn 1858–1983*, Process, London, 1996.

A.J. Cleveland, *History of the Norfolk and Norwich Hospital 1900–46*, Jarrold & Sons, Norwich, 1948.

H.M. Colvin, *A Bibliographical Dictionary of English Architects 1660–1840*, John Murray, London, 1954.

R. Cooter, *Surgery and Society in Peace and War*, Macmillan, Basingstoke, 1993.

M.A. Crowther, *The Workhouse System 1834–1929*, Methuen, London, 1981.

C. Davies (ed.), *Rewriting Nursing History*, Croom Helm, London, 1980.

A. Digby, *Pauper Palaces*, Routledge, London, 1978.

A. Digby, *Madness, Morality and Medicine: A Study of the York Retreat*, Cambridge University Press, 1985.

A. Digby, *From York Lunatic Asylum to Bootham Park Hospital*, Borthwick Paper, 69, York, 1986.

A. Digby, *The Evolution of British General Practice 1850–1948*, Clarendon, Oxford, 1999.

R. Dingwall, A.M. Rafferty and C. Webster, *An Introduction to the Social History of Nursing*, Routledge, London, 1988.

K. Doerner, *Madmen and the Bourgeoisie*, Blackwell, Oxford, 1981.

T.D. Dormandy, *The White Death: A History of Tuberculosis*, Hambledon, London, 1999.

J.C. Drummond and A. Wilbraham, *The Englishman's Food*, Jonathan Cape, London, 1964.

P. Fennell, *Treatment without Consent*, Routledge, London, 1996.

M. Foucault, *Madness and Civilisation*, Tavistock, London, 1967.

W. Hamish Fraser, *A History of British Trade Unionism 1700–1998*, Macmillan, Basingstoke, 1999.

D. Gittins, *Madness in its Place: Narratives of Severalls Hospital 1913–1997*, Routledge, London, 1998.

E. Goffman, *Asylums*, Penguin, Harmondsworth, 1961.

L. Hall, *Sex, Gender and Social Change in Britain since 1980*, Macmillan, Basingstoke, 2000.

A. Hardy, *Health and Medicine in Britain since 1860*, Palgrave, Basingstoke, 2000.

J. Harris, *Private Lives, Public Spirit: Britain 1870–1914*, Penguin, Harmondsworth, 1993.

D. Healy, *The Antidepressant Era*, Cambridge, Mass., Harvard University Press, 1997.

M. Jackson, *The Borderland of Imbecility*, Manchester University Press, 2000.

C.B. Jewson, *Jacobin City*, Blackie, Glasgow, 1975.

K. Jones, *Asylums and After*, Athlone, London, 1993.

K. Jones, *Lunacy, Law and Conscience 1744–1845*, Routledge, London, 1955.

J. Ledd (ed.), *Care in the Community: Illusion or Reality?*, Wiley, Chichester, 1997.

I. Loudon (ed.), *Western Medicine*, Oxford University Press, 1997.

I. Loudon, J. Horder and C. Webster (eds), *General Practice under the NHS 1948–97*, Oxford University Press, 1998.

R. Lowe, *The Welfare State in Britain since 1945*, Macmillan, Basingstoke, 1993.

C. McCall, *Looking Back from the Nineties: An Autobiography*, Gliddon, Norwich, 1994.

R. McGrew, *Encyclopaedia of Medical History*, Macmillan, London, 1985.

J. Melling and B. Forsythe (eds), *Insanity, Institutions and Society 1800–1914*, Routledge, London, 1999.

MIND, *Mental Health Yearbook*, 1981–2.

P. Nolan, *A History of Mental Health Nursing*, Chapman & Hall, London, 1993.

J. Pettigrew, R. Reynolds and S. Rouse, *A Place in the Country: Three Counties Asylum 1860–1998*, South Beds. Community Health Care Trust, 1998.

J.V. Pickstone (ed.), *Medical Innovations in Historical Perspective*, Macmillan, Basingstoke, 1992.

F.N.L. Poynter (ed.), *The Evolution of Hospitals in Britain*, Pitman Medical, London, 1964.

L. Prior, *The Social Organisation of Mental Illness*, Sage, London, 1993.

C. Rawcliffe, *Medicine and Society in Later Medieval England*, Sutton, London, 1995.

C. Rawcliffe and R.G. Wilson (eds), *The History of Norwich*, Hambledon, London, 2004 (forthcoming).

H. Richardson (ed.), *English Hospitals 1660–1948*, Royal Commission on the Historical Monuments of England, Swindon, 1998.

B. Robb (ed.), *Sans Everything: A Case to Answer*, Nelson, London, 1967.

A. Scull (ed.), *Madhouses, Mad-doctors and Madmen*, University of Pennsylvania, Philadelphia, 1981.

A. Scull, *The Most Solitary of Afflictions*, Yale University Press, New Haven, 1993.

V. Skultans, *Madness and Morals: Ideas on Insanity in the Nineteenth Century*, Routledge, London, 1975.

G. Searle, *Eugenics and Politics in Britain 1900–14*, Science in History Series, Leyden, 1976.

P. Sedgewick, *Psychopolitics*, Pluto, London, 1982.

E. Shorter, *A History of Psychiatry*, Wiley, New York, 1997.

E. Showalter, *The Female Malady: Women, Madness and the English Culture 1830–1980*, Virago, London, 1985.

L.D. Smith, *Cure, Comfort and Safe Custody*, Leicester University Press, 1999.

J. Taylor, *Hospital and Asylum Architecture in England 1840–1914*, Mansell, London, 1991.

J. and D. Taylor, *Mental Health in the 1990s; From Custody to Care?*, Office of Health Economics, London, 1989.

M. Thompson, *The Problem of Mental Deficiency*, Clarendon, Oxford, 1998.

D. Tomlinson and J. Carrier (eds), *Asylum in the Community*, Routledge, London, 1996.

N. Virgoe and T. Williamson (eds), *Religious Dissent in East Anglia*, Centre of East Anglia Studies, UEA, Norwich, 1993.

C. Webster, *The National Health Service: A Political History*, Oxford University Press, 1998.

R. White, *The Effects of the National Health Service on the Nursing Profession 1948–1961*, King's Fund, London, 1985, pp 120–43.

J.M. Winter, *The Great War and the British People*, Macmillan, London, 1986.

Articles from 1948

R. Adair, B. Forsythe and J. Melling, 'A danger to the public? Disposing of pauper lunatics in late-Victorian and Edwardian England', *Medical History*, 42, 1998, pp. 1–25.

J. Andrews, 'Notes on mental health care and prophylaxis in late 19th century Britain', *Health Care Discussion Papers*, 1, Oxford Brookes, 1998, pp. 14–34.

P. Bartlett, 'The asylum and the Poor Law: the productive alliance', in Melling and Forsythe (eds), *Insanity, Institutions*, pp. 48–67.

L. Bryder, 'The First World War: healthy or hungry?', History Workshop, 24, 1987, pp. 141–55.

J. Busfield, 'The female malady? Men, women and madness in nineteenth-century Britain', *Sociology*, 28, 1994, pp. 259–77.

M. Carpenter, 'Asylum nursing before 1914; the history of labour', in C. Davies (ed.), *Rewriting Nursing History*, Croom Helm, London, 1980, pp. 123–46.

S. Cherry, 'The role of a provincial hospital; the Norfolk and Norwich Hospital 1772–1880', *Population Studies*, XXVI, 2, 1972, pp. 291–306.

S. Cherry, 'Responses to sickness: health care in modern Norwich', in C. Rawcliffe and R.G. Wilson (eds), *The History of Norwich*, Hambledon, London, 2004 (forthcoming).

S. Cherry and B. Ross, 'The Norfolk and Norwich Hospital and the establishment of the NHS 1939–55', in D. Ralphs (ed.), *The Norfolk and Norwich Hospital 1946–2000* (forthcoming).

R. Cooter, 'War and modern medicine', in Bynum and Porter (eds), *Encyclopaedia History of Medicine*, Vol. 1, pp. 1536–73.

J.L. Crammer, 'Extraordinary deaths of asylum inpatients during the 1914–18 war', *Medical History*, 36, 1992, pp. 430–41.

J.L. Crammer, 'English asylums and English doctors: where Scull is wrong', *History of Psychiatry*, 5, 1994, 1, pp. 103–15.

A. Dally, 'Psychiatric treatment in the twentieth century', *Social History of Medicine*, 13, 2000, 3, pp. 547–54.

B. Forsythe, J. Melling and R. Adair, 'Politics of lunacy: central state regulation and the Devon Pauper Lunatic Asylum 1845–1914', in Melling and Forsythe (eds), *Insanity, Institutions*, pp. 68–92.

A.J. Goldstein, 'Psychiatry', in Bynum and Porter (eds), *Encyclopaedia History of Medicine*, Vol. 2, pp. 1350–72.

R. Hodgkinson, 'Provision for pauper lunatics 1834–71', *Medical History*, 10, 1966, pp. 138–54.

K. Jones, 'The culture of the mental hospital', in Berrios and Freeman (eds), *British Psychiatry*, Vol. 1, pp. 17–28.

K. Jones, 'Law and mental health: sticks or carrots?', in Berrios and Freeman (eds), *British Psychiatry*, Vol. 1, pp. 89–101.

Kingsley Jones, 'Insulin coma treatment in schizophrenia', *Journal of the Royal Society of Medicine*, 93, March 2000, pp. 147–9.

M. Linklater, 'A tale of ordinary madness', *Observer Review*, 26 Feb. 2001.

I. MacAlpine and R. Hunter, 'The "Insanity" of King George III: a classic case of porphyria', *British Medical Journal*, 8 January 1966.

L. Massie, 'The role of women in mental health care in 19th century England', *International History of Nursing Journal*, 1, 1995, pp. 39–51.

H. Merskey, 'Shell-shock', in Berrios and Freeman (eds), *British Psychiatry*, Vol. 2, pp. 245–67.

National Schizophrenia Fellowship, 'Forgotten army', *Guardian Society*, 6 June 2001.

M. Neve, 'Medicine and the mind', in Loudon (ed.), *Western Medicine*, pp. 232–48.

R.C. Olby, 'Constitutional and hereditary disorders', in Bynum and Porter (eds), *Encyclopaedia History of Medicine*, Vol. 1, pp. 412–37.

J.V. Pickstone, 'Psychiatry in district general hospitals', in Pickstone (ed.), *Medical Innovations*, pp. 185–99.

R. Porter, 'Was there a medical enlightenment in England?', *British Journal of Eighteenth Century Studies*, 5, 1982, pp. 49–63.

R. Porter, 'History of psychiatry in Britain', *History of Psychiatry*, 2, 1991, 3, pp. 271–9.

J. Raftery, 'The decline of the asylum or the poverty of a concept', in Tomlinson and Carrier (eds), *Asylum in the Community*, pp. 18–30.

J. Saunders, 'Quarantining the weak-minded: psychiatric definitions of degeneracy and the late-Victorian asylum', in Bynum, Porter and Shepherd (eds), *Anatomy of Madness*, Vol. 3, pp. 273–95.

A. Scull, 'Rethinking the history of asylumdom', in Melling and Forsythe (eds), *Insanity, Institutions*, pp. 295–315.

A. Scull, 'Psychiatry and its historians', *History of Psychiatry*, 2, 1991, 3, pp. 239–50.

L. Smith, 'The county asylum in the mixed economy of care', in Melling and Forsythe (eds), *Insanity, Institutions*, pp. 33–47.

M. Stone, 'Shellshock and the psychologists', in Bynum, Porter and Shepherd (eds), *Anatomy of Madness*, Vol. 2, pp. 242–71.

G. Thornicroft and G. Strathdee, 'Mental health', *British Medical Journal*, 303, 1991, pp. 410–12.

T. Turner, 'Public profile of the Medico-Psychological Association c. 1851–1914', in Berrios and Freeman (eds), *British Psychiatry*, pp. 3–16.

A. Walk, 'Mental hospitals', in Poynter (ed.), *Evolution of Hospitals*, pp. 123–46.

J. Walton, 'The treatment of pauper lunatics in Victorian England: the case of Lancaster Asylum 1816–70', in Scull (ed.), *Madhouses*, pp. 166–97.

J. Walton, 'Casting out and bringing back in Victorian England: pauper lunatics 1840–70', in Bynum, Porter and Shepherd (eds), *Anatomy of Madness*, Vol. 2, pp. 132–46.

C. Webster, 'Psychiatry and the early NHS: the role of the Mental Health Standing Advisory Committee', in Berrios and Freeman (eds), *British Psychiatry*, pp. 103–16.

J. Welshman, 'Rhetoric and reality: community care in England and Wales, 1948–74', in Bartlett and Wright (eds), *Outside the Walls*, pp. 204–26.

M. Winston, 'The Bethel at Norwich: an eighteenth century hospital for lunatics', *Medical History*, 38, 1994, pp. 27–51.

D. Wright, 'The discharge of pauper lunatics from county asylums in mid-Victorian England', in Melling and Forsythe (eds), *Insanity, Institutions*, pp. 93–112.

Index